Anatomy of
OROFACIAL
STRUCTURES

Anatomy of
OROFACIAL
STRUCTURES

RICHARD W. BRAND, B.S., D.D.S., F.A.C.D.

Associate Dean for Student Services and Professor of Anatomy,
Department of Biomedical Sciences,
Washington University School of Dental Medicine,
St. Louis, Missouri

DONALD E. ISSELHARD, B.S., D.D.S., F.A.G.D.

Private Practice, St. Louis, Missouri

FOURTH EDITION

with **706** illustrations

The C. V. Mosby Company

ST. LOUIS · BALTIMORE · PHILADELPHIA · TORONTO   1990

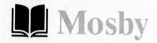

Editor: Robert W. Reinhardt
Assistant editor: Melba Steube
Project manager: Trish Tannian
Book and cover design: Gail Morey Hudson
Production: John Casey

FOURTH EDITION

Previous editions copyrighted 1977, 1982, 1986

Printed in the United States of America

The C.V. Mosby Company
11830 Westline Industrial Drive, St. Louis, Missouri 63146

Library of Congress Cataloging in Publication Data

Brand, Richard W. 1933-
    Anatomy of orofacial structures/Richard W. Brand, Donald E.
Isselhard.—4th ed.
        p.   cm.
    Includes bibliographical references.
    ISBN 0-8016-3505-5
    1. Teeth—Anatomy.   2. Mouth—Anatomy.   3. Head—Anatomy.
4. Neck—Anatomy.   I. Isselhard, Donald E.   II. Title.
    [DNLM: 1. Stomatognathic System—anatomy & histology.   WU 101
B817a]
    QM311.B78   1990
    611'.31—dc20
    DNLM/DLC
    for Library of Congress   89-13149
                                CIP

CL/DC/DC 9 8 7 6 5 4 3

We dedicate this book to our families

To my wife **Marie** *and*
Rodger, Holly, Gina, and **Robert**

Richard W. Brand

To my wife **Annette** *and*
Kerstin, Nissa, Michele, and **Tara**

Donald E. Isselhard

Preface

As we arrive at the fourth edition of this book, we are grateful for the input we have received from so many instructors and students, making suggestions that they feel would improve the text. Because this book was written for students beginning their study of the anatomical science of the head and neck, we have consistently tried to begin at a very basic level. We have also realized that the needs of the various dental programs vary as much as the backgrounds of the students. For this reason we have always chosen a middle ground, realizing that some instructors will have to supplement the material in the book, whereas others will choose not to study some areas. We still believe that the major key to the success of this book is the integrated coverage of the three areas of dental anatomy, oral histology, and head and neck anatomy. None of the areas was designed as a complete reference text, and we have tried to list more complete references at the end of each section of the text.

We have continued to present objectives at the beginning of each chapter and review questions at the end to help students determine their comprehension of the material. The new words in each chapter are in boldface type, and their definitions may be found in the glossary.

One new chapter has been included on developmental anomalies, and material has been added to the chapters on occlusion, the oral cavity, the development of the orofacial complex, and the temporomandibular joint.

The flash cards of the permanent dentition at the end of the book have been well received from the very beginning. In the third edition these cards were printed on heavier stock paper and were perforated for easier removal. Due to numerous requests, we have added cards for the primary dentition. We hope you will find them useful. The multiple choice questions at the end of the second through fourth parts of the book seem to be well received as a review for the various certifying examinations that the students have to take. We hope they continue to prove useful for you and would appreciate any comments on other areas to be included within those questions.

We hope that all who use this book will find it helpful. We thank the many persons who have sent us comments, suggestions, and criticisms and hope that all who use this text will feel free to communicate with us concerning any aspect of the book.

We would like to thank Dr. Christo Popoff for his original illustrations, Vicki Moses Friedman and Marcy Hoffman Hartstein for their original illustrations in the second, third, and fourth editions, Mr. Ed Gill for providing clinical photographs for the third and fourth editions, and Dr. Thomas Schiff and Dr. Samir El-Mofty for providing illustrations for the new chapter in this fourth edition. We also wish to thank Bonnie J. Trodden, R.D.H. of the University of Manitoba for her help and suggestions in the third edition. Finally, we would like to thank the many authors and publishers who have given their permission to use their illustrations in this book.

Richard W. Brand
Donald E. Isselhard

Contents

INTRODUCTION

1

Oral Cavity

OBJECTIVES

- To describe the boundaries and sub-boundaries of the oral cavity and the structures found there
- To define the terms vestibule, oral cavity proper, mucobuccal fold, frenum, alveolar mucosa, gingiva, exostoses, torus palatinus, and torus mandibularis
- To define the landmarks in the floor of the mouth and the hard and soft palate and the structures that form them

As students involved in all aspects of the dental profession you will be concentrating your studies on the head and neck, and, more specifically, the structures that make up the oral cavity. It is imperative that you are extremely familiar with the normal makeup and structures of this area. Therefore this chapter has been set forth to serve as an introduction to your studies of the head and neck.

The oral cavity begins the digestive system and, at its posterior end, forms a common pathway with the respiratory system. The oral cavity begins at the lips and extends posteriorly to the area of the **palatine tonsils,** which are usually referred to as the tonsils. These tonsils lie on the sides of the throat between two folds of tissues, one in front and one in back, called the **tonsillor pillars.** It is at this point that the oral cavity ends and the area behind, or posterior, to it becomes known as the **oral pharynx,** which is a shared pathway of the digestive system, from the oral cavity to the esophagus, and the respiratory sys-

tem, from the nasal cavity to the larynx, trachea, and lungs. When considering the oral cavity it is proper to divide it into two parts: (1) the vestibule, which is the space between the lips or cheeks and the teeth (in an edentulous person, or one without teeth, it would extend between the lips and cheeks and the alveolar ridges where the teeth were at one time) and (2) the oral cavity proper, which is the area from the teeth or alveolar ridges back to the area of the palatine tonsils.

VESTIBULE

In considering the vestibular area, you should begin by examining the lips. The lips are the junction between the skin of the face, which is a dry epithelium, and the mucosa of the oral cavity, which is a moist epithelium. Between these two areas lies a transitional zone of reddish tissue known as the **vermilion zone** of the lip. The skin of the upper lip has an indentation at the midline known as the **philtrum,** which is derived from the embryonic medial nasal processes (Fig. 1-1). It is at the lateral junction of this philtrum that a cleft lip would be seen.

Anterior and Posterior Borders

By elevating the mandible so that the teeth are in contact and then retracting the lips and cheeks, you can see the vestibule. Anteriorly it is bounded by the lips **(labia)** and laterally by the cheek **(bucca).** A finger placed in the posterior portion of the vestibule will be impeded by two obstacles—the bony anterior border of the ramus of the mandible and the soft tissue. The

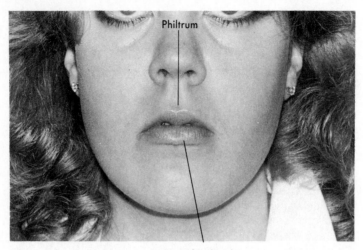

Philtrum

Vermilion border

Fig. 1-1   Vermilion zone of lips and philtrum of upper lip.

cheek is formed, to a great extent, by the buccinator muscle, covered with skin on the outside and moist mucous membrane on the inside. This muscle extends from the corners of the mouth to join with the muscles of the throat wall. As it passes backward, it crosses in front of the mandibular ramus from a lateral position to a medial position; this limits the posterior extent of the vestibule. As you run your finger in the upper posterior vestibular space, you can feel the ridge of bone that is the beginning of the anterior part of the zygomatic arch (cheekbone). Run your finger along the cheek area of the vestibule. Can you feel the landmarks and structures just mentioned?

Superior and Inferior Borders

The point at which the mucosa of the lips or cheeks turns to go toward the gingival, or gum, tissue is known as the mucobuccal or mucolabial fold. The mucosa lying against the alveolar bone is loosely attached and movable and known as alveolar mucosa. The point at which it becomes tightly attached to the bone is the beginning of the gingiva. This is known as the mucogingival junction (Fig. 1-2).

Pull outward on the lips or corners of the mouth and you will see that there are several areas where the tissue is attached in folds to the alveolar mucosa. At the midline in both the upper and lower lips there is a fold of tissue known as the **labial frenum.** The upper frenum is usually more pronounced than the lower, but problems may occur with either one. The attachment of the upper (maxillary) frenum may extend up to the crest of the alveolar ridge and even over the ridge. This band of tissue is so firm that the erupting central incisors might not penetrate it but be pushed aside slightly so that a space would exist between them. This space is known as a **diastema** (Fig. 1-3, *A*). Correction of a diastema usually involves the surgical removal or cutting of the frenum tissue between the teeth. After this, the teeth will generally move together into normal contact. This procedure is best done when a person is young.

The mandibular labial frenum seldom extends up between the teeth, but there are times when it extends close enough to the gingiva that it may contribute to gingival recession in that area by pulling downward on the tissue when the lip is tensed (Fig. 1-3, *B*).

Maxillary
labial
frenum

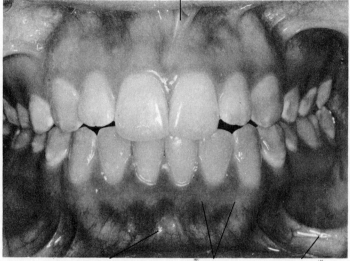

Mandibular labial frenum   Mucogingival   Mucobuccal fold
junction

Fig. 1-2 View of vestibule. There is change in color at mucogingival junction. Maxillary labial frenum is more evident than mandibular labial frenum. Mucobuccal folds are quite evident.

There are also less well-defined frenula in the maxillary and mandibular canine areas. Although these are not so well developed, they still have to be taken into consideration in the construction of a denture. If a groove is not reproduced in the **flange** or *edge* of the denture at that point, the appliance will cause irritation and possible ulceration of the frenular tissue.

Clinical Manifestations of the Vestibule

As we continue to consider the structure of the vestibule in relation to clinical dentistry, it is interesting to notice what happens to the vestibule when the mouth is opened wide. Place the teeth together, with the lips and cheeks relaxed. Position your index finger in the superior and posterior part of the vestibule adjacent to the maxillary third molar area. Now open the mouth wide. You can feel your finger being pushed anteriorly out

of the area. This is the **coronoid process** of the mandible moving into that vestibular space. The presence of the coronoid process can be of clinical consideration for several reasons.

In radiology, for example, you can take two periapical films of the maxillary molar area, one using a **bisecting angle** with the mouth in an open position, and the other using a **paralleling technique** with the mouth closed on a film-holding device. You will note the presence of the coronoid process on the film held by the patient. On the film taken with a holding device and the mouth closed, the coronoid process does not impinge on the space. The coronoid process may also cause some problems when you are trying to take maxillary study models. With the mouth open wide, the coronoid process may tend to push on the posterior part of the tray and cause it to move forward, making it difficult to obtain a

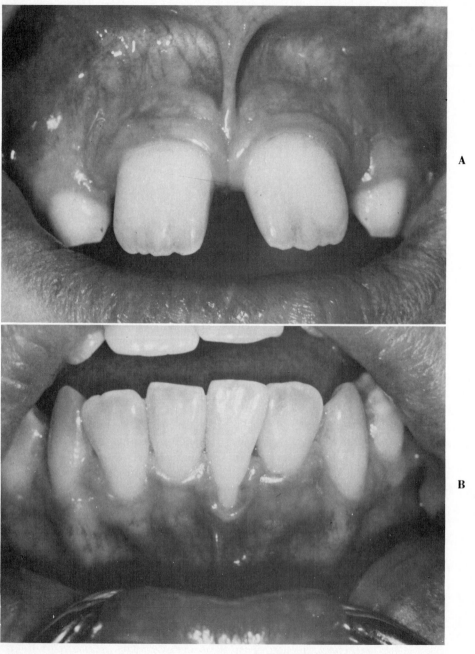

Fig. 1-3 **A,** Notice how labial frenum extends between maxillary teeth, causing separation, or diastema. **B,** Notice how mandibular labial frenum attaches close to area of gingival recession and contributes to that condition. (Courtesy Dr. David Vandersall.)

good impression of the third molars and the maxillary tuberosity region.

Study the texture of the inner surface of the lip. Pull the lower lip down and stretch it. Notice the small drops of fluid on the lip, indicating the openings of small salivary glands. These, of course, are also found in many other areas of the oral cavity, as indicated in Chapter 10.

The lips, cheeks, and retromolar pad areas posterior to the mandibular molars are also the most frequent sites of misplaced **sebaceous glands** frequently known as **fordyce granules.** These glands are normally associated with hair follicles, which would only be found on skin. In about 60% to 80% of the population, some sebaceous glands may be located on mucosa in these other areas. They appear as yellowish granular structures embedded in the skin. Look for these harmless glands in your own mouth.

Another condition found on the buccal cortical plate of the vestibule in a large portion of the population are small bony growths called **exostoses.** These are normally of no consequence unless they become tender from brushing in the area or unless dentures are being constructed. Under these circumstances they may have to be removed.

ORAL CAVITY PROPER

As the mouth is opened, you can see the oral cavity proper. First examine the roof of the mouth and study the hard and soft palates.

Hard Palate

Read or review Chapter 11 on the osteology of the skull for extent and makeup of the hard palate. There are transverse ridges of epithelial and connective tissue found in the anterior portion of the hard palate known as **rugae.** During speech and mastication, the tongue contacts these rugae. They are covered with keratinized epithelium and are frequently burned by hot foods. There is a singular bulge of tissue at the midline immediately posterior to the central incisors known as

the **incisive papilla.** Beneath this papilla is the incisive canal, which carries the nasopalatine nerve to the soft tissue lingual to the maxillary anterior teeth. This is a point of injection for anesthetizing the area. At the posterolateral part of the hard palate opposite the second and third molars are two openings in the bone, the greater palatine foramina, for the rest of the nerves to the hard palate. This area is also an injection site (Figs. 1-4 and 1-6).

The tissue beneath the palatal epithelium varies from region to region in the palate. In the midline of the hard palate the connective tissue is rather thin, and the palate feels very hard and bony in that part. In the anterolateral part of the hard palate the connective tissue contains fat cells, and overall the tissue is thicker than at the midline. In the posterolateral portion, the fat cells are minimal, but there are numerous minor salivary glands that secrete mucus. The soft palate also contains these mucus-secreting minor salivary glands.

The shape and size of the hard palate vary from individual to individual. It may be wide or narrow, have a high, arching curvature or vault, or be quite flat in its contours. Not infrequently, there may be some excess bone growth in the midline of the hard palate. This is referred to as a **torus palatinus** (Fig. 1-5). It may grow to varying sizes and is generally only a problem when construction of a denture is necessary. Under these circumstances, a denture cannot be accurately adapted to the palate area, and proper retention cannot be achieved without surgically removing the growth.

Soft Palate

The junction of the hard and soft palates forms a double curving line, with the **posterior nasal spine** of the palatine bone being the primary landmark at the midline (Figs. 1-4 and 1-6). The soft palate stretches back from the hard palate and in a relaxed state has an arching form from one side to the other. The most posterior portion at the midline is a downward projection known

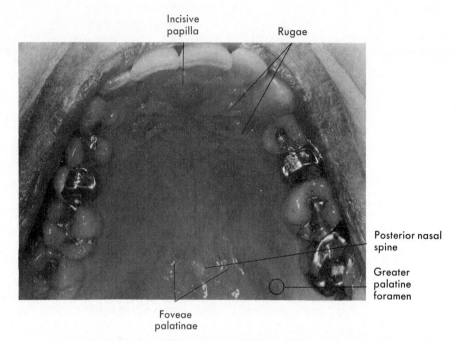

Fig. 1-4 View of palate. *Circle,* Position of greater palatine foramen. See incisive papilla and rugae as well as area of posterior nasal spine indicating end of hard palate.

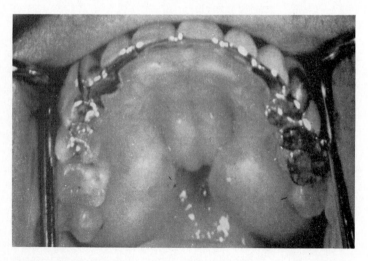

Fig. 1-5 Typical torus palatinus. Notice slightly constricted area where it attaches to hard palate. (Bhaskar: Synopsis.)

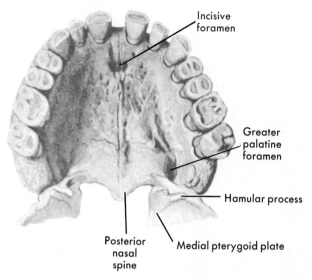

Incisive
foramen

Greater
palatine
foramen

Hamular process

Medial pterygoid plate

Posterior
nasal
spine

Fig. 1-6 Hard palate. Notice how posterior area curves toward posterior nasal spine. Laterally, notice hamular process of medial pterygoid plate. (DuBrul.)

as the **uvula.** In speech and swallowing, the soft palate moves into various positions. When a person speaks or swallows, the oral cavity is closed off from the nasal cavity. To do this, the muscle that elevates the soft palate **(levator veli palatini)** pulls it upward and backward until it contacts the posterior throat **(pharyngeal)** wall.

In Chapter 3, on development of the face and oral cavity, the cleft lip and palate are mentioned. These are rather drastic or outstanding medicodental problems and are being treated more and more by the dental profession. Another variation of cleft palate is the **short palate.** The soft palate may look normal, but when it is elevated during swallowing or speech, it does not contact the posterior pharyngeal wall and the patient produces a nasal or cleft speech sound. With a dental appliance and speech therapy this problem can be corrected with gratifying results.

Lateral Borders

The lateral borders of the oral cavity proper are bounded primarily by the teeth and associ-

ated mucosa. In the posterior lateral part of the oral cavity the boundary is the palatine tonsil and its associated **pillars.** The more prominent fold behind the tonsil, extending from the soft palate downward into the lateral pharyngeal wall is referred to as the **posterior pillar,** or **palatopharyngeal arch** or **fold.** Immediately in front of the palatine tonsil is the **anterior pillar,** or **palatoglossal arch** or **fold** (Fig. 1-7).

Posterior Borders

Just posterior to the mandibular third molar is a small elevation of tissue known as the **retromolar pad** (Fig. 1-8). This structure is a consideration in denture construction and occasionally in local anesthesia.

The posterior extent of the oral cavity is the space between the left and right tonsils known as the **fauces.** Looking into the oral cavity you can see the tongue and soft palate. If you depress the tongue with a tongue blade and ask the patient to say "ahhhh," it will elevate the soft palate and enable examination beyond the oral cavity into the oral pharynx. The posterior pharyngeal wall can indicate the health status of the patient's throat.

Tongue and Floor of Mouth

Tongue. Chapter 9 contains descriptions of structures on the tongue such as filiform, fungiform, vallate, or circumvallate papillae, and the roughened lateral surface of the tongue opposite the vallate papillae, which represents rudimentary foliate papillae. These foliate papillae should be carefully examined in a routine oral examination, since it is a difficult area to see and might hide early signs of oral cancer. There may also be enlargements of lymphoid tissue at the base of the tongue, which are referred to collectively as the lingual tonsils.

If you ask the patient to elevate the tongue, you will see that the underside, or ventral side, of the tongue has many blood vessels close to the surface. Extending from an area near the tip of the tongue down to the floor of the mouth is a fold of tissue known as the **lingual frenum,** or

Uvula   Posterior   Anterior
         pillar   pillar

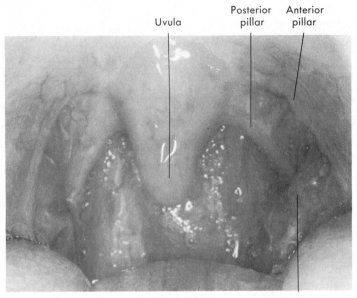

Tonsil

Fig. 1-7 Here one sees various posterior palatal structures.

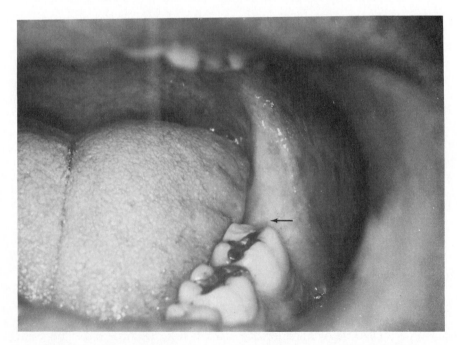

Fig. 1-8 Arrow indicates retromolar pad behind mandibular third molar.

frenulum. If this frenum is attached close to the tip of the tongue and is rather short, the tongue will have limited movement. This condition is known as **ankyloglossia,** or, as it is commonly called, **tongue-tie,** or being **tongue tied.**

Floor of mouth. At the base of the frenum there is a small elevation on each side known as the **sublingual caruncle.** This is the opening for two of the major salivary glands. Extending from the sublingual caruncle back along the floor of the mouth on either side is a fold of tissue known as the **sublingual fold.** Along the anterior and middle parts of this fold can be found a number of small openings of the multiple ducts of the sublingual salivary gland. This fold of tissue also marks the paths of a number of structures as they run forward in the floor of the mouth (Fig. 1-9).

There may frequently be some bony swellings on the lingual surface of the mandible at the ca-nine area. These are similar in nature to the pal-atal tori and are referred to as **mandibular tori** (Fig. 1-10). They may present a problem in radiology, since correct film placement may become difficult and sometimes painful to the patient. If the patient requires a lower denture, it may be necessary to remove these mandibular tori to eliminate undercuts, or improper contours, that would make denture construction difficult. The same condition can present problems when you are trying to take study models. The flange of the tray may strike the area and cause irritation.

The floor of the mouth is supported by the paired mylohyoid muscles, which form a sling from the mylohyoid line on one side to the same line on the other. Contraction of these muscles raises the tongue and floor of the mouth (see Chapters 11 and 13). If you look in a mirror while raising the tongue as high as possible, you will see the movement and get an idea of where

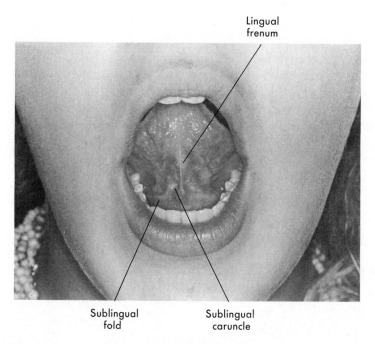

Lingual frenum

Sublingual fold

Sublingual caruncle

Fig. 1-9 Sublingual region demonstrating lingual frenum, sublingual caruncles, and sublingual folds.

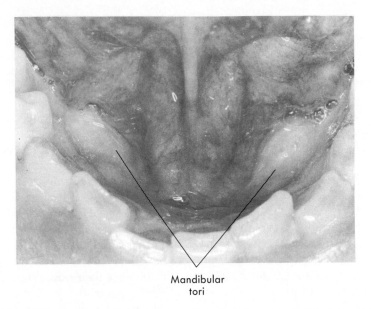

Mandibular
tori

Fig. 1-10   Another sublingual view demonstrating mandibular bony tori.

the mylohyoid muscle is attached to the mandible. This area of attachment is important in denture construction and determines how far into the floor of the mouth the denture flange will extend.

The oral tissue beneath the tongue in the floor of the mouth is the thinnest in the oral cavity and therefore quite sensitive to trauma. Of course, any of the oral tissues may be traumatized, but some are more resistant than others. Some of the common injuries you will see in the dental office may relate to hot foods and liquids. Potato chips or bony foods may cause cutting injuries to various areas of the oral cavity, especially the gingiva. *Be aware that these tissues may be readily injured!*

CLINICAL SIGNIFICANCE OF ORAL CAVITY

Although many other chapters in this book will refer to the oral cavity, it is important to stress that all who use this book need to be aware of the need for a solid background in the normal anatomy of the oral cavity. It is the responsibility of everyone who views the intraoral anatomy of the patient to be aware of what the normal anatomy of the oral cavity looks like, whether they be the dental assistant, laboratory technologist, dental hygienist, or dentist. Legally the dentist bears the primary responsibility for much of the diagnosis and treatment of the patient, but everyone should be on the lookout for anything that appears abnormal.

Frequently we think about the effects of oral diseases on other parts of the body and we consider the spread of dental infections, oral cancers, and the like. However, we must never lose sight of the fact that problems in other parts of the body may show up, early or late in the disease state, in the oral cavity. Early stages of measles show up as spots in the oral cavity. Many types of cancer from other parts of the body may spread to the oral cavity. A young child may be brought to the office because he or she has bleeding gums. The child may have good oral hygiene and the tissues may not appear too abnormal and yet the gums, or gingiva, bleed readily upon brushing. One should seriously consider having blood tests run because bleeding gingival tissues are one of the possible early signs of leukemia. A reddened, painful tongue may be a sign of vitamin deficiencies, and we now know that there are oral lesions that may be associated with AIDS. As you can readily imagine, this list is not meant to be the least bit comprehensive; rather it is meant to reinforce the fact that the entire dental team has the responsibility to be observant as they work within the oral cavity. We all owe our patients the very best care and concern we can provide, and a good solid knowledge of the normal anatomy of the oral cavity will enable any member of the team to spot something that does *not* appear to be normal and have the dentist follow up on the area of concern.

Therefore, as we go on through the various parts of this book, let us be ever mindful of doing the very best we can to understand the normal anatomy as fully as possible so that we can therefore recognize that which does not appear to be normal.

REVIEW QUESTIONS

1. What is the vestibule?
2. Do the frenum attachments of the lip contain muscles?
3. What are the divisions of the palate and what are the transverse ridges in the anterior palate called?
4. Where and what is the posterior nasal spine?
5. Which muscle supports the floor of the mouth?
6. What and where is the sublingual caruncle?
7. What makes up the anterior and posterior pillars and what lies between them?
8. What are the fauces?
9. What are the two parts of the oral cavity and what are their boundaries?
10. Why is knowledge of normal anatomy of the oral cavity so important?

ORAL HISTOLOGY AND EMBRYOLOGY

2

Basic Tissues

OBJECTIVES

- To describe a cell and its components
- To define the function of epithelium and name its various types
- To describe the origin of glands and the ways in which they may be classified
- To describe the components and functions of general connective tissues
- To describe briefly the structure of bone and the two ways in which it is formed
- To describe briefly the components and origin of blood cells and their function
- To discuss the three types of muscles—their functions and locations
- To discuss the neuron—its parts and function

This chapter on the basic tissues of the body is in no way meant to be a complete discussion; rather it is an introduction to the very basic concepts and structure of these tissues.

The body is composed of four basic tissues: **epithelium, connective tissue, muscle,** and **nervous tissue.** Some may ask, "What is a tissue?" An explanation may be that a tissue is an accumulation of cells, fibers, crystals, or fluids. Any one, or all, might compose a tissue. Then a similar question might be, "What is a **cell?**" This should be the starting point for discussing basic tissues.

CELL STRUCTURE

A cell can be thought of as a bag of fluid. The wall of this bag is called the **cell membrane.** Its function is to keep the fluid inside and foreign materials out, unless they are necessary. In Fig. 2-1 notice that the area inside the cell membrane is a fluid medium known as **cytoplasm.** Also, there are other components inside this cell. Looking through an average microscope, you would probably be able to distinguish only one structure—the **nucleus.** The nucleus is the master control of the cell. It contains those two now famous substances **DNA** and **RNA,** which control the operation of the cell.

Looking through a microscope, which can enlarge the inside of the cell even more, such as an electron microscope, you can see other parts of the cell. Most of these parts, for example, the nucleus, are referred to as **organelles.** This means small functioning parts. They allow the cell to remain alive and able to carry out its particular function.

Some of the more important organelles will be mentioned. The first are small, usually oblong structures known as **mitochondria.** These little organs are responsible for energy production and for the rate at which the cell uses energy, more commonly called the **metabolism** of the cell. If these mitochondria are injured, the cell will not be able to function and may die.

Another little organ is called the **endoplasmic reticulum,** which refers to a network within the fluid of the cell. The endoplasmic reticulum is a series of interconnecting tubules in the cell that are responsible for the manufacture of various products to be used inside or outside the cell. Some endoplasmic reticulum has small granules of RNA on the outside and is referred to as rough endoplasmic reticulum. It is responsible for the production of **protein** material. One example of

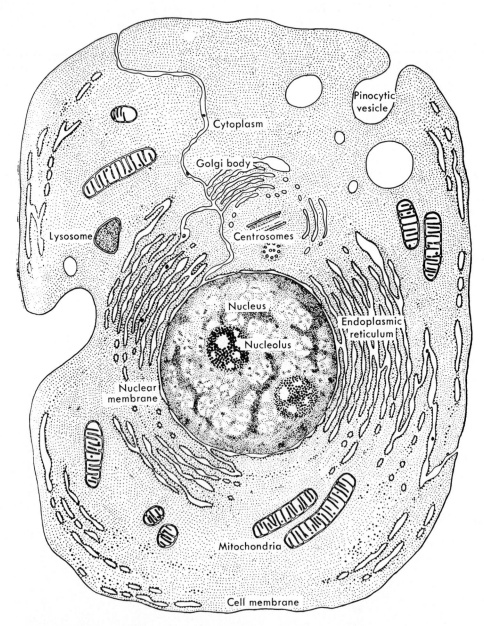

Fig. 2-1 Drawing of cell showing all basic components, except for lipid or glycogen inclusions. (Brachet J: The living cell, Sci Am 205:51, 1961. ©1961 by Scientific American, Inc. All rights reserved.)

the type of protein material produced is some components of saliva made by the cells of the salivary glands. Once this protein material is produced, it is frequently necessary to "package" it, as one would do in a shipping room.

There is another small organ in the cell that takes care of this "packaging"; it is known as the **Golgi apparatus.** In this area a thin membrane or wall surrounds the produced material so that it can be moved around the cell without mixing with the fluid of the cell and later can be pushed out of the cell.

One other organelle found in many cells is called a **lysosome.** This is a rather circular structure that acts as a scavenger for the cell. If any small parts of the cell die, or if the cell takes in some kind of foreign material from outside itself, this lysosome will digest the substances like a glorified vacuum cleaner. The one problem with this organelle is that it contains some very pow-

erful digestive **enzymes** to perform its job, and if it is injured, the enzymes will leak out and consume the cell. The person who discovered these organelles called them "suicide bags."

Organelles are intermixed in many cells with what are referred to as **cellular inclusions.** This term indicates that these "inclusions" are not really a functioning part of the cell but rather something that is stored in the cell to be used at a later time and possibly another place. These may include little spheres of fat, known as **lipid droplets,** or small units of a sugarlike compound, known as **glycogen.** Both are storage forms of energy. When the body requires this energy, they will be released from the cell to travel to other parts of the body and be used as needed (Fig. 2-2).

This is only a very brief discussion of cells and their components. As we continue, a number of different types of cells with different functions

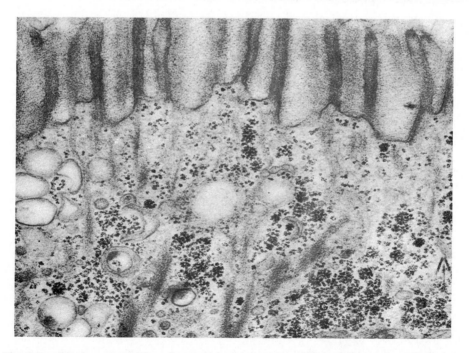

Fig. 2-2   Black spots in this cell are glycogen granules. Although there are no lipid droplets here, they resemble circular areas to left of field. (Bevelander: Outline.)

will be explored. In many ways these cells are similiar and have similiar structures, but there are some differences, which will be covered.

One final point should be mentioned at this time regarding the general size of the cells. Although they vary in size, the average is about 0.01 to 0.005 mm in diameter.

We will now take a brief look at the following four basic tissues of the body: epithelial tissue, connective tissue, muscle tissue, and nerve tissue.

EPITHELIAL TISSUE

Epithelium is a group of cells that covers the body, seen as skin, or lines the inside of the tubes or cavities of the body. An example of these lining layers is the inside of blood vessels or the digestive tract, as well as the lining of the chest and abdominal cavities. Glands, such as salivary and liver, also originate from epithelium. Shapes of these epithelial cells differ, and they are arranged in a variety of relationships. Because of these differences, each type of epithelium has a different name. Now to consider the different types.

Epithelium is classified according to the number of its cell layers—(1) simple, or single-layered, and (2) stratified, or multiple-layered, epithelium. Simple epithelium denotes one layer of cells resting on the underlying tissue.

Simple Epithelium

Simple squamous epithelium. The word "squamous" means 'flat' or 'platelike.' If you looked at the surface of **simple squamous epithelium,** it would look like a collection of fried eggs poured together in a big pan (Fig. 2-3, *A*). If you cut down through this epithelium and then looked at it from the side, it would look like an overdone fried egg cut right through the yolk (Fig. 2-3, *B*). Looking at it from this side view, you can imagine that such a thin layer would not be an extremely protective type of structure but might be thin enough for some materials to pass

through it between the cells. This type of epithelium is found lining the lungs, blood vessels, abdominal cavity, and small fluid-carrying tubes known as **lymphatic vessels.** Simple squamous epithelium allows for the exchange of oxygen and carbon dioxide between the lining and the blood vessels of the lungs.

Simple cuboidal or simple columnar epithelium. As the names indicate, **simple cuboidal** and **simple columnar epithelium** is cuboidal or rectangular. Again, these kinds of cells are one layer thick, but observe that one layer is much thicker than the squamous layer (Fig. 2-4). They are found in a number of areas in the body. The columnar cells are found lining the digestive tract, and the cuboidal cells are found in the ducts of various glands—kidney, salivary glands, **pancreas,** and others. When these cuboidal, or columnar, cells are packed together to form small ducts, they tend to form a pyramid shape (Fig. 2-5) and are frequently referred to as **pyramidal cells.**

If one looks at the arrangement of these kinds of cells, it is apparent that on two sides the cells adjoin, whereas on the other two visible sides one rests on some underlying tissue and the other end faces a free border, or **lumen,** of a duct. The side facing the underlying tissue is referred to as the **basal end** of the cell. Facing the free surface is the side frequently referred to as the **apical end** of the cell. This terminology makes sense when you look at a pyramidal cell and see that the apical end is the apex of the pyramid and the basal end is the base of the pyramid. Later we will discuss cells that secrete or give off a product from their apical end.

Pseudostratified columnar epithelium. The term **pseudostratified columnar epithelium** means falsely layered epithelium, or epithelium that looks like more than one layer. Viewed under a microscope, it appears that there are several rows of nuclei, indicating that there are more than one row of cells. However, on closer examination it is evident that all the cells reach all the way down to the underlying tissue. Some

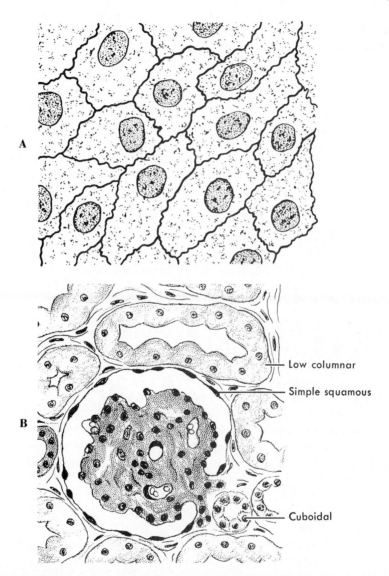

A

B

Low columnar

Simple squamous

Cuboidal

Fig. 2-3 **A,** Superior view of simple squamous epithelium. **B,** Cross section of simple squamous, simple columnar, and simple cuboidal epithelium. Notice shape. (Bevelander: Outline.)

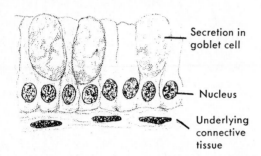

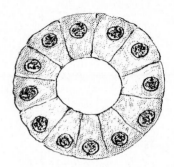

Fig. 2-4 Simple columnar epithelium with single-celled glands (goblet cells) interspersed. Simple cuboidal epithelium cells are more square. (Bevelander: Outline.)

Fig. 2-5 Columnar cells forming tube, or duct, pushed into pyramidal pattern. Apical end is narrower than basal end. Secretions come from apical end. (Bevelander: Outline.)

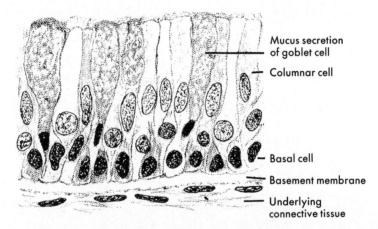

Fig. 2-6 Representation of pseudostratified columnar epithelium from trachea. Notice goblet cells intermixed. There appears to be more than one row of cells, but there is only one because all cells rest on basement membrane. (Bevelander: Outline.)

of the cells are very short, but others begin on the underlying tissue with a very narrow stem and then bulge out once they reach the upper part of the cell layer. This type of epithelium is seen in several areas of the body, but the most prominent is the upper respiratory tract. In the respiratory tract, as well as in other places, the epithelium has small single-celled glands called **goblet cells** intermixed with the epithelium (Fig.

2-6). These glands secrete a mucous substance and lubricate the surface of the epithelium for a number of functions.

Along with the goblet cells, this epithelium also has small hairs, known as **cilia,** which are capable of a waving, beating motion. These cilia get mucus on them from the goblet cells and then trap contaminants in the air passing through the respiratory passage. These trapped particles are passed along from cilium to cilium by means of the beating motion until they reach the nasal opening or the opening of the oral cavity where they are removed from the body.

Stratified Epithelium

There are three varieties of multiple-layered, or stratified, epithelium, only two of which are seen in any quantity.

Stratified cuboidal, or stratified columnar, epithelium. A type of epithelium not commonly found is **stratified cuboidal,** or **stratified columnar, epithelium.** It consists of two rows of cuboidal or columnar cells on top of one another and is generally only found forming large ducts of glands.

Transitional epithelium. "Transitional" indicates change, and that appropriately describes **transitional epithelium.** It changes in thickness and appearance as the need arises. Composed of multiple layers of cells and varying in thickness, it is found in the urinary system, with the primary concentration in the urinary bladder. When the bladder is empty, the epithelium is relaxed and there are about eight to ten layers, with the

deepest layers being composed of rather cuboidal cells and the surface layers, inside the bladder, somewhat more flattened but with rounded bulging nuclei (Fig. 2-7). When the bladder is full, the epithelium is stretched and may appear to be only three to five layers thick. The deepest cell layers appear somewhat more flattened, and the surface layers, as well as the nuclei, are extremely flattened. This change in appearance accounts for the name "transitional" and represents a very functional arrangement of cells.

Stratified squamous epithelium. The most common type of epithelium is **stratified squamous epithelium.** As skin it covers the body and also makes up the mucosa of the oral cavity and esophagus. In a discussion of this type of epithelium, it seems appropriate to consider the similarities in different areas.

STRATUM BASALE, OR STRATUM GERMINATIVUM. A single layer of cuboidal cells that rests on the underlying connective tissue is known as **stratum basale,** or **stratum germinativum.** It is in this layer that the cells divide and form more cells to maintain the supply and replace those that are lost.

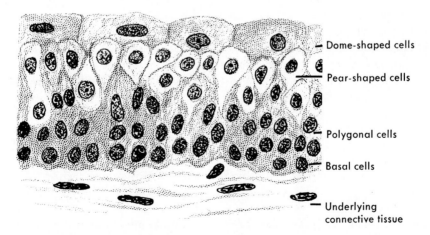

Dome-shaped cells

Pear-shaped cells

Polygonal cells

Basal cells

Underlying connective tissue

Fig. 2-7 Relaxed transitional epithelium of bladder. There seem to be about seven rows of cells. When this epithelium is stretched, surface cells flatten and there are then three to five rows of cells. (Bevelander: Outline.)

STRATUM SPINOSUM. As more cells form in the basal layer, they become displaced because of the crowding; thus they are pushed out of the basal layer into the layers above them toward the surface. The **stratum spinosum** varies in the number of rows of cells, from two or three to ten or more. In this layer the cells are no longer cuboidal but seem to be star shaped, or having many small points; hence the adjective "spinosum." The cells continue to be pushed toward the surface by the newly forming basal cells, and eventually they reach the next layer.

STRATUM GRANULOSUM. Not clearly seen in many areas of the mucosa of the oral cavity, **stratum granulosum** is particularly evident in thick skin. When seen, it appears as two or three layers of rather flattened cells, which contain granules, or spots, within the cytoplasm of the cell. These granules are made up of a material called **keratohyalin** and will eventually cause the cell to die when the amount of **keratin** becomes great enough.

STRATUM CORNEUM. The term "corneum" is the same as the term "keratinized." It means 'horn-like,' resembling the tissue of the fingernail. In many instances **stratum corneum** is misnamed because the top layers of cells are not always dead. Three different situations can be seen in this layer: (1) the cells may be alive and the epithelium referred to as nonkeratinized stratified squamous epithelium; (2) the cells on the surface may be in the process of dying and referred to as partly, or **parakeratinized,** stratified squamous epithelium; or (3) the cells on the surface can be dead and referred to as keratinized stratified squamous epithelium (Fig. 2-8).

The thickness of this upper dead layer varies, depending on the amount of trauma or rubbing the tissue is subjected to. As you know, working with a shovel or rake will eventually cause a callus to form. This is a result of a thickening of the stratum corneum, as well as a thickening of the stratum spinosum. The cells are continually produced in the lowest layer of the epithelium, the **basal layer,** and move up through the other layers until they reach the surface, where they are shed. This process can be understood when one sits in a tub of hot water for a while without using soap and watches a ring develop around the tub. This ring is not readily visible but can be felt. The primary component of this ring is dead epithelial cells, which **slough** off and float to the edge of the tub. Just think of the mechanism that regulates the rate of cells produced with the rate of those lost and that adjusts itself to meet any changes. Without this control we would either have skin as thick as an elephant or have no skin whatsoever!

Another important mechanism relating to cell replacement in skin has to do with pigment in the skin and changes in that pigment level. Immediately beneath the basal layer of cells in all persons are cells called **melanocytes,** which produce a pigment, or color, called **melanin.** These cells, when stimulated by **ultraviolet rays** from a sunlamp or the sun, produce more pigment. It is picked up by the epithelial cells and carried to the surface. As this happens, the skin darkens. After the person is no longer subjected to these ultraviolet rays, the pigment level is reduced, the cells containing it are eventually lost, and the skin lightens in color.

Glands

Most of the glands of the body are developed from epithelium. As the epithelium develops, some of the basal cells begin to grow downward into the connective tissue beneath it. As they grow downward, they form a tube of epithelial cells. When they have reached a certain depth, these tubes form a number of little bulblike or tubelike processes on their ends, which are generally referred to as **acini,** or **tubules,** respectively. Glands can be classified in a number of ways.

Distributive mechanisms. A distributive mechanism is the manner in which the secretory products are carried away from the gland. There are **exocrine** glands, whose products are carried away by ducts leading from the gland. Then there

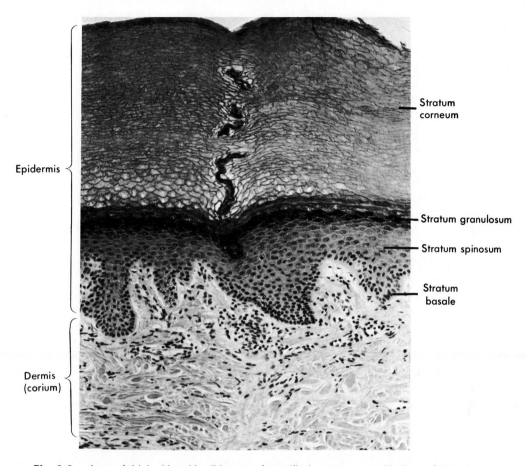

Fig. 2-8 Area of thick skin with all layers of stratified squamous epithelium. Cells of stratum corneum have no nuclei, indicating that they are dead. (Bevelander: Outline.)

are **endocrine** glands, whose ducts are lost after the gland develops and whose products are carried away from the gland in the bloodstream. Salivary glands are an example of exocrine glands.

Secretory mechanisms. A secretory mechanism is the manner in which the product is secreted from the gland. In **holocrine** glands the entire cell dies and the secretion is lost when the cell membrane breaks up. The secretory products of **merocrine** glands pass through the cell wall without allowing any cell cytoplasm to escape. This is how the salivary glands secrete, without any loss of cytoplasm.

Arrangement of components. Exocrine glands have secretory and excretory portions. The secretory portion is composed of the cells that actually secrete and modify the substance being produced by the gland. The excretory portion is the duct system that carries the product to the surface. The arrangement of these components varies from a simple tubular gland, which is just a straight tube, to a **compound tubuloalveolar** gland, of which salivary glands are an example. A compound gland has numerous levels of branching in its duct system, similar to the branches of a tree. A tubuloalveolar portion has tubelike secre-

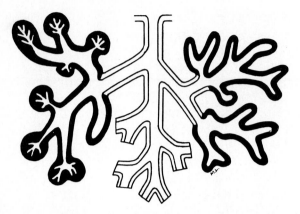

Fig. 2-9 Representation of compound tubuloalveolar glands. There are branchings of ducts and dark tubular endpieces with rounded ends. (Bevelander: Outline.)

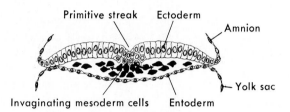

Fig. 2-10 Cross section through flat plate of cells of 16-day embryo. There are three germ layers and mesoderm originating from ectoderm. (Langman.)

tory parts, with a rounded alveolus or acinus at the end (Fig. 2-9).

Products. Salivary glands produce the following types of secretions:

1. **Serous** secretion—A thin watery substance
2. **Mucous** secretion—A thicker, more viscous substance
3. **Seromucous** secretion—Produced by many of the glands that have both types of cells, in varying quantities, within the same gland.

Embryonic Origin

The next point to consider, which concerns the other basic tissues as well, is embryonic origin. You know that an individual begins development from a single cell, the fertilized ovum. From this one cell, the following occur. The ovum divides into two cells, and the two into four, and so on. This multiplication forms a ball of cells, inside of which the embryo begins to form. At first it is an elongated flat structure, made up of two layers of epithelial cells. The outer layer of epithelial cells are called the **ectoderm** layer, meaning 'cells developing on the outside.' The inner layer of epithelial cells is called the **entoderm,** or 'cells developing on the inside.' Eventually some cells of the outer (ecto-

derm) layer work their way in between these two layers and become the **mesoderm,** or middle layers. All the other cells of the body develop from these three layers. Different kinds of epithelium may come from any one of these three germ layers—the skin from ectoderm, the epithelium of the digestive tract from entoderm, and the squamous lining of the abdominal cavity from mesoderm (Fig. 2-10).

CONNECTIVE TISSUE

The name "connective tissue" seems self explanatory in that it indicates something that holds or connects parts of the body together, and to some extent this is true. However, since blood is classified as a component of connective tissue, this definition may be confusing. All the various types of connective tissue originate from mesoderm. Connective tissues can be divided into the categories of general connective tissue and more specialized connective tissue, such as cartilage, bone, and blood.

General Connective Tissue

General connective tissue is composed of cells, fibers, and the fluidlike material referred to as **ground substance.** It is subdivided into irregular connective tissue, which is found primarily beneath epithelium, and regular connective tissue, such as **tendons** and **ligaments.**

Irregular connective tissue. If we examine the epithelium, for example, the skin on an arm, we can feel that it is quite movable. The epithelium has no blood vessels, and yet its cells are active and therefore must have a nutrient source somewhere. The answer is in the connective tissue immediately below the skin, or epithelium. As mentioned earlier, this tissue is composed of cells, fibers, and ground substance. There are many different types of connective tissue cells, but for our purposes one of the most important cells is the fibroblast. The suffix *-blast* will appear frequently; it means 'sprout.' Therefore the word "fibroblast" refers to one of the cells that "sprouts," or forms, fibers. These are known as **collagen** fibers. They are nonelastic and function by holding the epithelium to the underlying muscles or bone, holding bones together, or attaching muscles to bone. The collagen fiber is also the fiber that attaches the tooth to its socket.

Another type of cell found in the connective tissue is a rather primitive cell of mesodermal origin called the **mesenchymal cell.** This is the first cell seen when mesoderm develops in the early embryo. This cell has the potential of changing into a number of other cell types, including fibroblasts, which were just mentioned. The presence of mesenchymal cells in the tissue allows for replacement of some components of connective tissue that are lost through injury. There are cells present in the connective tissue that produce antibodies to fight off or resist certain substances entering the body. Other cells, called **macrophages,** act as scavengers and devour dying cells and bacteria.

Along with these other cells found in connective tissue are other fibers in different areas. One, a **reticular fiber,** is primarily seen as a framework for a number of organs. The other is an **elastic fiber,** which as the name indicates, stretches and then returns to its original length.

Irregular connective tissue is so named because its fibers run in all directions. Also running in this irregular connective tissue are the nerves and blood vessels that supply the area (Fig. 2-11).

The third major component of connective tis-

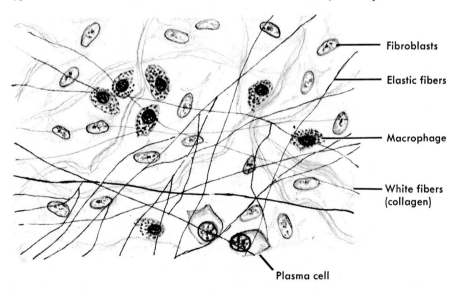

Fibroblasts

Elastic fibers

Macrophage

White fibers (collagen)

Plasma cell

Fig. 2-11 Irregular connective tissue with fibroblasts, collagen fibers (white fibers), and other cells of connective tissue. Invisible ground substance holds all together. (Bevelander: Outline.)

sue, the ground substance, can be thought of as a gluelike substance that holds the cells and fibers together.

Regular connective tissue. The term "regular connective tissue" simply means that the collagen fibers run parallel with one another, with fibroblasts squeezed in between. These regular connective tissues are found as tendons, which attach muscle to bone, and ligaments, which attach bone to bone.

Special Connective Tissue

Let us now consider the somewhat more specialized components of connective tissue—cartilage, bone, and the blood vascular system.

Cartilage. **Cartilage** is a noncalcified supporting component of the body. It is made up of cells called **chondroblasts** or **chondrocytes,** fibers of either collagen or **elastin,** and a ground substance. There are three types of cartilage—**fibrocartilage, elastic cartilage,** and **hyaline cartilage.**

Fibrocartilage contains a great deal of collagen fibers and functions as a cushioning substance. It is found in such areas as intervertebral discs between vertebrae of the spinal column and in later years the temporomandibular joint of the jaw.

Elastic cartilage contains elastic fibers, and the cartilage is therefore very flexible. It is found in the firm but flexible part of the ear, as well as in the epiglottis over the larynx.

The third type, hyaline cartilage, is firmer than the other two and contains smaller amounts of collagen fibers. It can be seen in an adult in such areas as the larynx, or voice box, trachea, and certain parts of bones. During a person's development from the embryonic stage into adulthood, many of the areas that originate as hyaline cartilage later change into bone. It is also this hyaline cartilage that allows the bones of the arms and legs to grow in length.

Bone. We know that bone is a hard substance. But what makes it hard? Bone is made up of cells called **osteoblasts** (meaning 'bone-formers') or **osteocytes** (meaning 'bone cells'), as well as col-

lagen fibers and ground substance. It also has microscopic crystals of a substance called **hydroxyapatite.** These crystals of calcium and phosphorus are found packed into the ground substance and fibers in between the cells, giving bone its hardness. If a bone is placed in an acid substance, the crystals will dissolve and only the other three components will be left. Then what happens? Consider the following experiment in which a chicken bone is placed in vinegar. After a few days the bone can be bent into a pretzel shape. The vinegar is acetic acid and dissolves the crystals, leaving the bone flexible.

INTRAMEMBRANOUS FORMATION. How does bone form? One way is by **intramembranous bone formation.** This means formation within tissue. The bone forms in regular connective tissue by some of the primitive mesenchymal cells becoming osteoblast cells. This cell secretes ground substance, collagen fibers, and then hydroxyapatite crystals. The crystals grow and pack more tightly together, and the forming bone hardens. Most of the bone growth in the head area is of the intramembranous type (Fig. 2-12).

ENDOCHONDRAL FORMATION. The second way in which bone forms is called **endochondral bone formation.** The prefix *endo-* means 'within' and *chondral* refers to 'cartilage.' In this type of bone formation, cartilage is first formed and then invaded by bone cells, which replace the cartilage with bone (Fig. 2-13). As mentioned earlier, this is the mechanism in the ends of long bones of the extremities that causes the growth of an individual. In certain very important areas of the bottom of the skull the bone growth is endochondral.

BONE STRUCTURE. Once bone has developed, it all tends to appear the same microscopically. It is covered on the outside with a double layer called the **periosteum.** The outer layer is fibrous, and the inner layer is composed of cells that become osteoblasts and can form bone. In the center of bone is a cavity, generally referred to as the **marrow cavity.** This space serves as a site of blood cell production. Later in life the marrow

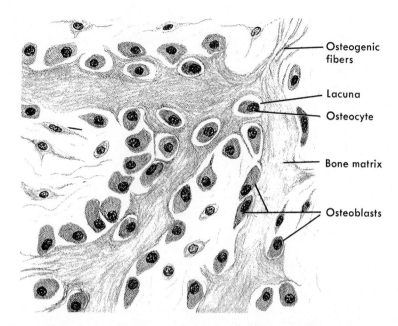

Osteogenic fibers

Lacuna

Osteocyte

Bone matrix

Osteoblasts

Fig. 2-12 Intramembranous bone formation. Osteoblasts secrete components and become trapped in mix. They are then referred to as osteocytes. Space occupied by these osteocytes is referred to as a lacuna. (Bevelander: Outline.)

cavity in many bones changes into storehouses for fat. The hard structure in between the periosteum and the marrow cavity known as cortical bone has numerous blood vessels running through it to keep it vital, or alive. Around these blood vessels are gathered many trapped bone cells, referred to in their trapped state as osteocytes. This arrangement of blood vessels and osteocytes is referred to as a **haversian system** (Fig. 2-14).

The haversian system is a series of blood vessels running parallel to one another. Because of this blood supply in bone, we refer to it as being a "vital," or alive, tissue. As bone grows, these blood vessels lying on the surface of the bone go through a series of changes whereby the bone surrounds the blood vessels. We now have a hollow tube in the bone with a blood vessel in the middle. The bone cells, osteoblasts, lining this tube begin to secrete bony layers and entrap

themselves as osteocytes. These layers continue building and fill in the tube right up to the blood vessel. Fig. 2-14 shows each of these haversian systems as a circular structure running through the bone. These longitudinal blood vessels are connected with other blood vessels running perpendicular to them traveling through openings known as **Volkmann's canals.** Blood enters the surface of the bone through a "nutrient artery." These arteries interconnect with one another bringing blood to the inside of the bone. Within the haversian system nutrients are passed on to the entrapped osteocytes closest to the blood vessel, and they in turn pass it on to the cells farther from the blood vessels. Blood is also carried into the marrow spaces where blood cells are manufactured and passed on out of the bone.

The area between these haversian systems also has entrapped bone cells and layers known as **interstitial lamellae.** These are parts of older haversian systems that have been partly destroyed and replaced by newer systems. Bone is also deposited on its surface by the **periosteum,** which is the fibrous and cellular layer on the surface of bone that provides new bone cells to the surface. These layers formed by the periosteum are known as periosteal, or **circumferential, lamellae.** On the inside, adjacent to the marrow spaces there are layers produced known as **endosteal** lamellae.

These haversian systems are best seen in cross section of long bones of the arms or legs (Fig. 2-14). These same systems do exist in the flat bones and some irregular-shaped bones of the skull.

It is important that bone be nourished with blood because it is a constantly changing structure. A perfect example is orthodontic treatment. The moving of teeth is only possible because bone is able to change and remodel itself as the

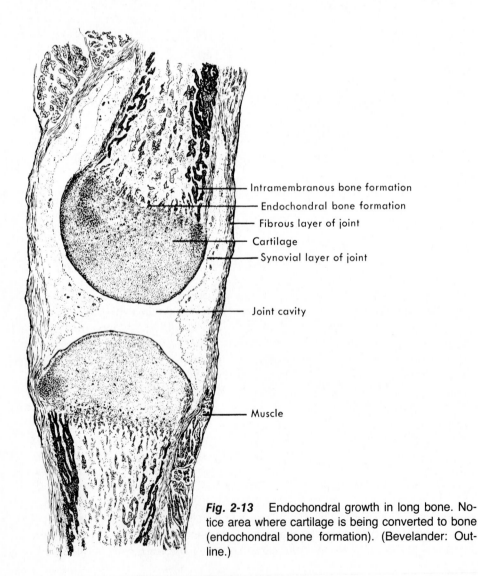

— Intramembranous bone formation
— Endochondral bone formation
— Fibrous layer of joint
Cartilage
— Synovial layer of joint

Joint cavity

Muscle

Fig. 2-13 Endochondral growth in long bone. Notice area where cartilage is being converted to bone (endochondral bone formation). (Bevelander: Outline.)

tooth moves. Cells called **"osteoclasts"** will be referred to in its remodeling process. The suffix -*clast* means 'something that destroys,' and, as you know, the prefix *osteo-* means 'bone': thus 'bone-destroying cells.' So osteoblasts and osteoclasts work together to change bone constantly as stresses are placed on it.

Blood. Blood is also considered a special connective tissue. The vessels that carry it, as well as the heart, are part of one of the organ systems of the body, known as the cardiovascular system, along with the respiratory, digestive, and other systems. Blood is made up of two components:

the fluid part and the cellular part. The fluid is called **plasma** and is similar in composition to the fluid that is found between the cells of the body.

The cellular part is divided into **red blood cells, white blood cells,** and **platelets.** Every cubic millimeter of blood contains 4.5 to 5 million red blood cells. Red cells are unusual in that they have no nucleus in their mature state. They are described as **biconcave discs,** in that they are very thin in the middle and thick at the edges. They have an iron-containing element known as **hemoglobin.** Hemoglobin has the ability to at-

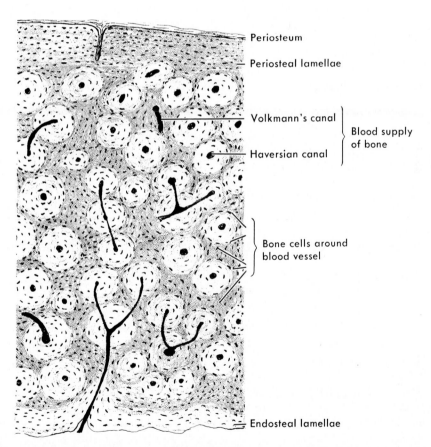

Periosteum

Periosteal lamellae

Volkmann's canal

Haversian canal

Blood supply of bone

Bone cells around blood vessel

Endosteal lamellae

Fig. 2-14 Section through portion of long bone of an extremity. At top is periosteum and below is beginning of marrow area. *Dark circles and lines,* Passages for blood vessels of haversian system. *Small dots,* Osteocytes. (Bevelander: Outline.)

tach oxygen molecules to its structure and carry it from the lungs to the cells where it is needed. It also has the ability to carry the waste product carbon dioxide from the cell and back to the lung for elimination. These cells have a life-span of about 4 months. They are eliminated by the spleen, located in the upper left abdominal area, when they are worn out.

Any significant decrease in the number of red blood cells, or their ability to carry oxygen, brings on a condition known as **anemia.** There are several types of anemia—one of them is brought on by a deficiency of vitamin B_{12} and another by the lack of iron in the body. These are **acquired** deficiencies. There is an **inherited** anemia found primarily in blacks in whom the red blood cell is C shaped, rather than round, and lacks sufficient hemoglobin. This is known as **sickle cell anemia.** There is still a significant death rate from sickle cell anemia.

White blood cells are much less numerous than red, numbering only 8,000 to 10,000 per cubic millimeter of blood. These white blood cells are divided into two groups by the presence or absence of granules in their cytoplasm. Those with granules are referred to as **granulocytes** and those without are **agranulocytes,** meaning 'without granules.'

GRANULOCYTES. Granulocytes have three varieties based on the staining properties of their granules.

Neutrophils. Of white blood cells, 50% to 70% have granules that do not stain readily and are therefore referred to as **neutrophils.** They live only about 2 days. During that time they function as **phagocytes.** They kill and devour bacteria. When bacteria enter the body where they are not normally found, they set up an **inflammatory reaction.** The four signs of inflammation are redness, warmth, swelling, and pain. The redness and warmth are attributable to more blood being sent to that region. The swelling and pain are attributable to an increase in **intercellular fluid.** This increase in fluid between the cells is caused by blood plasma that leaks from the smallest of blood vessels, the capillaries and small veins, or venules, of the area. As the fluid leaks out of the blood vessels, so too do the neutrophils. They move to the area of the invading bacteria and begin devouring them.

Eosinophils. Of white blood cells, 1% to 4% are stained red with a dye known as eosin. These **eosinophils** function to help combat **allergic reactions** and inflammatory reactions.

Basophils. Of white blood cells, 0.5% are stained blue with a basic stain and are known as **basophils.** These cells, along with connective tissue cells known as **mast cells,** contain a substance known as **histamine.** This substance is released in reaction to an **allergenic** substance. Histamine causes fluid to leak from blood vessels, and the local tissues swell. To decrease this swelling we use a drug that combats this histamine reaction and is therefore known as an **antihistamine.** This combats the action of the histamines and stops the leakage of the vessels, and the swelling decreases.

AGRANULOCYTES. There are two types of white cells that have no granules and are therefore referred to as agranulocytes. They are the **lymphocytes** and **monocytes.**

Lymphocytes. Of white blood cells, 20% to 40% are lymphocytes. They are found in the circulating blood and in **lymphoid tissues,** such as lymph nodes, spleen, and tonsils. There are two different types of lymphocytes, both having to do with providing **immunity** for an individual. One of these lymphocytes produces a cell known as a **plasma cell.** This cell is also associated with immune responses and is readily seen in tissue where there have been long-lasting infections.

Monocytes. Of white blood cells, 2% to 8% are monocytes. Monocytes become macrophages in acute inflammation. In these cases one sees neutrophils, lymphocytes, and monocytic macrophages in inflamed tissues. Monocytes fuse together in multiplication and form osteoclasts, which are large, multinucleated cells that destroy bone and other hard tissues of the body such as dentin, cementum, and possibly enamel.

During the disease process, the number of white blood cells increases, mainly neutrophils and lymphocytes. **Leukemia** is a disease of white blood cells in which one type of white cell starts multiplying rapidly, choking out the production of red blood cells. Most blood cells are produced in bone marrow, as well as the spleen, thymus, lymph nodes, and tonsils, where lymphocytes are formed. We frequently read of persons who have bone-marrow transplants. They are first treated with drugs that kill their own marrow, which is defective, and then receive new marrow, which, it is hoped, will produce a normal blood cell population.

PLATELETS. There are 250,000 to 350,000 platelets per cubic millimeter of blood. Platelets are a membrane-bound particle of a larger cell called a **megakaryocyte,** which is found in bone marrow. These platelets play an important role in the clotting of blood. When platelets reach a broken blood vessel, they may break and release a substance called **serotonin,** which causes blood vessels to contract, similar to other **vasoconstrictors,** such as **epinephrine,** that we use in dental anesthetic agents. Other platelets simply stack up in the leakage area and help begin forming what will eventually be a blood clot. Today there is a process known as **pheresis** in which blood is removed from a donor's arm, run through a centrifuge, which separates out the platelets, and run back into the donor's other arm. This provides the platelets that are necessary for leukemia patients who have clotting problems. Platelets exist for only 8 or 9 days, and so they are replaced within the week. It is possible to be a pheresis donor almost once a week.

MUSCLE TISSUE

The third basic tissue is found throughout the body. There are three types of muscle tissue—**skeletal, cardiac,** and **smooth.** All muscle tissue,

through its contraction, or shortening in length, accomplishes work.

Skeletal Muscle

The most widely studied muscle is skeletal muscle, also known as striated **voluntary muscle.** The term "striated" refers to the striped appearance of the muscle fibers under a microscope. The word "voluntary" means that the contraction, or shortening, of the muscles is under the willful control of the person or animal. A skeletal muscle, such as the biceps in the upper arm, is made up of thousands of individual muscle fibers, or muscle cells. Each of these skeletal muscle cells has hundreds of nuclei, which is rather unusual. This cell is referred to as a **myofiber,** *myo-* meaning 'muscle.' Each fiber, in turn, is made up of many smaller components of the cell—**myofibrils.** In between the myofibrils are the usual components of cells, such as the mitochondria and endoplasmic reticulum. These myofibrils also have the striated, or striped, appearance descriptive of skeletal muscle. It was originally believed that myofibrils were the smallest component of muscle and that for the muscle to contract it was necessary for these fibrils to be shortened. Later it was found that the myofibrils were made up of two smaller **myofilaments** called **actin** and **myosin.** The thinner actin filaments slightly overlap the thicker myosin filaments, and a chemical reaction causes the two filaments to slide over one another. The overall fiber shortening takes place by this sliding mechanism. This whole process is repeated hundreds of times in a single fibril.

There are hundreds of light and dark staining bands in a fibril. The light band is called the **I band,** and the dark band is called the **A band.** Halfway through the I band is a thin dark line, which is called the **Z line.** The distance between two Z lines is called a **sarcomere,** and within one sarcomere are all the components of this sliding filament mechanism of skeletal muscle (Fig. 2-15).

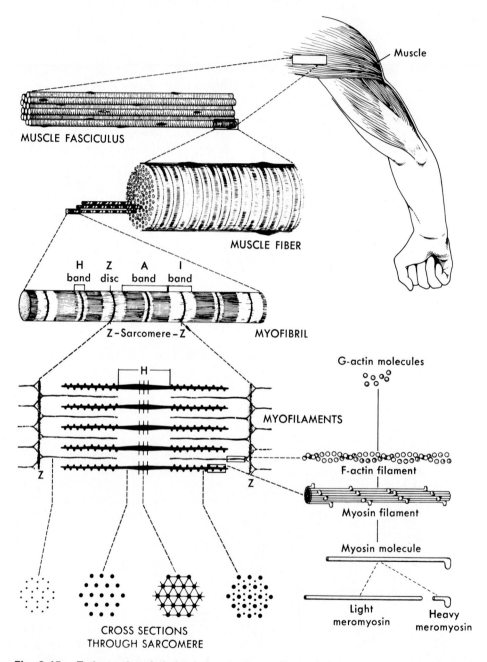

MUSCLE

MUSCLE FASCICULUS

MUSCLE FIBER

H band   Z disc   A band   I band

Z – Sarcomere – Z   MYOFIBRIL

H

MYOFILAMENTS

Z   Z

CROSS SECTIONS
THROUGH SARCOMERE

G-actin molecules

F-actin filament

Myosin filament

Myosin molecule

Light meromyosin   Heavy meromyosin

Fig. 2-15 Entire realm of skeletal muscle tissue, from whole muscle to components of sarcomere. Thin and thick filaments slide over one another in contraction. (Bloom and Fawcett; drawing by Sylvia Colard Keene.)

Cardiac Muscle

Heart muscle, or cardiac muscle, is also re-ferred to as striated **involuntary muscle,** mean-ing it has striping similar to the skeletal muscle. The term "involuntary" means that control of the heart is not under willful control of the individ-ual but rather is regulated automatically by the body. Cardiac muscle differs from skeletal mus-cle in that it has only one or two nuclei per cell and the muscle cells or fibers branch as they meet one another (Fig. 2-16). The heart muscle is also unusual in that it has specialized muscle cells, **Purkinje's fibers,** that act like nerves in the heart and conduct messages through the heart to help it contract, or beat, properly.

Smooth Muscle

Smooth muscle is the third kind of muscle tis-sue, also known as nonstriated involuntary mus-cle. This means that it does not have stripes and cannot be willfully controlled. These muscle fi-bers are found lining such areas as the digestive tract (where they move the food through the tract), in blood vessels (where they regulate the flow of blood to different parts of the body), and in many other organs. Smooth muscle has actin and myosin filaments as seen in the other two kinds of muscle; however, these filaments are not neatly arranged, and as a consequence the muscle fibers do not appear striped (Fig. 2-17).

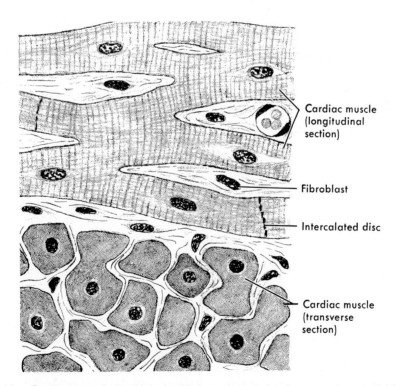

Cardiac muscle (longitudinal section)

Fibroblast

Intercalated disc

Cardiac muscle (transverse section)

Fig. 2-16 Cardiac muscle is striated, with branches and only one or two nuclei in each cell. Heavy dark line running across fiber is intercalated disc, the point at which two cells join. (Bevelander: Outline.)

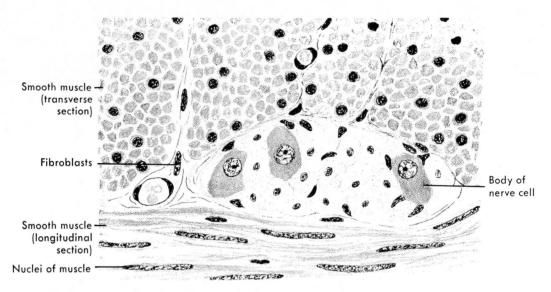

Smooth muscle (transverse section)

Fibroblasts

Smooth muscle (longitudinal section)

Nuclei of muscle

Body of nerve cell

Fig. 2-17 Smooth muscle cut in transverse (cross) section and longitudinal section. Notice that nuclei are in center and fiber is only as wide as nucleus. Also notice elongation of smooth muscle fibers. (Bevelander: Outline.)

NERVOUS TISSUE

Nervous tissue (or the nerves of the body) serves as the communicating system of the body. Messages are carried from the outer parts of the body toward the brain and these are called sensory, or **afferent,** messages. They provide information for the brain, and it reacts accordingly. The messages leaving the brain for distant parts of the body are referred to as motor, or **efferent,** messages: they usually cause some kind of action to take place.

The cell of the nervous system is called the **neuron.** There are three parts to the neuron: the **cell body,** the **axon,** and the **dendrite.** A neuron functions to carry a message by passing a small electrical current along the cell wall. This current does not have a message in it, only a wave of electricity. It is the brain itself that converts the electricity to information based on the type of neuron carrying the message, where it is from, and at times the relation to a past experience. Neurons carry messages generally in only one direction. The wave of electricity passes from the dendrite to the cell body and out along the axon. When it gets to the end of the axon, it contacts the dendrite or cell body of the next neuron and passes the message or impulse along that neuron until it reaches its destination. Thus there are neurons carrying messages to the brain and other neurons carrying messages from the brain (Fig. 2-18).

Many of these nerve cells, or neurons, have a protective covering around their axons. This protective covering is called a **myelin sheath.** Therefore some nerves are referred to as **myelinated** nerves. This myelin sheath plays a very important role in some nerves when it is present. For example, consider a lower tooth extraction in which the lip and jaw in that area are numb after the surgery. In many instances the numbness disappears after a period of time. Following is a simplified explanation of what may occur.

The dendrite is injured and part of it may die. When it dies, it dissolves but may leave the pro-

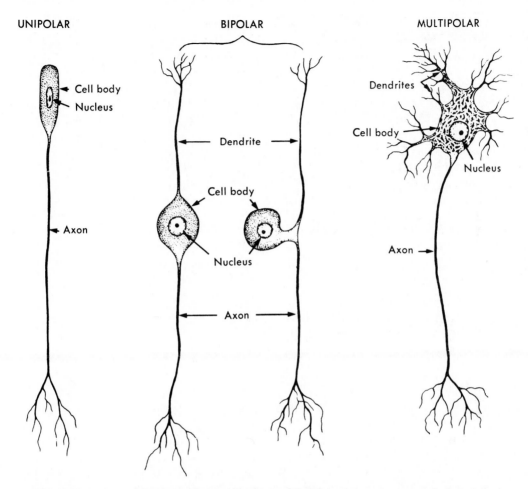

UNIPOLAR

Cell body
Nucleus
Axon

BIPOLAR

Dendrite
Cell body
Nucleus
Axon

MULTIPOLAR

Dendrites
Cell body
Nucleus
Axon

Fig. 2-18 **Some different shapes of neurons. Multipolar is most commonly found. Impulse passes from dendrites and cell body down along axon to meet with another neuron. (Ham.)**

tective myelin sheath in place. The nerve, or more accurately the dendrite, regrows down this remaining tube until it reaches the point it once supplied sensation to; then the numbness disappears. If the myelin sheath is damaged, there is a good possibility that when the dendrite starts to regenerate, it will be unable to locate the old area, which will remain numb.

These neurons are found in the nerves that run out into the body, as well as in the spinal cord and brain. Most nerves have neurons carrying messages both ways. Frequently it takes two or three neurons in a chain to relay the message to the brain and another two or three to transfer it from the brain back to the various parts of the body.

See Chapter 19 for additional discussion on the nervous system.

REVIEW QUESTIONS

1. Name the parts of the cell and their general functions.
2. Define epithelium.
3. Which is the most common type of epithelium?
4. How do the epithelial cells in skin arise, and what happens to them?
5. Where do glands come from?
6. How are glands classified?
7. Name the embryonic germ layers. Which layer or layers do epithelium come from?
8. Name the components of general irregular connective tissue.
9. How do cartilage and bone differ?
10. What makes bone hard?
11. What is the haversian system?
12. What are the divisions of blood cells?
13. What are the functions of each of the white blood cells and platelets?
14. Where do we find hemoglobin and what is its function?
15. Name the three types of muscle tissue and give examples of their locations.
16. Define or describe the following:
    a. Myofiber
    b. Myofibril
    c. Myofilament
17. What is a sarcomere?
18. How does skeletal muscle contract?
19. What are the parts of a neuron?
20. Define afferent and efferent.
21. What is a myelin sheath?
22. In what direction does an impulse, or message, travel in a neuron?

3

Development of Orofacial Complex

OBJECTIVES

- To list the developmental stages of the human from fertilization to birth
- To list the embryonic structures that form the face and discuss the approximate age of formation
- To discuss the mechanism involved in the development of the upper lip
- To name the structures involved in the formation of the palate and the timing of its development
- To describe the mechanism involved in the development of the palate
- To describe the other structures arising from the pharyngeal arches
- To discuss the embryonic structures involved in the development of the cleft lip and palate

EMBRYOLOGIC STAGES

From the time of fertilization of the ovum until full-term development is reached, the developing human goes through the following three stages:

1. Fertilization through 2 weeks is the period of the ovum.
2. Weeks 3 through 8 is the period of the embryo.
3. Weeks 9 through 36 is the period of the fetus.

During the period of the ovum the cells are differentiating into the tissues that will form the three germ layers of the body: ectoderm, mesoderm, and endoderm, as well as the surrounding membranes that protect and nourish the human as it develops.

PREFACIAL EMBRYOLOGY

One can begin to see the early features of the face developing by the embryonic age of 3 weeks. By that time the embryo has gone from a flat disk-like structure consisting of the three germ layers from top to bottom, ectoderm, mesoderm, and endoderm, to a structure that is elongated, has a developing spinal cord and brain, and has a body wall. The body wall is relatively hollow with the exception of the fact that there is a tube closed at its upper and lower ends running up the middle of the body cavity whose lining has developed from endoderm. This tube is the developing digestive tract and is divided into three parts. The upper part is the **foregut,** which forms the digestive tube from the throat region to the duodenum. The middle portion is the midgut, which forms the small intestine. The lower portion is the hindgut, which forms the large intestine.

By the time the embryo is about 3 weeks old, it is approximately 3 to 4 mm from the top of the head to the tail area (Fig. 3-1). Even at that small size, the forerunners of the structures that are going to form the face can be seen. Fig. 3-1 is a lateral view of the embryo, and several important features can be seen. There is the umbilical cord (shown cut here), which attaches the embryo to the placenta embedded in the wall of the uterus. The heart bulge appears as it does because at this time it originally develops in an extremely anterior position and pushes out on the upper body wall, which will later become the thorax. As the thorax and its ribs develop, the heart will assume a position inside the thoracic cage and will no

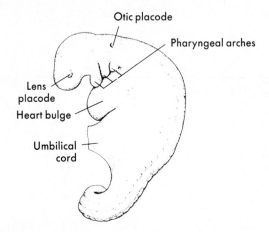

Fig. 3-1 Lateral view of 3- to 4-week-old embryo showing cardiac bulge, three pharyngeal arches, and developing eye and ear.

longer bulge outward. Finally, there are three ridges of tissue, the **pharyngeal arches,** that can be seen bulging out laterally. Eventually six of these arches will develop. The fifth one, however, will degenerate and form nothing of any consequence. The ones closest to the head end are the largest, and those further down are smaller in size.

For a better understanding of the structure of these pharyngeal arches it is necessary to look at a longitudinal section through this embryo, which divides it into equal halves (Fig. 3-2). Although this is only the upper half of the embryo, you can see the foregut. At this time the tube is still closed at the top and bottom. Eventually the bottom end of the tube will break down and become the anal opening, and the upper end will break down and connect with the primitive oral depression known as the **stomodeum.** The point in Fig. 3-2 where the foregut region and the stomodeum share a common wall is known as the **buccopharyngeal membrane.** This membrane is found in the location that corresponds to the region between the palatine tonsils and an area about two thirds of the way back from the tongue. During the fourth embryonic week this membrane breaks down, and the connection between the oral cavity and the digestive tract is established. The pharyngeal arches we saw in Fig. 3-1 are actually U-shaped bars of tissue. The open end of the U faces posteriorly and surrounds the upper end of the foregut and part of the primative oral cavity.

FACIAL DEVELOPMENT

The upper two of these pharyngeal arches, aside from being numbered with roman numerals I and II, are also known respectively as the

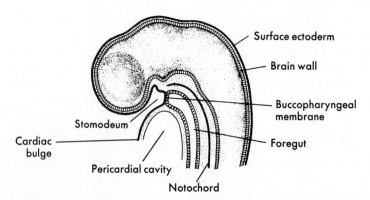

Fig. 3-2 Longitudinal section through 3-week embryo. Notice relationship between stomodeum, buccopharyngeal membrane, and foregut. (Langman.)

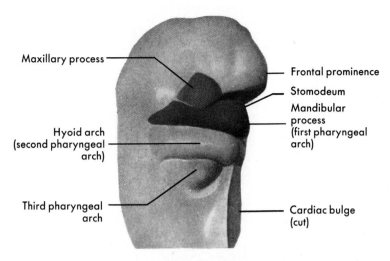

Maxillary process

Frontal prominence

Stomodeum

Mandibular process (first pharyngeal arch)

Hyoid arch (second pharyngeal arch)

Third pharyngeal arch

Cardiac bulge (cut)

Fig. 3-3   Lateral view of 3-week embryo. Notice frontal prominence of forehead region and first three pharyngeal arches. Also observe that mandibular arch is now divided into maxillary and mandibular processes.

mandibular and **hyoid arches.** The mandibular arch begins to show some growth from its posterior end on the upper surface. When that begins to happen, the mandibular arch can be subdivided into **mandibular processes** and **maxillary processes** (Fig. 3-3). The mandibular processes will form the mandible, and the maxillary processes will form most of the maxillae and the palatine bones, which form the hard palate in the roof of the mouth.

In the anterior view of a 3-week embryo, notice the forehead area, known as the **frontal prominence,** stomodeum (primitive oral cavity), and mandibular process of the mandibular arch (Fig. 3-4). During the fourth embryonic week some changes can be seen. First, two small depressions form low on the frontal prominence. These are the **nasal pits,** the beginning of the nasal cavities. The areas on either side of these nasal pits are the **medial** and **lateral nasal processes** (Fig. 3-5). From the side of the head, notice that the maxillary processes are starting to enlarge slightly and seem to be growing toward the midline. By the sixth week, the two medial nasal pro-

cesses and the two maxillary processes have formed the upper lip (Fig. 3-6). The lateral nasal process takes no part in forming the upper lip. Also about this time the nasal pits deepen until they open into the primitive oral cavity (Fig. 3-7).

The medial nasal and maxillary processes begin to fill in the groove that lies between them. There is an increase in the connective tissue of the upper lip in the area of the groove, and the groove fills in and slowly disappears. This process is known as **migration.** If this migration fails to take place, as development continues, the tissues will be stretched and will tear. This results in a separation between the medial nasal process and maxillary process known as a **cleft lip.** This takes place by the sixth embryonic week if it happens.

PALATAL DEVELOPMENT

The formation of the palate, or roof of the mouth, involves the same processes: the right and left maxillary processes and the medial nasal processes. The medial nasal processes form a

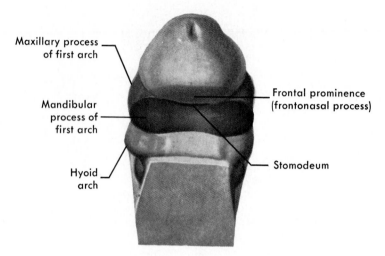

Fig. 3-4 Frontal view of 3-week embryo. Notice that maxillary process is just barely visible. (Bhaskar: Orban's.)

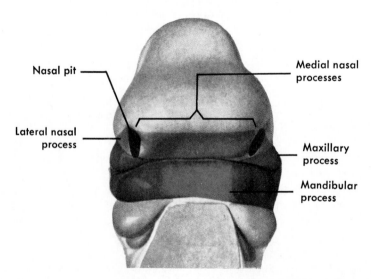

Fig. 3-5 Four-week embryo. Lower end of frontal prominence has divided into medial and lateral nasal processes. Also there is forward growth of maxillary process. (Bhaskar: Orban's.)

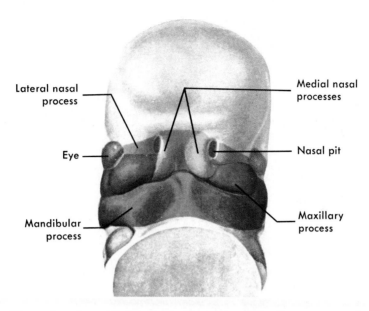

Fig. 3-6   Six-week embryo. Medial nasal processes and maxillary processes are filling in groove to form upper lip. (Bhaskar: Orban's.)

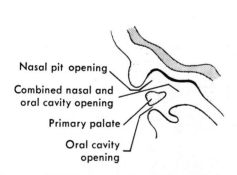

Fig. 3-7   Sagittal section through head at nasal pit area during sixth week, showing nasal pit opening into primitive nasal cavity area. There is only one chamber for oral and nasal cavities at this time. (Langman.)

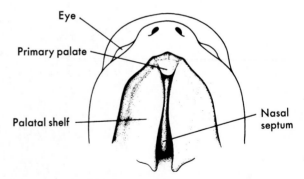

Fig. 3-8   Inferior view of primitive oral cavity of 7-week embryo. Notice V-shaped growth of primary palate (premaxilla) and beginning growth of palatal processes of maxillae. (Langman.)

block of tissue that includes the area of the maxillary central and lateral incisors, as well as a small V-shaped wedge of tissue lingual to these teeth back to the **incisive foramen;** this is also known as the **primary palate** or **premaxilla** (Fig. 3-8). The medial nasal processes also help to form the nasal septum, a wall that divides the nasal cavity into right and left halves.

The remainder of the hard and soft palate develops from the maxillary processes. This action begins at about the sixth and a half to the seventh week with the growth of the medial nasal processes into what is known as the primary palate. This primary palate eventually will be the bony area that includes the maxillary central and lateral incisors and running back to the incisive papilla referred to in Chapter 1. From the maxillary processes inward toward the midline, small

ledges of epithelial covered tissue start to grow and form the **palatal shelves,** or the palatal processes of the maxilla. As they grow inward, they tend to become trapped beneath the developing tongue (Fig. 3-9). Fortunately, at this time the face is growing in a downward and forward direction, and the tongue moves downward, pulling out from between the palatal processes. They move into a horizontal position and come into contact first with the primary palate, then, more posteriorly, with one another as well as the downward growing nasal septum (Fig. 3-10)

What should happen next is the breakup of these contacting epithelial layers because of the influence of chemicals produced by the cells. When this happens, the connective tissue beneath the epithelium on either side flows together and fuses. If viewed microscopically, this

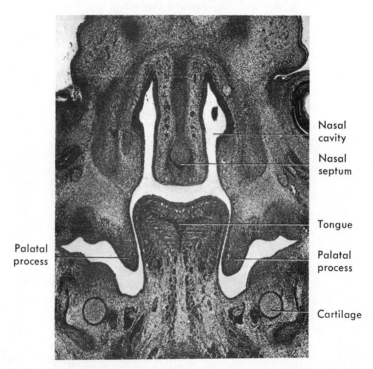

Fig. 3-9 Frontal section of 8-week embryo. Palatal processes are trapped beneath tongue. (Bhaskar: Orban's; courtesy P. Gruenwald.)

area would show that not all the epithelial cells break up; rather, a few of them remain embedded in the connective tissue. These cells are referred to as **epithelial rests.** It is possible that, at a later time, these clumps of epithelial cells will begin to multiply and form a sac of cells known as a **cyst.** This cyst may grow and distort the tissues around it, and it generally should be removed.

The two maxillary processes fuse with the primary palate during the seventh to eighth week and then fuse with one another, first in the anterior region and then moving on backward, just like a zipper being zipped from front to back. This process is completed by the eleventh week. If a **cleft palate** is going to develop, it will begin somewhere between the seventh and the eleventh week. If it occurs early, the entire palate will be open, or cleft; if it happens near the eleventh week, only the soft palate, or the uvula will be affected (Fig. 3-11).

OTHER STRUCTURAL DEVELOPMENT INSIDE THE PHARYNGEAL ARCHES

There are a number of important structures that develop from these pharyngeal arches. To understand these structures better, make a cut from left to right, down through the head and the pharyngeal arches (Fig. 3-12). If you remove the front half and view it from behind, you see a series of bulges with depressions between them (Fig. 3-13). The depressions on the outside are known as pharyngeal grooves or clefts, and the depressions bulging outward on the inside are known as pharyngeal pouches. In Fig. 3-13 you

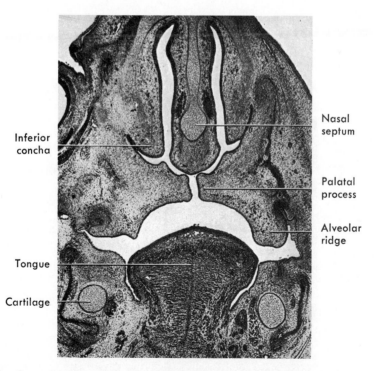

Inferior concha

Nasal septum

Palatal process

Alveolar ridge

Tongue

Cartilage

Fig. 3-10   Same section as in Fig. 3-9 at late 8 or early 9 weeks. Notice downward movement of tongue and palatal processes now in horizontal position contacting nasal septum. (Bhaskar: Orban's; courtesy P. Gruenwald.)

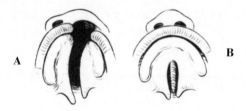

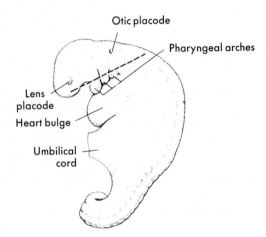

Fig. 3-11 **A,** Cleft lip and palate formed during seventh or eighth week. **B,** Cleft palate probably formed during ninth or tenth week. Notice difference in extent of clefts. (Ross and Johnston.)

Fig. 3-12 Duplicate of Fig. 3-1 with a dotted line marking a cut made from left to right through pharyngeal arches.

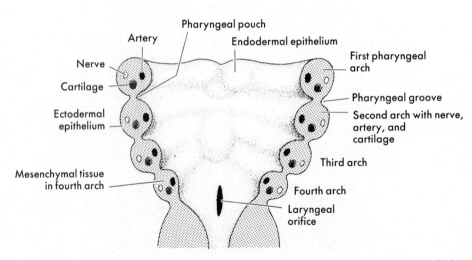

Fig. 3-13 Drawing of pharyngeal arches removed with cut seen in Fig. 3-12 and viewed from behind showing four of the five arches. Notice external grooves and internal pouches.

can see each of the arches numbered. In each of these arches is a bar of cartilage, an artery, a cranial nerve, and mesodermal tissue. Specific structures will develop from each one of these arches; bone, cartilage, and muscles. For example, the cranial nerve of the first arch is the fifth cranial nerve, or trigeminal nerve, and the cranial nerve of the second arch is the seventh cranial nerve, or the facial nerve. In later chapters on muscles of the head and neck you will read that the muscles of mastication are supplied by the fifth cranial nerve and the muscles of facial expression are innervated by the seventh cranial nerve. This tells you that the muscles of mastication arose from the first arch, since they are supplied by the fifth cranial nerve, and the muscles of facial expression arose from the second arch, since they are supplied by the seventh cranial nerve.

In the next figure (Fig. 3-14) you are looking at one side of the cut seen in Fig. 3-13. The upper groove and pouch form the eardrum and auditory tube leading into the back nose region. The second pouch forms the tonsils, and the pouches below that form some of the **endocrine glands,** such as the **parathyroid** and **thymus** glands. If you look at the middle portion of Fig. 3-13, you will see the region where the tongue and **thyroid gland** develop. In the next views (Fig. 3-15) you

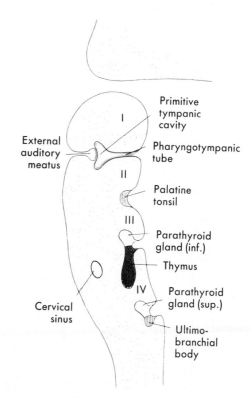

Fig. 3-14 Later view of one side of Fig. 3-13. All but first external groove have been covered over. Notice other structures arising from pouches.

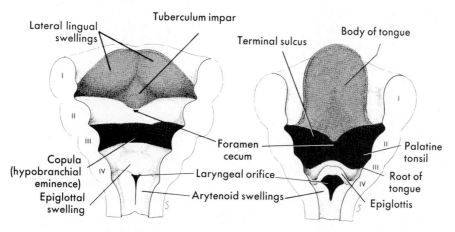

Fig. 3-15 Various structures that go into formation of tongue and epiglottis.

can see a number of structures that go into making up the tongue, the basic ones being the **lateral lingual swellings, tuberculum impar,** and the **copula.** You also can see a small depression in the middle of the tongue known as the **foramen cecum.** This is the point where the thyroid gland begins to develop and then migrates downward to eventually lie in the lower front neck region. The timing for these structures varies somewhat, but it takes place over several months. One other important structure arises from this early oral cavity area. In the roof, or top of the oral cavity, there is an upward growth of tissue that breaks loose from the oral cavity and comes into contact with a downward growth of tissue from the brain. This upward growth is known as **Rathke's pouch** and forms a part of the **pituitary gland,** which is the master control gland for the **hormones** of the body. For further information you should consult a text such as *Langman's Medical Embryology.*

Cleft Lips and Palates

Although clefts were mentioned earlier, it seems appropriate to include here a discussion of clefts, the frequency of them, some of the terminology, and finally treatment, including the role of the dentist. Cleft lips and palates happen in about one in every 700 to 1,000 births in the United States. The two most common types of cleft lips are the unilateral and bilateral clefts. A unilateral cleft lip is the lack of migration between one maxillary process with the medial nasal process. A bilateral cleft lip occurs when neither maxillary process migrates with the medial nasal process (Fig. 3-16, *A* and *B*).

The cleft palate has similar terms. A unilateral cleft palate occurs when one palatal process fuses with the nasal septum, resulting in an opening from the oral cavity into one side of the nasal cavity. A bilateral cleft palate exists when neither palatal process fuses with the opposing process or the nasal septum. This leaves an opening from the oral cavity into both sides of the nasal cavity (Fig. 3-16, *C*).

The cleft lip can usually be treated surgically with good results. A cleft palate is first treated surgically as much as possible. The dentist can make an appliance to fill in the rest of the gap in the roof of the mouth, and then a speech therapist can retrain the person in proper speech patterns.

One final thing to consider in studying cleft lips and palates is the relationship between the timing of the occurrences and their potential causes. We noted that the cleft lip developed during the third to sixth week after fertilization, and the cleft palate starts six and a half to eleven weeks after fertilization. It is known that there are hereditary factors involved in the development of clefts and that if they exist in a family lineage they will occur with a little greater frequency in that family. Two other main factors are drugs and environmental factors. If a pregnant woman is on various kinds of drugs, both legal and illegal, or if she is in a polluted environment that may have

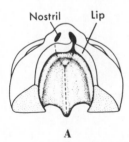
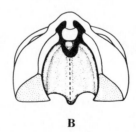
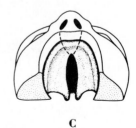

A   **B**   **C**

Fig. 3-16   **A,** Unilateral cleft lip. **B,** Bilateral cleft lip. **C,** Bilateral cleft palate. (Langman.)

harmful particles in the air, her child may stand a greater risk of suffering birth defects, such as clefts. A woman may be using potentially harmful drugs at a time when she is not yet aware that she is pregnant. Because these deformities develop so early, it is important that a woman who may be pregnant be cognizant of the danger she is placing on that unborn child by using harmful drugs.

REVIEW QUESTIONS

1. During which embryonic weeks do the lips form?
2. What is the buccopharyngeal membrane, and when does it rupture?
3. Which processes form the upper lip?
4. Which processes form the hard and soft palates, and when do they form?
5. What are epithelial rests, and what might they do in later life?
6. What are unilateral and bilateral cleft lips and palates?
7. When do cleft lips and palates form?
8. What are some other structures that form from the oral cavity and pharyngeal arch areas?
9. What are the differences in the mechanism between the development of the upper lip and the palate?

4

Dental Lamina and Enamel Organ

OBJECTIVES

- To define dental lamina and tell in what embryonic week it is first seen and define successional lamina
- To describe bud, cap, and bell stages and the various layers found in each
- To describe dental papilla and dental sac and their functions

DENTAL LAMINA

The first signs of tooth development are seen during the sixth embryonic week. At that time the embryonic **oral** (stratified squamous) **epithelium** begins thickening.

This thickening oral epithelium is known as the **dental lamina.** It is U shaped and is found in a position corresponding to the future arch-shaped arrangement of the upper and lower teeth. This thickening does not begin all at once throughout the mouth but is first seen in the anterior midline, slowly spreading posteriorly toward the molar region (Fig. 4-1).

Again, starting at the midline and spreading posteriorly, there is a continued thickening in 10 areas of the dental lamina of the upper arch and 10 of the lower arch. These 20 localized thickenings correspond to the position of the future primary dentition. They will form the enamel of the future teeth. It is important to stress that this enamel develops from the oral epithelium, which comes from the outer embryonic germ layer known as ectoderm. In oral pathology you will probably study about a condition called ecto-dermal dysplasia, in which there is poor development of structures arising from ectoderm, for example, skin, hair, sweat and sebaceous glands, and the enamel of teeth. Since they all have a common ectodermal origin, this allows you to understand why the enamel is affected as well as the skin and other structures in this disease.

ENAMEL ORGAN
Bud Stage

The initial budding off from the dental lamina at 10 areas in each arch is referred to initially as the **bud stage** (Fig. 4-2). At first it looks like a blob of cells from the dental lamina of the oral epithelium projecting deeper into the underlying connective tissue. The cells in the middle of this bud come from the outer, or superficial, layers of the oral epithelium, whereas the cells in the periphery of the bud come from the deep, or basal, layers of the oral epithelium. This bud seems to be stretching out from the dental lamina as it grows. As development continues, the deepest part of the bud becomes slightly concave, or pushed in. It is at this point that the developing enamel organ goes from the bud stage into the **cap stage.**

Cap Stage

As the **enamel organ** comes into the cap stage it consists of three components: outer enamel epithelium, inner enamel epithelium, and stellate reticulum.

Outer enamel epithelium. The outermost part of the structure of the cap stage is the **outer enamel epithelium (OEE).** It is a direct continu-

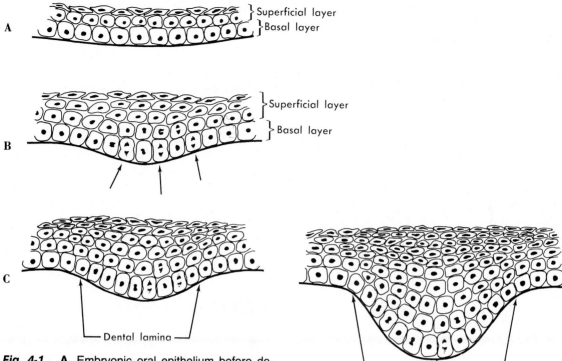

Fig. 4-1   **A,** Embryonic oral epithelium before development of dental lamina. Notice thickness of superficial layers of cells and basal layer of cells. Embryonic connective tissue lies beneath embryonic oral epithelium. **B,** Thickening of superficial layer and multiplication of cells at arrows in basal layer. **C,** Further advancement in completed thickening of dental lamina.

Fig. 4-2   Bud stage. Notice further downward extension of cells of oral epithelium to form bud. Stretching out of cells is still considered part of dental lamina.

ation of the basal, or deep, layer of oral epithelium. These are low columnar cells.

Inner enamel epithelium. The cells that outline the concavity in the deepest part of the cap stage compose the **inner enamel epithelium (IEE).** These cells are continuous with the outer enamel epithelial cells and also come from the basal, or deep, layer of the oral epithelium.

Stellate reticulum. The cells between the IEE and the OEE compose the **stellate reticulum.** These cells originate from the superficial layers of the oral epithelium. Although they may resemble embryonic mesodermal cells, they are really

ectodermal cells, as are other parts of the enamel organ (Fig. 4-3). As the concavity of the deep part of the cap grows more pronounced, the **bell stage** is reached.

Bell Stage

The differentiation between the cap and bell stages is made when a fourth layer appears in addition to the three already mentioned. The **stratum intermedium** is several layers of flattened squamous cells lying between the IEE and the stellate reticulum (Fig. 4-4).

As the development continues in the bell

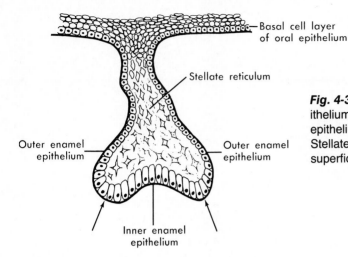

Basal cell layer of oral epithelium

Stellate reticulum

Outer enamel epithelium

Outer enamel epithelium

Inner enamel epithelium

Fig. 4-3 Cap stage. Basal layer of cells of oral epithelium is continuous with inner and outer enamel epithelium. *Arrows,* Dividing point of IEE and OEE. Stellate reticulum can be seen as a continuation of superficial layers of oral epithelium.

stage, two processes occur. First, the future outline, shape, or form of the crown of the tooth is being determined by the way in which the cell layers expand as the enamel organ grows. Second, there are changes in the various cells, particularly the IEE cells, that will lead to the production of enamel. (See also Chapter 5.)

Function of the Four Layers of the Enamel Organ

1. Basically the OEE can be considered a protective layer for the entire enamel organ.
2. The cells of the IEE elongate and change internally to become responsible for actual enamel formation. (See also Chapter 5.)
3. The stellate reticulum functions as a cushioned protection for IEE cells and also plays some role in nourishment by allowing vascular fluids to move between the loosely packed cells and bring nourishment to the stratum intermedium.
4. The cells of the stratum intermedium probably help provide nourishment for IEE cells (future ameloblasts) by changing vascular fluids into a more readily utilizable form.

SUCCESSIONAL LAMINA

In the developing primary teeth the dental lamina develops an extension off each tooth to the lingual side (Fig. 4-4). This extension is known as the **successional lamina.** These successional laminas go through a bud, cap, and bell stage just like the primary teeth and form the permanent incisors, canines, and premolars. The permanent molars develop from a posterior growth of the dental lamina.

DENTAL PAPILLA AND DENTAL SAC

The **dental papilla** is a small area of condensed cells arising from mesoderm and located next to the IEE. It is first seen in the late bud stage and grows and becomes more pronounced as it goes through the bell stage. This structure forms the dentin and pulp of the tooth.

The **dental sac** constitutes several rows of flattened cells that surround part of the dental papilla and part of the enamel organ. This also arises from mesoderm and forms the cementum of the tooth, the periodontal ligament, and some alveolar bone (Fig. 4-5).

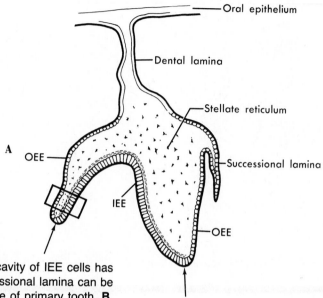

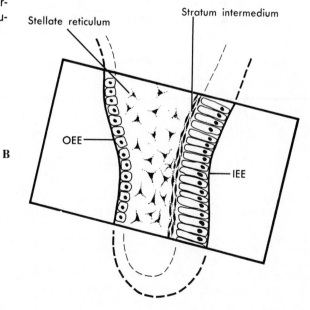

Fig. 4-4 Bell stage. **A,** Concavity of IEE cells has increased in bell stage. Successional lamina can be seen developing to lingual side of primary tooth. **B,** Enlargement of outlined section of **A.** There are several layers of flattened cells, which are stratum intermedium, as well as IEE, OEE, and stellate reticulum.

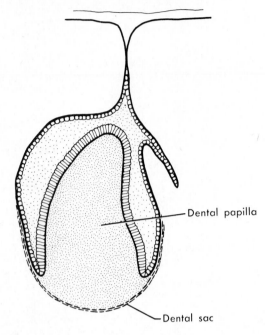

Fig. 4-5 Condensed cells, which make up dental papilla, as well as flattened layers of dental sac, which surrounds part of dental papilla and part of enamel organ.

REVIEW QUESTIONS

1. When is the first sign of tooth development, that is, the dental lamina, seen?
2. Oral epithelium is an example of what type of epithelial arrangement?
3. The enamel organ comes from what germ layer?
4. What are the four layers of the enamel organ as seen in the bell stage?
5. What is the function of each of these layers?
6. Define successional lamina, dental papilla, and dental sac.

5

Enamel, Dentin, and Pulp

OBJECTIVES

- To discuss the changes in the inner enamel epithelial cells that allow them to become enamel-forming cells
- To discuss the interrelationship between enamel formation and dentin formation
- To describe the properties of enamel and the makeup of the enamel rod
- To define the following terms: striae of Retzius, hypoplastic enamel, hypocalcified enamel, enamel lamellae, enamel tuft, enamel spindle
- To describe the properties and components of dentin
- To differentiate primary, secondary, and reparative dentin
- To define the following terms: interglobular dentin, dead tracts, sclerotic dentin
- To describe the components and age changes of pulp
- To describe and classify pulp stones

A close relationship exists in the formation of enamel, dentin, and pulp. Remember that enamel develops from the enamel organ, which is derived from ectoderm, whereas dentin and pulp develop from the dental papilla, which is derived from mesoderm.

Dental papilla

During the bud stage the cells of the embryonic connective tissue deep to the bud resemble large multipointed cells known as mesenchymal cells. As the enamel organ goes into the cap stage, the mesenchymal cells adjacent to the cap become more rounded and condensed and are known as dental papilla cells. (Fig. 5-1). This condensation continues into the bell stage, during which further changes occur. It is at this point that the relationship between enamel and dentin formation becomes more obvious. Following is a list of events that occur during their formation.

1. During the bell stage the inner enamel epithelial cells become taller. They increase from 12 to 40 μm (μ)* in length. These taller cells are now referred to as **preameloblasts.**
2. The peripheral cells of the dental papilla adjacent to the preameloblasts become low columnar or cuboidal and are referred to as odontoblasts (Fig. 5-2).
3. The odontoblasts move away from the preameloblasts toward the center of the dental papilla and secrete behind them a **matrix** of mucopolysaccharide ground substance and collagen fibers.
4. The secretion of this dentin matrix causes the preameloblast to change its polarity (the nucleus moves from the center of the cell to the end nearest the stratum intermedium). This is attributable to the change in the route of nourishment of the preameloblasts. Up until this time the nourishment had been coming from the dental papilla directly to the cells adjacent to it. After the dentin matrix is laid down, this acts as a

---

*μm = micrometer = 1/1000 millimeter; μm (micrometer) and μ (micron) are synonymous.

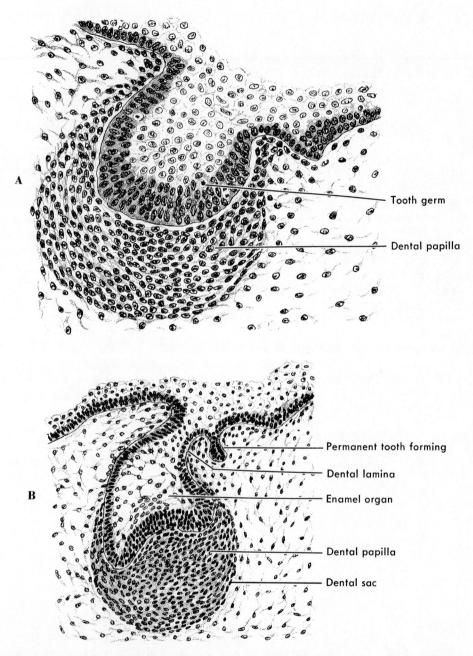

A

B

Tooth germ

Dental papilla

Permanent tooth forming

Dental lamina

Enamel organ

Dental papilla

Dental sac

Fig. 5-1 **A,** General condensation of dental papilla. **B,** Later stage. Condensation of cells in dental papilla is more pronounced. (Bevelander: Outline.)

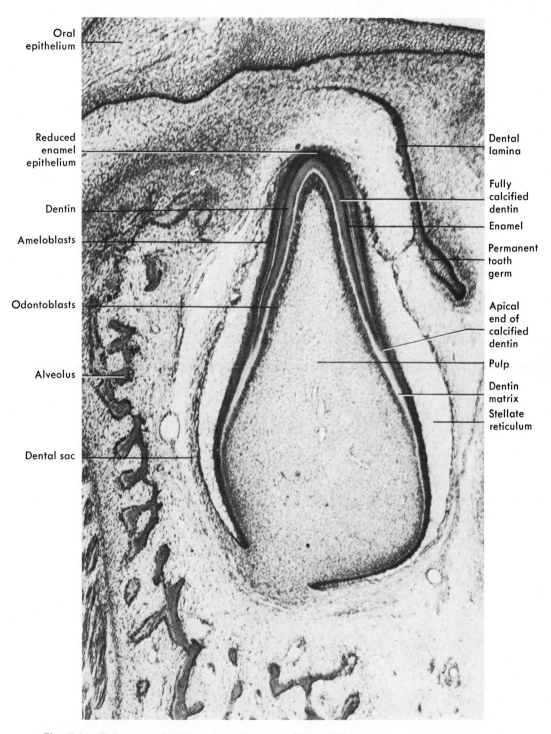

Oral epithelium

Reduced enamel epithelium

Dentin

Ameloblasts

Odontoblasts

Alveolus

Dental sac

Dental lamina

Fully calcified dentin

Enamel

Permanent tooth germ

Apical end of calcified dentin

Pulp

Dentin matrix

Stellate reticulum

Fig. 5-2 Enlargement of dental papilla area. Odontoblasts are becoming more columnar. Ameloblasts at tip of cusps have met outer enamel epithelium, forming reduced enamel epithelium. (Bevelander: Atlas.)

barrier between the dental papilla and the preameloblasts, and it becomes necessary to find a new route to provide nourishment to the cells. To do this, vascular channels begin to penetrate the enamel organ through the outer enamel epithelium. Fluid nutrients pass to the stellate reticulum, the stratum intermedium, and then the preameloblasts. The nuclear shift of these preameloblast cells relates to the nucleus's need to be closer to the nutrient supply. With the change in polarity, the cell is now referred to as an **ameloblast** and is ready to begin the secretion of enamel matrix.

5. The ameloblast lays down a matrix of mucopolysaccharides (ground substance) and organic fiber next to the dentin matrix, and the future **dentinoenamel junction** (DEJ) is formed. As the ameloblast secretes the matrix, it moves away from the dentin toward the outer enamel epithelium (Fig. 5-3).

6. The dentin begins to lay down crystals and calcify (crystals begin growing).

7. The enamel begins to lay down crystals and calcify (crystals begin growing).

This process is identical for all developing teeth. It is seen first in developing anterior teeth and later in posterior teeth. Within any single tooth this type of interrelationship is first seen at the tip of the cusp of a tooth and later spreads toward the cervical line. As you look at a developing tooth you may see enamel and dentin formation at the tip of a cusp and yet, near the cervical line, you will find that the odontoblasts have not yet differentiated and the cells of the enamel organ may still be at the inner enamel epithelial stage. They have not lengthened into preameloblasts.

All this development takes place in each tooth, whether primary or permanent. The permanent molars develop as a budding off of a posterior extension of the dental lamina, whereas the anterior permanent teeth and the permanent premolars develop from a budding off of the dental lamina of the primary teeth developing in that position. Regardless of the tooth, the steps of development are always the same.

ENAMEL COMPOSITION

Enamel is the hardest structure of the body. It is generally white but at times appears yellowish because of the reflection of the color of the underlying dentin. Enamel is about 96% inorganic in composition. This inorganic structure is composed of many millions of crystals of **hydroxyapatite,** the chemical formula of which is $Ca_{10}(PO_4)6\cdot2(H_2O)$. The other 4% of enamel is composed of water and an organic material that is fibrous in structure.

The basic unit of structure of enamel is called the **enamel rod.** This rod is a column of enamel that runs all the way from the dentinoenamel junction to the surface of the tooth. The rod is generally perpendicular to the dentinoenamel junction and to the surface (Fig. 5-4). There is much debate about how the enamel rod develops. The ameloblast is round or hexagonal in cross section, and the enamel rods, which fit together very tightly, are usually referred to as keyhole shaped (Fig. 5-5). The enamel is composed of two parts: the rod and rod sheath. The rod it-

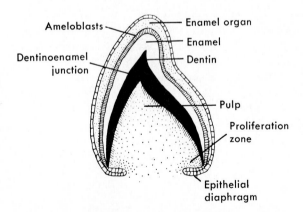

Fig. 5-3 Beginning of dentinoenamel junction (DEJ) formation. Ameloblasts have already moved away from dentinoenamel junction in upper section but have not in lower section. (Bhaskar: Orban's.)

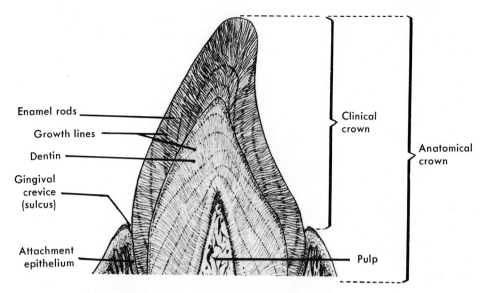

Fig. 5-4 Notice slight curvature of enamel rods and that ends of rods are perpendicular to dentinoenamel junction and outer surface of tooth. (Ham.)

self is made up of hydroxyapatite crystals. The **rod sheath** outlines the rod and contains most of the organic fibrous substance (Fig. 5-6).

DEVELOPMENT OF ENAMEL

At the end of the bell stage the ameloblasts lay down a substance known as the matrix, which is composed of the gluelike material, referred to as ground substance, and fibers. In a few days the ameloblasts deposit millions of crystals into the small area of matrix. It is important to remember that all the crystals that will ever be in that particular area of rod are laid down initially. This is referred to as the mineralization stage of calcification of the enamel rod (Fig. 5-7, *A*).

The second stage of calcification of the enamel rod is known as the maturation stage (Fig. 5-7, *B*). During this stage the crystals grow in size until they are tightly packed together. If the crystals do not grow to full size, the enamel crystals are less tightly packed together and the enamel is not 96% inorganic. Under these conditions the

enamel is said to be hypocalcified, or as some people say, "I have soft teeth." Clinically these areas appear very white and may tend to decay more readily without careful and proper care. The ameloblast produces this matrix and enamel at a rate of about 4 µm per day. Every fourth day there seems to be a change in the development of the rod, and a brownish line develops in the enamel. These lines are called the **striae of Retzius** and curve outwardly and occlusally from the dentinoenamel junction (Fig. 5-8). They can be seen in a longitudinal section of a tooth and can also be seen on the surfaces of a number of teeth. If you look at the labial surface of an anterior tooth you will see horizontal lines on the crown. These are known as **imbrication lines** and are surface manifestations of the striae of Retzius.

FATE OF ENAMEL ORGAN

As the ameloblast moves away from the dentinoenamel junction toward the outer enamel epi-

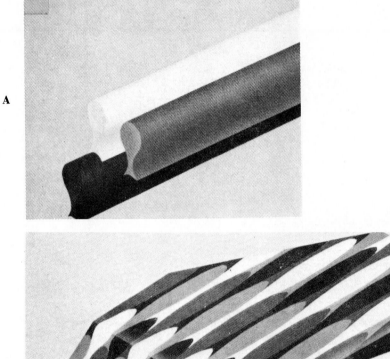

A

B

Fig. 5-5 **A,** Three enamel rods. **B,** Groups of rods and their relation to one another. Notice how different cutting angles change appearance. (Meckel et al.)

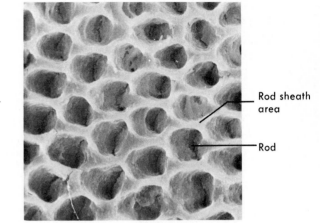

Rod sheath area

Rod

Fig. 5-6 Rod sheath area, which surrounds rod itself. (Bhaskar: Orban's; courtesy Dr. A.R. Boyde.)

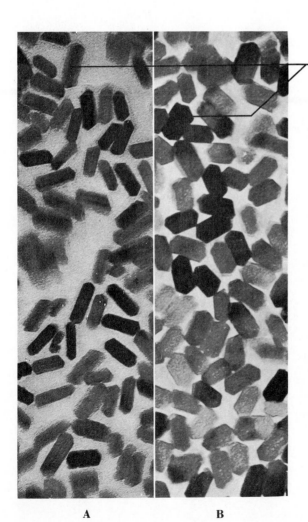

Crystals

Fig. 5-7 **A,** Mineralization stage of calcification. Notice spaces between crystals. **B,** Same magnification as **A** but showing maturation stage with crystal growth and increased density. (Bhaskar: Orban's.)

A B

thelium, it begins to compress the two layers in the middle—the stratum intermedium and the stellate reticulum. These two middle layers eventually lose their identity, and the ameloblasts contact the outer enamel epithelium (Fig. 5-2). This is the signal for the ameloblasts to cease formation of enamel. The final effort of the ameloblast is to lay down a protective layer over the enamel, called the **primary enamel cuticle,** or **Nasmyth's membrane.** This membrane covers the crown and remains there for many months after eruption until worn away by toothbrushing and other abrasion. It is this membrane that is stained green or yellow in the newly erupted teeth of young children, particularly in the cervical one third of the crown. It can be removed by polishing and the use of other instruments.

After the ameloblast produces the primary cuticle, it begins flattening out and blending with the outer enamel epithelial cells in what is called the **reduced enamel epithelium.** This reduced enamel epithelium produces an adhesive-like secretion called the **secondary enamel cuticle,** or **epithelial attachment,** which functions to hold the gingiva to the tooth. This epithelium adheres to the tooth and is known as the **attachment epithelium.** (See Chapter 7.)

ABNORMALITIES OF ENAMEL

There are a number of enamel abnormalities. Some are readily seen by clinical examination; others are confirmed by radiographic examination; and still others are seen only by histological examination of the sectioned tooth.

Hypocalcified Enamel

With **hypocalcified enamel,** spots or entire areas of the teeth appear white to whitish yellow in color. It is the result of insufficient growth of the enamel crystals or an insufficient number of crystals originally deposited in the matrix. Thus a less dense enamel is produced, which may decay more rapidly.

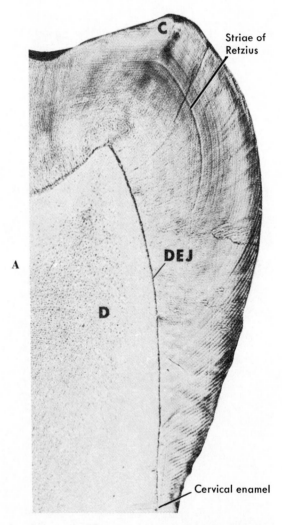

Fig. 5-8 **A,** Heavy black lines represent striae of Retzius. Notice their curving direction. (**A** and **B,** Provenza.)

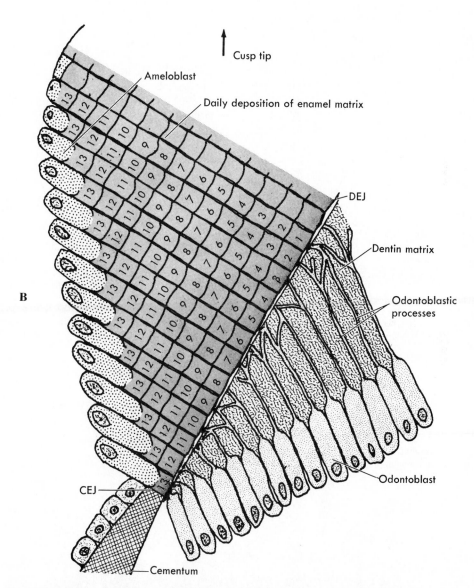

Fig. 5-8, cont'd **B,** Enlarged representation of several enamel rods. Segments are labeled according to day of formation. Enamel formation is most advanced at cusp tip.

Hypoplastic Enamel

The density of **hypoplastic enamel** is generally normal, but the enamel is thin. The enamel will have a more yellowish to grayish hue and may be seen radiographically as a thinner layer.

Enamel Lamellae

Cracks in the enamel caused by developmental problems or **trauma** are called **enamel lamellae.** The most common types are those caused by trauma. Clinically they appear as hairline cracks in the enamel. These may extend all the way through the enamel and even into the dentin. The less common type of lamella is a developmental defect and is the result of one or more ameloblasts ceasing enamel production and thus leaving a space between other enamel rods. These are usually seen histologically and not clinically. They also provide a potential pathway through the enamel for bacteria.

Enamel Tuft

A small area of hypocalcified enamel seen at the dentinoenamel junction and extending about one fourth to one third of the way through the enamel is an **enamel tuft.** It is not seen clinically but only in a histological section of tooth, and it has no great clinical significance.

Enamel Spindle

An **enamel spindle** is an odontoblastic process that becomes trapped between ameloblasts in early development and thus ends up with its process in enamel (Fig. 5-9). It is seen only histologically.

DENTIN COMPOSITION

The dentin is a hard yellowish substance. It is about 70% inorganic hydroxyapatite crystal; the remaining 30% is primarily organic, composed of collagen and mucopolysaccharide ground substance, as well as water. Dentin, in cross section, is composed of the following three distinct areas microscopically (Fig. 5-10):

1. **Dentinal tubule**—A long tube, running from the dentinoenamel junction or dentinocemental junction to the pulp. This tube

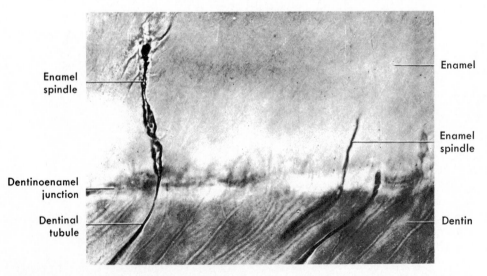

Fig. 5-9 Enamel spindle or odontoblastic process extension crossing dentinoenamel junction and lying in enamel. (Bhaskar: Orban's.)

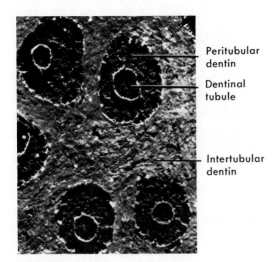

Fig. 5-10 Cross-sectional view of dentin. (Bhaskar: Orban's.)

Labels on figure: Peritubular dentin; Dentinal tubule; Intertubular dentin

is filled with a cellular extension of the odontoblast called the **odontoblastic process.**

2. **Peritubular dentin**—An area of higher crystalline content immediately surrounding the dentinal tubules.

3. **Intertubular dentin**—The bulk of the dentinal material.

These are all microscopic structures. Clinically, dentin appears to be solid.

FORMATION OF REGULAR DENTIN (PRIMARY DENTIN)

As the odontoblast begins to secrete dentin matrix at the future dentinoenamel junction or dentinocemental junction, it moves toward the pulp. The odontoblast differs from the ameloblast in that it leaves part of the cell behind and secretes matrix around it. In doing this, the cell wall stretches or lengthens so that part of the odontoblast stretches all the way from the dentinoenamel junction or dentinocemental junction inward to the periphery of the pulp (Fig. 5-11). The secreted matrix from adjacent odontoblasts

spreads peripherally until it meets with other dentin matrices and eventually forms intertubular dentin. As the intertubular dentin calcifies, the space that runs through it and is occupied by the odontoblastic process is referred to as the dentinal tubule. Later the odontoblastic process shrinks in diameter, and the space that it formerly occupied is filled with a more highly calcified dentin known as peritubular dentin (Fig. 5-10).

FORMATION OF SECONDARY AND REPARATIVE DENTIN

When the tooth erupts into the oral cavity, the dentin that has formed by that time is known as **primary dentin** or regular dentin. Dentin continues to be formed as either secondary or reparative dentin.

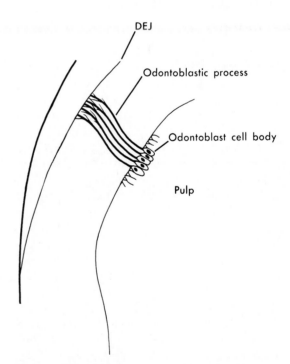

Labels on figure: DEJ; Odontoblastic process; Odontoblast cell body; Pulp

Fig. 5-11 Cell body of odontoblast with elongated odontoblastic process stretching from dentinoenamel junction (*DEJ*) to pulp.

Secondary Dentin

The layer formed inside the regular dentin is **secondary dentin.** It starts forming about the time the root formation is almost completed. It is formed by the same odontoblasts that formed the regular dentin. As the secondary dentin forms, it causes the overall size of the pulp chamber to decrease. This is most noticeable in radiographs of newly erupted permanent maxillary central incisors and in those of the same teeth that have been erupted for a number of years (Fig. 5-12). Newly erupted teeth have large pulp chambers and prominent pulp horns. As secondary dentin formation proceeds, a decrease in the size of the pulp canals, chambers, and pulp horns occurs. It is this process of secondary dentin formation that allows metal crowns to be constructed on teeth after they have been erupted for a few years. If this formation did not take place, the cutting of tooth structure for crowns would tend to injure the large prominent pulp horns and pulp chambers of teeth.

Reparative Dentin

Reparative dentin is formed in response to local trauma. There are very few if any dentinal tubules seen in this type of dentin, and it is located immediately beneath the area of trauma. This trauma is of several varieties: occlusal, mechanical, and chemical trauma.

Occlusal trauma is the condition that exists when one tooth or a part of that tooth is subjected to more occlusal stress than is normal. This usually relates to the cusp area of the tooth. The odontoblast layer beneath the cusp responds to the trauma by quickly producing dentin. This dentin, as was stated previously, has very few if any tubules. Under the microscope it looks very dense and unorganized.

Mechanical trauma is usually the result of cavity preparations in the tooth. Cavity preparations should extend through the enamel into the dentin. For every square millimeter of dentin that is cut there are 30,000 to 40,000 odontoblastic processes damaged. Most of this damage leads to the

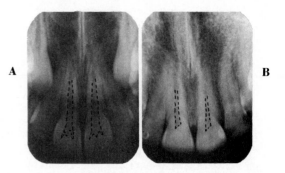

Fig. 5-12 Radiographs of maxillary central incisor of 8-year-old, **A,** and 43-year-old, **B,** persons. Notice prominence of pulp horns and chamber size of 8-year-old pulp compared with that of 43-year-old pulp.

death of the odontoblasts in that area. These odontoblasts are replaced with reserve mesenchymal cells from adjacent pulpal tissue. These cells change into odontoblasts and produce reparative dentin.

Chemical trauma is usually brought about by the carious process and usually in the form of acids produced by the bacteria responsible for the caries. We can also see chemical trauma sometimes produced by substances we use in filling teeth if we have not protected the cavity preparation. Radiographically, we can distinguish some of the causes. Occlusal trauma will result in reparative dentin being produced beneath the involved area, usually a cusp tip. Mechanical and chemical traumas will be in areas where there has been decay or cavity preparations such as grooves, cervical, or interproximal areas (Fig. 5-13).

ABNORMALITIES IN DENTIN

There are several abnormalities found in dentin. Because dentin lies beneath either enamel or cementum, most of the more common abnormalities cannot be seen without one sectioning the tooth and studying it with a hand lens or microscope.

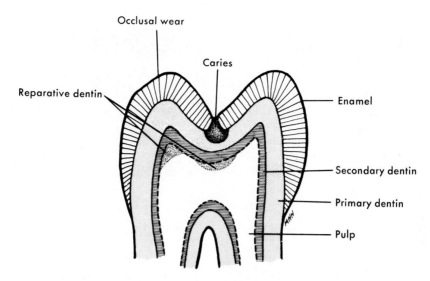

Fig. 5-13 Primary, secondary, and reparative dentin. Notice how secondary dentin has decreased size of entire pulp chamber, whereas reparative dentin is formed only beneath traumatic areas, such as carious region and area of occlusal wear.

Interglobular Dentin

In the process of calcification, some areas of poorly calcified dentin become entrapped. These poorly calcified areas are the **interglobular dentin.** They are found next to the dentinoenamel junction in the crown and the dentinocemental junction in the root. The root interglobular dentin is generally called the **granular layer of Tomes.**

Dead Tracts

Dentinal tubules that are empty because of the death of the odontoblasts that originally occupied them are known as **dead tracts.** These are not seen clinically, only microscopically. Because the tubules are empty, they provide a pathway to the pulp for the bacteria involved in decay. This means more rapid penetration of decay and insufficient time for reparative dentin to be formed.

Sclerotic Dentin

A condition in which the dentinal tubules are filled with a dentin material is called **sclerotic dentin.** The cause of this is related to occlusal trauma or decay. The odontoblastic processes in the area of trauma begin secreting matrix substance, and the tubules of the degenerating odontoblasts are filled. This has also been referred to as **transparent dentin.**

PULP

As mentioned before, the pulp develops from the mesodermal tissue of the dental papilla. As it develops, it will eventually consist of blood vessels, lymphatic vessels, nerves, fibroblasts, and collagen fibers, as well as other cells of connective tissue. As dentin grows inward, it compresses the inner tissue of dental papilla. At this point blood vessels, lymphatic channels, nerves, and connective tissue cells are evident. Many of the mesenchymal cells become fibroblasts and begin forming collagen fibers (Fig. 5-14). The nerves of the pulp are primarily sensory and transmit only one type of sensation—pain. There are some motor nerves that innervate the smooth muscle cells in the walls of the blood vessels and cause

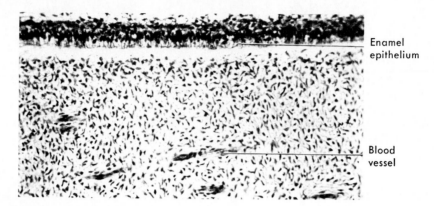

Fig. 5-14   Young pulp with mesenchymal cells and developing blood vessels. (Bhaskar: Orban's.)

them to constrict. This kind of reaction is important in vascular changes in the pulp caused by irritation to the tooth.

Young pulpal tissue is considered primarily cellular, with a lesser concentration of fibers. There are a number of cell types present. Aside from the fibroblasts mentioned above, there are macrophages, which will protect the pulp, and a large number of reserve mesenchymal cells. These cells are the kind we see in the dental papilla as the tooth starts to develop. These cells have the ability to form a number of different types of cells, including fibroblasts and odontoblasts. As the pulp ages, there are some of these cells that are used to form odontoblasts to replace those that are damaged. There are some of them that will change to fibroblasts and produce more collagen. When a tooth is young, the pulp has many cells and few fibers. These cells can aid in repair. As the pulp ages, more of these cells become fibroblasts and produce collagen. With the aging of the tooth, the pulp becomes smaller because of secondary and reparative dentin and less able to resist trauma because it loses its reserve cells. We hope this will help us to understand why young people are less susceptible to permanent pulpal damage. One last thing to keep in mind is that odontoblasts are an integral part of dentin, but they are also the peripheral cells of the pulp and that is the reason they are also discussed here (Fig. 5-15).

ABNORMALITIES IN PULP

There is one primary abnormality seen in pulp—structures known as **pulp stones.** They are small, circular, calcified areas found in the pulps of about 80% of older persons. With such a high rate of occurrence it might be questionable to identify them as abnormalities, but they are considered a pathological condition. There are several classifications of stones based on their origin and density. True pulp stones originate from odontoblasts and are very rare. False stones are the most common type and probably originate from dead cells with concentric layers of calcium phosphate around them. When studied under the microscope, they resemble an onion cut in cross section. Another classification of stones is referred to as diffuse calcifications; they are very tiny calcified structures found in groups.

Pulp stones are also classified according to their location. Free pulp stones are found in the middle of the pulp. Attached pulp stones are those that have become attached to the dentin in the periphery of the pulp. Embedded stones are those that were attached to the dentin and become surrounded by secondary dentin (Fig. 5-16).

Pulp stones usually do not affect the health of the pulp. The pulp can have a number of stones and still be vital. They may be seen as small globular **radiopacities** on radiographs. The only problem that may occur would be in the endodontic treatment of a tooth with numerous pulp stones. The stones may make it difficult to remove pulpal tissue with reamers and files.

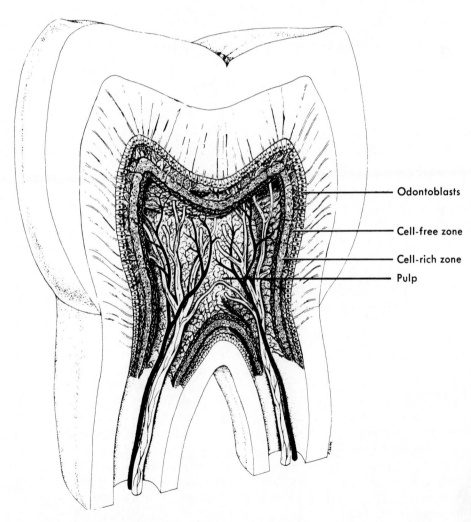

Odontoblasts

Cell-free zone

Cell-rich zone

Pulp

Fig. 5-15 Odontoblasts surrounding pulp as outer layer. (Bhaskar: Orban's.)

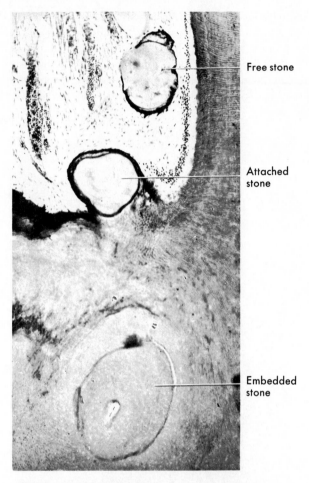

Free stone

Attached
stone

Embedded
stone

Fig. 5-16 Pulp stones in three stages: free, attached, and embedded. (Bhaskar: Orban's.)

REVIEW QUESTIONS

1. How do inner enamel epithelial cells change to become preameloblasts?
2. How do preameloblasts change to become ameloblasts?
3. What happens if enamel crystals do not grow to full size?
4. What is Nasmyth's membrane?
5. What are enamel lamellae?
6. What is the difference between secondary dentin and reparative dentin in terms of composition and location?
7. What are dead tracts and sclerotic (or transparent) dentin?
8. What happens to the pulp as it grows older?
9. What are pulp stones?
10. How do pulp stones affect the health of the pulp?

6

Root Formation and Attachment Apparatus

OBJECTIVES

- To discuss the role of the epithelial root sheath in root form and dentin formation
- To describe the fate of the epithelial root sheath
- To describe the beginning of cementum formation—the two varieties and where they are found
- To define and diagram alveolar bone and its components
- To define periodontal ligament and list its various groups and subgroups of fibers
- To describe briefly bone's reaction to pressure and tension and how this affects tooth movement

This chapter deals with the formation of the root—how its form is determined and developed, as well as the development of the cementum, periodontal ligament, and alveolar bone, collectively referred to as the **attachment apparatus.**

ROOT FORMATION

Root formation begins after the outline of the crown has been established but before the full crown is calcified. If you refer to Figs. 4-4 and 5-3 (bell stage), you will see that the point where the outer enamel epithelium becomes the inner enamel epithelium is located at the deepest part of the enamel organ and is known as the cervical loop. Also notice that there are no interposing layers of stellate reticulum or stratum intermedium as one sees higher up in the crown. These layers of OEE and IEE will now be referred to as

the **epithelial root sheath (Hertwig's epithelial root sheath).** The cells in these two layers start to undergo rather rapid **mitotic division** and grow deep into the underlying connective tissue—the beginning of root formation. As this deepening growth continues, it is important to keep in mind the relationship of the dental papilla and the dental sac to this epithelial root sheath. The dental papilla is on the inside, and the dental sac is on the outside (Fig. 6-1). As this downgrowth continues, the tip of the epithelial root sheath turns horizontally inward; this turned-in portion is known as the **epithelial diaphragm** of the root sheath. These two components guide the shape and the number of roots.

As you study Fig. 6-2, keep in mind that it is a two-dimensional representation of a three-dimensional object. To help you better see this three-dimensionally, visualize a paper cup. The rim of the cup represents the cervical line of the tooth, and the side of the cup is the epithelial root sheath. Next cut a round hole in the bottom of the cup, about two thirds the diameter of the cup. Now make a vertical cut through the middle of the cup and study the cut surface. The bottom of the cup that remains represents the epithelial diaphragm. The way in which this epithelial diaphragm continues to grow inward will determine whether the tooth will have one, two, or three roots. If you looked at the deep surface of the epithelial diaphragm, you would continue to see changes occurring. As the vertical epithelial root sheath continues to grow longer, forming root length, the horizontal epithelial diaphragm continues to grow inward toward the middle of the

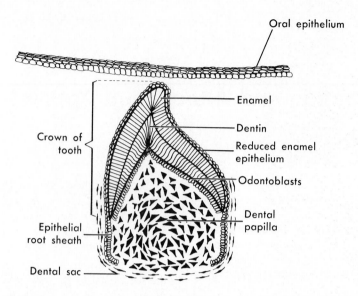

Fig. 6-1 Beginning root development. Epithelial root sheath interposed between dental papilla and dental sac.

tooth. If the entire circumference grows evenly, it will eventually form a single-rooted tooth. If two areas opposite one another grow inward more rapidly and meet, it will then separate into two columns of root formation to form a bi-rooted tooth. If three areas grow inward to meet, a trirooted tooth will be formed (Fig. 6-3). In multirooted teeth, the point where the epithelial diaphragm meets is the bifurcation or trifurcation of the tooth.

ESTABLISHMENT OF DENTINOCEMENTAL JUNCTION

We have briefly mentioned what guides the shape and form of the root and now will further consider the formation of the hard structures of the tooth. Fig. 6-1 shows the relationship of the epithelial root sheath to the dental papilla and dental sac. As the root sheath starts growing deeper into the tissue from the cervical line, it influences the peripheral cells of the dental papilla adjacent to it to differentiate into odontoblasts. This is similar to what happens in the

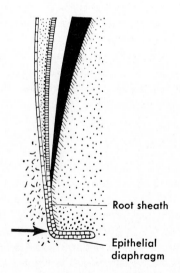

Fig. 6-2 Epithelial diaphragm is horizontal component of epithelial root sheath. Mitosis and growth of root sheath take place at point of arrow. (Bhaskar: Orban's.)

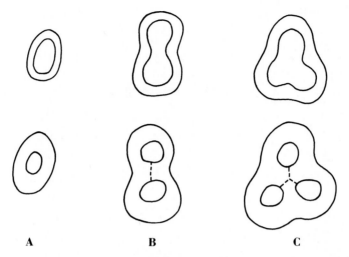

Fig. 6-3 Inferior view of epithelial diaphragm. **A,** Entire circumference of epithelial diaphragm grows inward, and single-rooted tooth will be formed. **B,** Epithelial diaphragm grows inward at two opposite areas and meets in middle, forming double-rooted tooth. **C,** Epithelial diaphragm grows inward at three areas and meets, forming three-rooted tooth.

crown of the tooth. Once dentin begins to form next to the epithelial root sheath, there is cellular influence that causes the root sheath to begin to break up. There is still some debate as to which cells cause this breakup. It may be the odontoblasts or it may be the cells of the dental sac on the outside. To picture this breaking up of the epithelial root sheath, imagine that the sheath originally is a solid wall of cells surrounding the developing tooth root. Later it seems riddled with holes like a piece of Swiss cheese. With the appearance of these holes there is no longer any barrier separating the odontoblasts and dentin on the inside from the cells of the dental sac on the outside. Some of the dental sac cells begin to differentiate into cementoblasts and begin to form cementum. This cementum is laid down against the previously formed dentin and establishes the dentinocemental junction (Fig. 6-4). Remember that the epithelial root sheath is perforated; therefore the cementoblasts that contact dentin are able to accomplish the transformation only in the areas where the sheath has broken

up. While this occurs, the remaining root sheath cells pull away from the dentin, and the cementoblasts contact all the dentin and establish the rest of the dentinocemental junction. Occasionally, some epithelial root sheath cells do not pull away and may differentiate into ameloblasts, forming a small glob of enamel. These are referred to as **enamel pearls** and are usually found in bifurcations and trifurcations of roots. Other defects occurring at this time may lead to the formation of **accessory root canals,** which make it difficult for the dentist to remove all pulpal tissue completely if the tooth has to be treated endodontically.

The remaining cells of the epithelial root sheath, after they have moved away from the dentin, are found in the periodontal space next to the tooth and are then referred to as the **epithelial rests of Malassez,** or just epithelial rest cells. If these cells begin dividing later in life, they may lead to the formation of cysts in the jaws similar in origin to the cysts mentioned in Chapter 3.

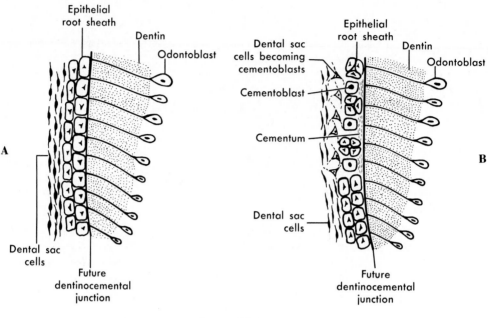

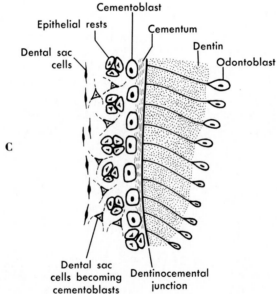

Fig. 6-4 **A,** Epithelial root sheath separates dentin from dental sac cells. **B,** Epithelial root sheath breaks up, and dental sac cells become cementoblasts. **C,** Epithelial root sheath moves away from dentin, and dentinocemental junction is formed.

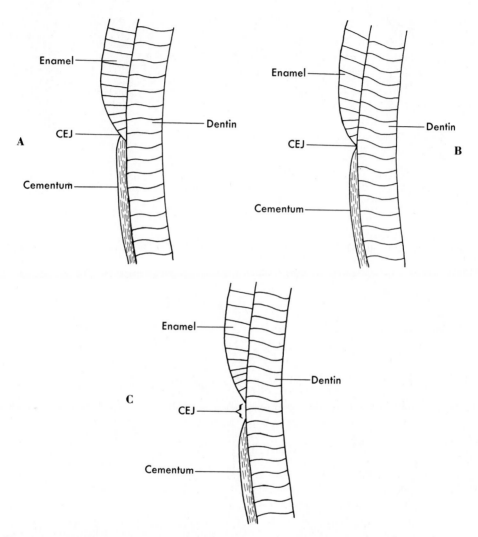

Fig. 6-5   Variations in cementoenamel junction. **A,** Cementum overlaps enamel. **B,** Cementum and enamel meet in sharp junction. **C,** Cementum and enamel do not meet and dentin is exposed.

CEMENTUM FORMATION

Cementum is a hard yellowish substance covering the root of the tooth. It is composed of about 45% to 50% inorganic hydroxyapatite crystals, and the remaining 50% to 55% is organic components and water. As in other hard substances, the organic component is primarily collagen fibers and mucopolysaccharide ground substance.

As cementum formation begins, it is first seen at the cervical line of the tooth, also referred to as the cementoenamel junction. As cementum is laid down, it may assume three different relationships with the enamel of the crown. In about 60% of the cases the cementum overlaps the enamel, and in 30% the cementum meets the enamel in a sharp junction. In the remaining 10% of the cases the cementum and enamel do not meet, thus leaving dentin exposed at the cervical line area. This type of relationship with exposed dentin may make the tooth very sensitive in that area if the patient develops gingival recession (Fig. 6-5).

As the cementoblast begins laying down cementum, it functions in somewhat the same way as the ameloblast, moving away from the dentinocemental junction and secreting matrix behind it. This type of secretion allows the cementum to form without entrapping any of its own cells. Such an arrangement is seen in the cervical two thirds of the root, but not usually in the apical one third, and is referred to as acellular cementum. In this arrangement all the cells remain on the surface of the cementum. As root formation, and therefore cementum formation, proceeds from the cervical line to the apex of the root, another type of cementum arrangement takes place. Toward the middle to apical third of the root, the cementoblasts, as they are secreting matrix, surround themselves and become entrapped, as do osteoblasts in bone formation. Histologically, then, examination of the tissue reveals numerous entrapped cells, which are referred to as **cementocytes.** Because of these cells, the tissue is referred to as cellular cementum. In the

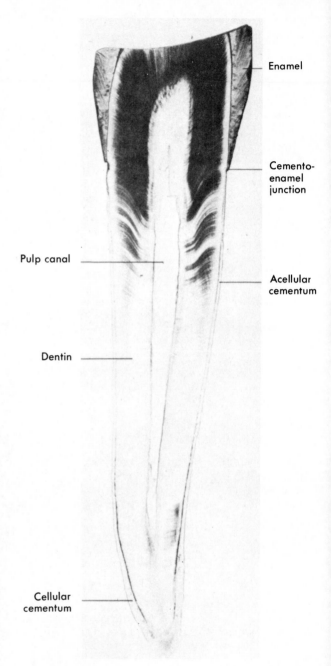

Fig. 6-6 Acellular cementum is found on cervical two thirds of root. Cellular cementum covers apical one third of root with overlapping near middle. (Bevelander: Atlas.)

middle third of the root, cellular cementum can be seen covering acellular cementum. Because of the presence of these cells, the cellular cementum is a more vital, or alive, tissue and is more responsive to remodeling of itself (Fig. 6-6).

As mentioned before, the outer layer of cementum is lined with cementoblasts, which are probably capable of cementum formation throughout a person's life. As the **periodontal ligament** forms, the ends of the periodontal fibers are surrounded by these cementoblasts and their secretion, and the cementum tissue hardens around the ends of the fibers, attaching them to the cementum. The parts of the periodontal ligament that are embedded in cementum are known as **Sharpey's fibers.** It should be stressed that Sharpey's fibers are the parts of the periodontal ligament that are surrounded by both cementum and alveolar bone (Fig. 6-7).

The cellular cementum at the apex of the root tends to increase in thickness with the passage of time and as a result of stress. This thickening is referred to as **hypercementosis** and, in general, causes no great problem to the tooth unless it becomes necessary to extract it. If so, the bulbous apex might make it necessary to remove the bone around the tooth, since it may be impossible to spread the socket wider (Fig. 6-8).

Cementum, like dentin, is a vital tissue in that it has the capacity to rebuild itself when it is in-

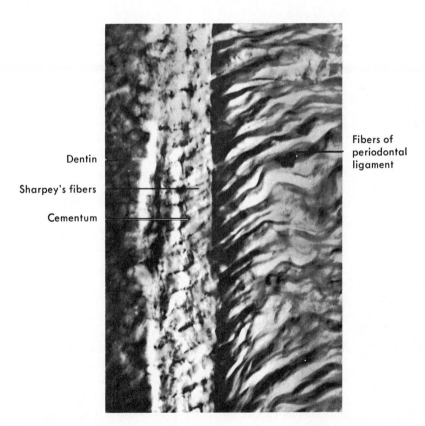

Dentin

Sharpey's fibers

Cementum

Fibers of periodontal ligament

Fig. 6-7   Sharpey's fibers. Ends of periodontal ligament become entrapped in cementum, and this entrapped part is called Sharpey's fiber. (Bhaskar: Orban's.)

jured. It is considered a vital tissue because it has, in some areas, entrapped cells, which must be maintained. These entrapped cells, known as cementocytes, have long cellular processes that point toward the surface of the tooth. The overall nourishment comes from the blood vessels of the periodontium. The cementoblasts on the surface of the cementum not only initially build cementum but also aid in rebuilding cementum when it is damaged.

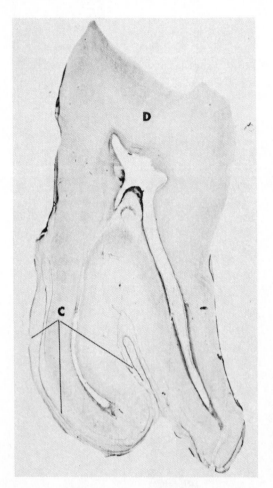

Fig. 6-8 Hypercementosis. Apex of root has become quite bulbous and can become trapped in socket by cementum overgrowth as indicated by lines. (Provenza.)

The same cell that destroys bone, the osteoclast, may also destroy or resorb cementum. Later in the chapter bone resorption is discussed. It is the same type of reaction that may be seen in cementum, except in cementum it proceeds at a much slower rate because the metabolic rate is lower in cementum. Therefore it is not affected by trauma as quickly as bone is.

ALVEOLAR BONE

By definition, **alveolar bone** is the bone of the upper or lower jaw that makes up the sockets for the teeth. More will be said later of the overall relation of alveolar bone to the rest of the bone in the jaw.

The composition of dried bone varies, depending on whether it is young or adult bone. Adult bone is about 65% inorganic crystal, and the 35% organic composition is about 31% collagen and 4% noncollagenous material. Alveolar bone originates by intramembranous development, as discussed in Chapter 2. It is mesodermal in origin, as are all types of connective tissue.

Alveolar bone is composed of three layers, as seen in cross section. The layer of compact bone on the buccal or lingual surface is referred to as the **cortical plate** of bone. It is typical bone, with a normal periosteum. The bone that forms the socket for the tooth is also a compact bone, but it does not have a normal periosteum. Although this is a compact layer, there are numerous holes in the bone that allow for the passage of blood vessels, connecting the deeper part of the bone with the vessels of the periodontal space. This layer is referred to as the **cribriform plate,** or **alveolar bone proper.** Radiographically, it is referred to as the **lamina dura.** The tooth socket is constantly being remodeled, and additional bone is laid down on the cribriform plate. This bone is referred to as **bundle bone** (Fig. 6-9, *B*). A thickened lamina dura is caused by bundle bone being laid down on the cribriform plate. In between the cortical plate and the cribriform plate is a layer of **spongy,** or **cancellous, bone** (Fig. 6-

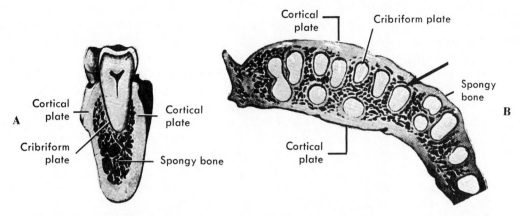

Fig. 6-9 Alveolar bone. **A,** Cross section through mandible. Cortical plate is on buccal and lingual sides with cribriform plate in socket. Spongy bone is in between. **B,** Longitudinal horizontal section through mandible. Notice thickened lamina dura at arrow. This is caused by bundle bone being deposited on cribriform plate. (Bhaskar: Orban's.)

9, *A*). This spongy bone is a bone marrow, as mentioned in Chapter 2. Remember that the cortical plate is only on the buccal and lingual sides; therefore a radiograph will not show the cortical plate but only the cribriform plate and the spongy bone. On a radiograph the crest of bone that joins two sockets is referred to as the interproximal **alveolar crest** of bone. The contours of this bony area are a good indicator of periodontal health (Fig. 6-10).

Like cementum, bone also has embedded parts of the periodontal ligament in it, and these are also referred to as Sharpey's fibers. Bone has a much higher metabolic rate than cementum does and therefore is much more responsive to stress. It is this difference that allows bone to change in response to stress; yet there is very little if any change in the cementum, since it is not so rapidly responsive.

PERIODONTAL LIGAMENT

The periodontal ligament also develops from the mesodermal cells of the dental sac. This happens after the cementum has begun forming. As

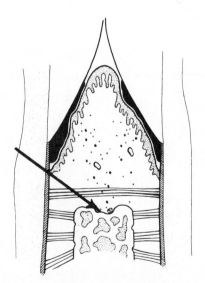

Fig. 6-10 Destruction of alveolar crest. *Arrow,* Blunted alveolar crest, indicative of periodontal disease. (Pawlak and Hoag.)

the dental sac cells begin to change, they first become fibroblasts and the fibroblasts form collagen fibers. At first these fibers are arranged around the tooth and parallel with the root surface. Some of the early arrangements of fibers are discussed in Chapter 7. About the same time the fibers are forming, the other components of the periodontal ligament are also starting to appear. Blood vessels, lymphatic vessels, nerves, and various types of connective tissue cells are seen. Remember that the nerves of the pulp can transmit only impulses of pain. The nerves of the periodontal space have pain fibers and fibers that allow one to feel light touch and pressure and probably heat and cold. When biting down on something hard produces a sharp pain, it is the nerves of the periodontal ligament that are stimulated, not the pulp of the tooth. After a person has had root canal work done on a tooth, it is still possible to feel pain at times; however, this is not from the pulpal area but from the peri-

odontal ligament. The blood vessels of the ligament space are branches of the vessels that go to the pulp, but they also have branches that penetrate the holes in the wall of the cribriform plate and join with the vascular channels in the spongy part of the alveolar bone; others come from the gingival blood supply.

As the fibers of the ligament form, they begin to arrange themselves in a definite pattern. When the fibers reach their final arrangement, they can be descriptively arranged into three groups: **gingival fibers, transseptal fibers,** and **alveolodental fibers.**

1. Gingival fibers
   a. Gingival fibers—Run from cementum into free and attached gingival area; tend to support gingiva
   b. Circular gingival fibers—Run around tooth in free gingiva and hold gingiva against tooth
2. Transseptal fibers—Run from the cemen-

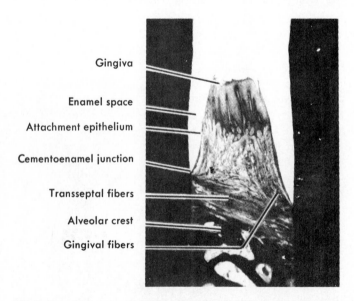

Gingiva

Enamel space

Attachment epithelium

Cementoenamel junction

Transseptal fibers

Alveolar crest

Gingival fibers

Fig. 6-11 Gingival and transseptal fibers. Transseptal fibers go from cementum of one tooth to cementum of next tooth. Gingival fibers extend from cementum up into gingiva. Circular gingival fibers (cut in cross section) circle tooth in free gingiva. (Bevelander: Outline.)

tum of interproximal portion of one tooth, across alveolar crest of bone to cementum of interproximal portion of adjacent tooth; tend to hold teeth in interproximal contact (Fig. 6-11)

3. Alveolodental fibers—Run from cementum to alveolar bone (Fig. 6-12)

   a. Alveolar crest group—Runs from cementum, slightly apically to alveolar crest of bone; help resist horizontal movements of teeth

   b. Horizontal group—Runs from cementum horizontally to alveolar crest; resist horizontal movement

   c. Oblique group—Runs from cementum coronally into alveolar bone; main fiber group for resisting occlusal stresses

   d. Apical group—Runs from apex of tooth into adjacent alveolar bone; resist forces trying to pull tooth from socket

   e. Interradicular group—Found only on multirooted teeth; run from alveolar crest of bone between roots of tooth to adjacent cementum; resist forces trying to remove tooth

Let us take another look at the total periodontal space and all of its associated structures. On one side we see the cementum of the tooth with cementoblasts lying on its surface. The embedded ends of the periodontal ligament (Sharpey's fibers) are embedded in the cementum lying perpendicular to the surface. Close to the surface of the tooth amid the periodontal fibers we see small clumps of epithelial cells, the epithelial rests of Malassez. On the other side of the periodontal space we see the compact bony layer, which is perforated in many places, the cribriform plate. Additional bone has been laid down as bundle bone, and there is a thickening of the lamina dura. Here also we see the embedded Sharpey's fibers of the periodontal ligament. All types of nerve fibers will also be found within this periodontal space. We also find fibroblasts, macrophages, and various blood cells and numerous open areas wherein one can see the well-developed pattern of blood vessels.

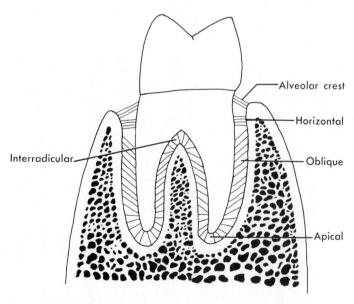

Alveolar crest

Horizontal

Interradicular

Oblique

Apical

Fig. 6-12 Diagram showing the five groups of alveolodental fibers. In single-rooted teeth there would be no interradicular fibers.

BONE REMODELING IN TOOTH MOVEMENT

What happens when a tooth is lost? Many times the tooth posterior to the missing tooth will tilt forward into the unoccupied space. This phenomenon has been referred to as mesial drift. The same type of movement can be accomplished in orthodontic tooth movement. Since the tooth fits into a socket, it is necessary to change the shape of that socket if the tooth is to be moved. In most tooth movement the tooth does not move bodily but tilts on an axis. This rotational point on a tooth is located about two thirds of the way down the root. If a tooth tilts mesially (Fig. 6-13), bone must be resorbed on the cervical two thirds of the mesial side and the apical one third of the distal side. This resorption is a result of the tooth causing pressure on the alveolar bone in these areas. However, as the tooth moves in that direction, there is tension on the periodontal fibers in the apical one third of the mesial side and the cervical two thirds of the distal side. This tension causes bone to build new bone, and the socket fills in at the area the tooth's root once occupied (Fig. 6-14).

Why does the bone change and remodel and the cementum usually does not? Remember that cementum has a low metabolic rate, whereas bone metabolism is much higher. Because of this, the bone reacts more quickly to stress and can remodel itself before the stress on the cementum causes any destruction. If the tooth is moved too fast in orthodontic treatment, it is possible that the fibers attaching tooth to bone will be torn out of their attachment, and before they can be reembedded, the tooth could conceivably be lost.

One of the important factors in bone remodeling is the compression of blood vessels when a tooth is moved. This compression decreases the blood supply in that area, and this change in blood flow aids in triggering the formation of the osteoclasts.

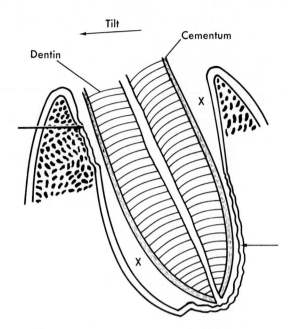

Fig. 6-13 Mesial drift. Tooth is tilted mesially and bone is destroyed at arrow. X, Areas once occupied by tooth.

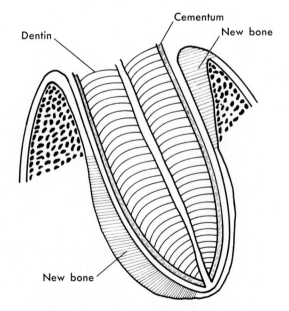

Fig. 6-14 Remodeling of bone. Hash marks indicate new bone formation following tooth movement.

REVIEW QUESTIONS

1. The epithelial root sheath develops from what earlier structures?
2. What happens to the epithelial root sheath after root dentin starts to form?
3. What are epithelial rests, and what might happen to them later in life?
4. What are the two types of cementum, and where are they found on the root?
5. What are Sharpey's fibers?
6. What are the layers of alveolar bone?
7. What are the various periodontal fiber groups, and what are their functions?
8. What is mesial drift?
9. What causes bone resorption and apposition (remodeling)?

7

Eruption and Shedding of Teeth

OBJECTIVES

- To name the three stages of active tooth eruption and the points at which each one begins
- To discuss the fate of the epithelial layers covering the crown of the tooth
- To name four forces in tooth eruption and to tell which one most likely has the greatest influence
- To discuss briefly what causes the shedding of primary teeth
- To diagram or describe the origin and position of the permanent teeth as compared with the deciduous teeth
- To list and describe the factors that lead to a retained primary tooth

ACTIVE TOOTH ERUPTION

The term "active tooth eruption" implies the emergence of a crown into the oral cavity. In general, however, the term refers to the total life span of the tooth, from the beginning of crown development until the tooth is lost or the individual dies. This eruptive process is usually divided into three categories, or stages, and although there may be some difference in the terminology, they refer to the same mechanism.

Preeruptive Stage

The **preeruptive stage** begins as the crown starts to develop. Recall that the dental lamina formation—bud, cap, and bell stages, as well as the calcification of the crown—takes place in the connective tissue beneath the oral epithelium. During this time the bone of the maxilla or mandible surrounds the developing primary tooth in a U-shaped crypt, or beginning socket (Fig. 7-1).

The eruptive movement associated with the preeruptive stage is of two varieties—spatial and excentric. In spatial movement, the crown develops while the bottom of the socket fills in with bone and the crown is pushed toward the surface. There is also a similar facial movement that accompanies jaw growth. In excentric, or off-center, growth the crown of a tooth does not grow in a perfectly symmetrical pattern. As the crown enlarges, it grows more in one area than in another, and so the tooth seems to be moving because the center of the tooth is shifting. This can be visualized when one blows up a small round balloon to a diameter of 3 to 4 inches. Put a mark on the center of the balloon and continue to blow it up to a diameter of 8 to 10 inches. Again mark the center of the balloon. Since the balloon walls are not of equal thickness, it expands more in one area than in another. Thus the center of the balloon moves from the original marking. This same principle can be applied to the developing crown. It appears to have moved, since the center point of the developing crown has shifted. This is the activity of the preeruptive stage. It involves crown growth and some movement toward the surface as the crypt fills in.

Eruptive Stage

The **eruptive stage,** or **prefunctional eruptive stage,** begins with the development of the root. In an earlier chapter the development of the root and Hertwig's epithelial root sheath were dis-

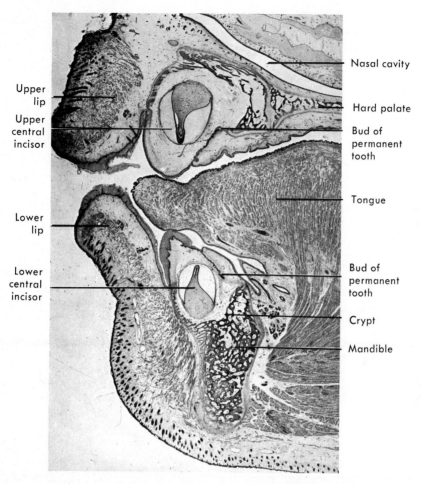

Upper lip

Upper central incisor

Lower lip

Lower central incisor

Nasal cavity

Hard palate

Bud of permanent tooth

Tongue

Bud of permanent tooth

Crypt

Mandible

Fig. 7-1   Primary mandibular and maxillary incisors developing in recess or "crypt" of bone, which forms socket. Depth of crypt builds up from osteoclastic activity at its base and increases in height to form future alveolar bone. (Bhaskar: Orban's.)

cussed. The root develops in a crypt of bone. As it begins forming, osteoclasts deepen the crypt by taking away bone at the bottom to accommodate for the increase in root length. While root length continues to grow, the tooth begins to move toward the surface of the oral cavity. As it approaches the oral cavity, the alveolar bone is growing to keep pace with it. But, in time, the tooth moves faster than the growing alveolar bone and approaches the surface of the oral epithelium and breaks into the oral cavity.

As mentioned earlier, the crown of the tooth is surrounded by reduced enamel epithelium. As the tooth moves to the surface, this reduced enamel epithelium moves with it until it pushes the connective tissue out of the way or causes it to disintegrate. The reduced enamel epithelium then contacts the oral epithelium. These two layers fuse into one layer—the **united oral epithelium.** The tooth breaks through this layer and emerges into the oral cavity. It is believed that this breakdown of epithelium is caused by an enzyme probably produced by the reduced enamel epithelium. This stage continues until the erupting teeth meet the opposite teeth.

Causes of eruption. What causes this eruption? What are the forces involved? Much work has been done concerning this problem, and much more needs to be done. Following are several theories.

GROWTH OF ROOT. It has been said that the increase in root length forces the tooth into the oral cavity. Two things would tend to disprove this. Experiments have been done in which Hertwig's root sheath has been destroyed and root growth has been stopped or inhibited yet the tooth has still erupted. On the other hand, third molars have grown roots to full length but the teeth have not erupted.

GROWTH OF PULPAL TISSUE. At one time it was believed that the continued growth of pulpal tissue and its compression by the inward growth of dentin caused pulpal tissue to be squeezed or forced out of the apex of the tooth, causing an opposite reaction that forced the tooth toward the surface. This sounds quite plausible, except that some erupting teeth have had endodontic treatment. Even after the pulp was removed, the tooth continued to erupt.

BONE DEPOSITION IN ALVEOLAR CRYPT. There is bone deposition seen at the base of the alveolar crypt, and yet this is not constant. There are times when the base of the crypt undergoes resorption to allow for the growth of the root.

PERIODONTAL LIGAMENT. A number of experiments have been done in an effort to eliminate the possibility of the above three forces affecting the eruption of a tooth. The teeth, however, continued to erupt. Many now believe that the periodontal ligament may be responsible for tooth eruption. Although the exact mechanism is unknown, this is the most likely answer.

Posteruptive Stage

The **posteruptive stage** begins when the teeth come into occlusion and continues until they are lost or death occurs. This posteruptive stage functions in several ways. First, as the mandible continues to grow and increase the space between the maxilla and mandible, the teeth will continue to erupt to maintain a balance in the arches. Second, as the teeth wear occlusally because of prolonged masticatory stress and wear, they will continue to erupt to maintain tooth contact. Third, because there is interproximal wear, there will be a slight mesial eruptive force that keeps the teeth in contact. This is frequently referred to as mesial drift. Last, if an opposing tooth is lost, the tooth may continue to erupt in what is generally referred to as **supraeruption.** Some authorities will still consider the last as a part of the eruptive stage. It can cause serious problems in the replacement of the missing tooth, since the supraerupted tooth makes it difficult to establish the normal occlusal plane.

SHEDDING OF PRIMARY DENTITION

As mentioned before, the 20 permanent teeth that follow the primary teeth develop as offshoots of the primary dental lamina. Recall that the anterior permanent teeth develop apically and lingually to the primary teeth (Fig. 7-2), whereas the permanent premolars develop between the roots of the primary molars (Fig. 7-3). Regardless of its position, the fact that the permanent tooth is there and its root is developing causes the permanent tooth to move toward the surface, putting pressure on the root of the primary tooth. It is believed that this pressure causes osteoclasts to form and begin resorbing the primary tooth root. This resorption is intermittent and not constant. This is the usual manner in which resorption occurs, but there may be other factors involved. Although most primary teeth would be retained if a permanent tooth did not develop, it is still possible to see a primary tooth undergo root resorption in the absence of a permanent tooth and a primary tooth retained in the presence of a permanent tooth. Therefore, although the pressure of a developing tooth is a major factor in resorption of primary teeth, it is not the only factor. There is much to be learned!

RETAINED PRIMARY TEETH

There are several reasons why primary teeth are retained beyond their normal time for **exfoliation.** Here we are not really considering a general delayed eruption that you may see in some patients because of retarded growth patterns but are considering the case where one or two teeth are retained well beyond the expected period of time for them to be lost.

The reasons for this are several. First, there may be no permanent successor, and the tooth remains. Second, there may be **ankylosis** of the tooth. This is a condition where the alveolar crest of bone fuses in the cervical area with the cementum of a resorbing root. Although virtually all the root may have been resorbed, the tooth remains firmly in place. This prevents the permanent tooth below from erupting. This may remain that way for years, and yet, when you re-

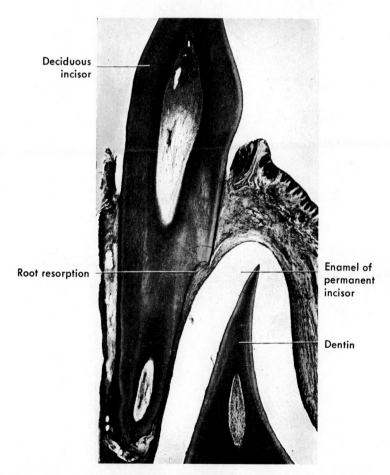

Deciduous incisor

Root resorption

Enamel of permanent incisor

Dentin

Fig. 7-2   Permanent anterior tooth lying lingual and apical to its deciduous predecessor, causing resorption of that tooth. (Bhaskar: Orban's.)

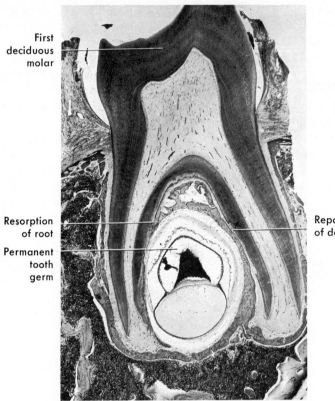

First deciduous molar

Resorption of root

Permanent tooth germ

Repaired resorption of dentin (X)

Fig. 7-3   Notice position of permanent posterior tooth lying between roots of primary tooth. (Bhaskar: Orban's.)

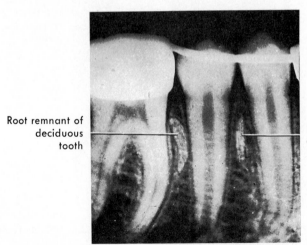

Root remnant of deciduous tooth

Root remnant of deciduous tooth

Fig. 7-4   Radiograph shows remnants of roots of deciduous molar still embedded in bone because of lack of resorption. (Bhaskar: Orban's; courtesy Dr. G.M. Fitzgerald.)

move the ankylosed tooth, the permanent tooth will generally begin to erupt. The last reason for a retained primary tooth is if the permanent tooth does not erupt in its normal position and therefore does not cause resorption of the primary tooth root or roots and the tooth remains.

Another problem associated with shedding of teeth is unresorbed root fragments. This condition is usually but not always associated with a malaligned primary or permanent tooth. If the root tip of a primary tooth is not in the path of eruption of a permanent tooth, the cervical portion of the root may be resorbed, leaving the apical part still embedded in the jaw (Fig. 7-4). They may remain there for some time and eventually may work their way to the surface and be removed. These retained root tips are seen in radiographs from time to time.

■ ■ ■

The time schedule of eruption and shedding is varied. In general, the posterior teeth go through a slower process than the anterior teeth do. Not only will the length of time for eruption vary, but also its beginning or ending time will vary from one person to another. As pointed out earlier, there is a range for normal eruption time, and only when this period is exceeded is there cause for concern. (See Chapter 24.)

REVIEW QUESTIONS

1. What are the three stages of active tooth eruption? When do they begin and end?
2. What are the possible theories of tooth eruption, and what is its most likely cause?
3. What causes the breakdown of the connective tissue between the erupting tooth and the oral epithelium?
4. What is the position of the permanent teeth in relation to their deciduous predecessors?
5. What is ankylosis? What problems may it cause? How is it treated?
6. Give three causes of retained primary teeth.

8

Oral Mucous Membrane

OBJECTIVES

- To name the three categories of mucosa and discuss where they are found
- To name the three stages of keratinization of stratified squamous epithelium and to discuss where these different types are found
- To discuss the factors that affect the mobility of various types of mucosa
- To describe the typical clinical picture of normal gingiva
- To describe some of the changes that are seen in diseased gingiva
- To describe the four stages of passive eruption

DIVISIONS OF MUCOUS MEMBRANE

The lining of the oral cavity is referred to as oral mucosa, or oral mucous membrane. It is a stratified squamous epithelial arrangement that runs from the margins of the lips posteriorly to the area of the tonsils. Although this same epithelium is found posterior to this point, it is part of the oral pharynx and not the oral cavity. This oral mucous membrane is divided into three categories:

1. **Specialized mucosa**—Mucosa on the upper surface, or **dorsum, of the tongue;** discussed in detail in Chapter 9.
2. **Masticatory mucosa**—Comprises the gingiva and hard palatal tissue; undergoes trauma or compression during mastication.
3. **Lining,** or general, **mucosa**—All other oral mucosa.

Mucous membrane is composed of stratified squamous epithelium and connective tissue. Recall that stratified squamous epithelium can have various characteristics on its surface (Fig. 8-1).

1. **Keratinized**—Having layers of dead cells, without nuclei, on its surface.
2. **Parakeratinized**—Some dead cells on the surface without nuclei and some cells that appear dying and have slightly shriveled nuclei.
3. **Nonkeratinized**—Cells on the surface all tending to have nuclei that appear fairly healthy and normal.

The lining mucosa is nonkeratinized to parakeratinized under most circumstances. The bottom, or basal, layer of cells rests on the underlying connective tissue, with a basement membrane in between. Although this underlying connective tissue contains some rather well-developed collagen fibers, it is still loose enough to allow the overlying epithelium to be fairly movable. Also allowing for this mobility is the way in which the epithelium and the connective tissue interdigitate, or relate to one another.

As seen in Fig. 8-2, there is a definite interdigitation between the epithelium and the connective tissue. In this illustration the ridges appear to interdigitate between the two; however, looking at a three-dimensional representation (Fig. 8-3), you can see that there are not only ridges of connective tissue but also pegs of connective tissue projecting up into the epithelium. The length of these ridges and connective tissue pegs determines how tightly the epithelium attaches to the underlying connective tissue and therefore how movable the epithelium is. Remember that the

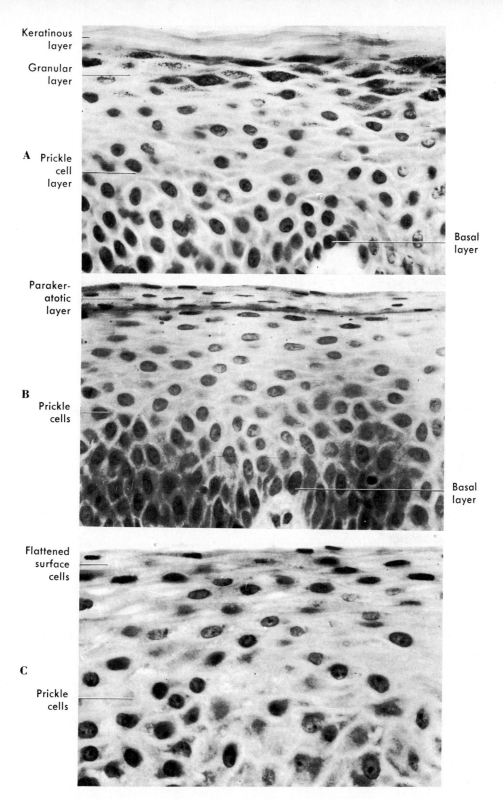

Fig. 8-1 **A,** Keratinized epithelium. Notice thick layer at top without any sign of nuclei. These are dead cells. **B,** Parakeratinized epithelium. Although nuclei are present even at top, there is less and they appear flattened and shriveled. **C,** Nonkeratinized epithelium. See how nuclei are obvious even at top. (Bhaskar: Orban's.)

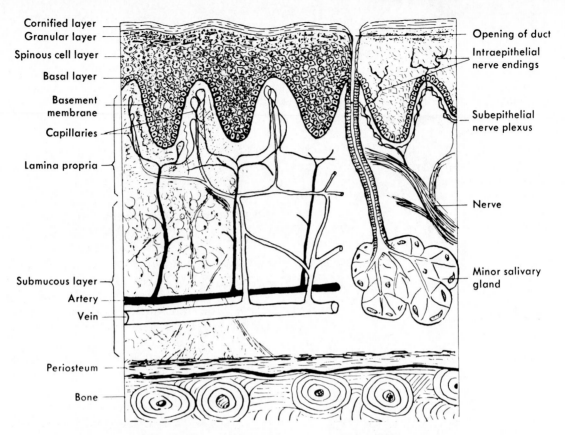

Fig. 8-2 Epithelium-connective tissue junction in two-dimensional representation. Notice interdigitation of what seem to be ridges of each. (Bhaskar: Orban's.)

Labels (top left to bottom):
Cornified layer
Granular layer
Spinous cell layer
Basal layer
Basement membrane
Capillaries
Lamina propria
Submucous layer
Artery
Vein
Periosteum
Bone

Labels (right):
Opening of duct
Intraepithelial nerve endings
Subepithelial nerve plexus
Nerve
Minor salivary gland

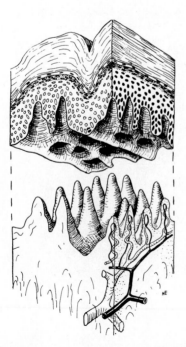

Fig. 8-3 In three-dimensional representation connective tissue pegs project up from ridges into epithelium. (Elias and Pauly.)

connective tissue is attached to underlying bone in some areas or to fatty or muscle tissue in other areas.

The lining mucosa tends to have poorly developed epithelial-connective tissue interdigitations and therefore is rather movable on the underlying tissue. Notice also that this degree of mobility is influenced as well by the attachment of the connective tissue to the tissue lying beneath it. The lining mucosa includes the mucosa of the cheeks, lips, soft palate, floor of the mouth beneath the tongue, and undersurface, or ventral surface, of the tongue, as well as the alveolar mucosa, which is the movable tissue immediately adjacent to the gingiva.

MASTICATORY MUCOSA

Masticatory mucosa is the mucosa of the gingiva and hard palate. During mastication, food is forced off the teeth and onto the gingiva around the necks of the teeth. The pressure of the food on this tissue causes it to become parakeratinized or keratinized. Food in the hard-palate area and the slight pressure of the tongue rubbing on the palate also cause this area to be parakeratinized or keratinized, depending on the amount of trauma.

What is the appearance of this gingiva and palatal mucosa? First, we shall consider the gingiva.

The gingiva is divided into two regions, the **free gingiva (marginal gingiva)** and the **attached gingiva.** These two combine to form the peak of gingiva that extends coronally between the teeth, which is known as the **interdental papilla** (Fig. 8-4). The part of the interdental papilla that is apical to the contact area is known as the **col** and is nonkeratinized.

Looking closely at the teeth and gingiva, you will find that there is a very shallow groove, or sulcus, around the tooth. The average depth of this sulcus, measured with a periodontal probe is about 2 mm (Fig. 8-5). The stratified squamous epithelium lining this sulcus is nonkeratinized, and at the bottom of the sulcus the epithelium is continuous with the cells that attach to the tooth, known as the **attachment epithelium (junctional epithelium).** In cases of periodontal disease the sulcus deepens either as a result of the free gingiva swelling or as a result of the attachment epithelium breaking down or moving farther apically on the tooth. One can frequently see the extent of the free gingiva because there may be a shallow groove on the gingival surface that corresponds to the depth of the free gingiva. This is called the free gingival groove.

The interdental papilla is an extremely important part of the gingiva. In a healthy state it fills the area between the teeth up to their contact areas. It prevents food from becoming lodged or

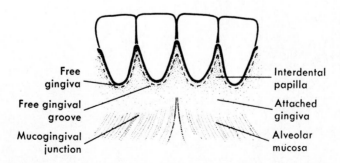

Fig. 8-4 Free gingiva and free gingival groove, which divides it from attached gingiva. Notice stippled appearance of gingiva compared with alveolar mucosa. (Pawlak and Hoag.)

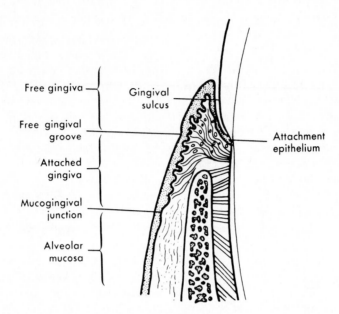

Fig. 8-5 Gingival sulcus and tissues that form it. Notice area of attachment epithelium at bottom and free gingival groove that marks depth of sulcus. (Pawlak and Hoag.)

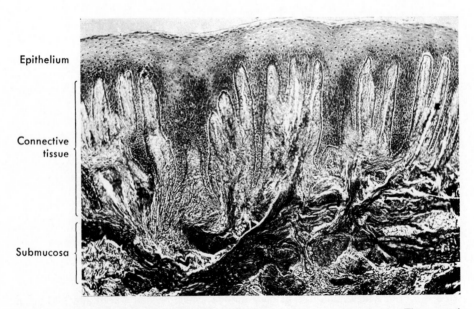

Fig. 8-6 Long interdigitations between epithelium and connective tissue. These make masticatory mucosa immovable. (Bhaskar: Orban's.)

impacted between the teeth during mastication. It is also one of the earliest areas involved in periodontal disease, when it tends to become swollen and blunted. As this happens, the lack of original contour causes it to be further irritated during mastication, and the problem becomes more complicated. For that reason it is an important area to study and check for swelling, blunting, reddening, and so on, as disease indicators.

The remainder of the gingiva is referred to as the attached gingiva. It derives its name from the fact that it is tightly attached to the underlying connective tissue and bone (Fig. 8-4). In a healthy state the gingiva usually has a stippled, or dimpled, appearance. This is caused by the connective tissue fibers attaching epithelium to the underlying bone. In periodontal disease, one of the first signs of gingival problems is a loss of stippling. This is initially caused by swelling, or **edema,** of the gingival tissues.

Where the attached gingiva meets the **alveolar mucosa** there is a change in color and a loss of the stippling because the epithelium is not attached tightly to the bone in this alveolar mucosa.

In the maxillary arch, the lingual gingiva does not change into alveolar mucosa but is directly continuous with the masticatory mucosa of the hard palate. This palatal mucosa, as was mentioned before, is generally the area of thickest mucosa in the oral cavity and the most likely to be keratinized.

In this area of masticatory mucosa the interdigitations between connective tissue and epithelium are rather long and narrow and therefore help to make the epithelium very adherent and relatively immovable (Fig. 8-6). Remember that it is within this connective tissue that the blood vessels, nerves, small salivary glands, and some fatty deposits are found.

PASSIVE ERUPTION

In Chapter 7 we discussed active eruption and how the tooth broke through the mucosa and into the oral cavity. There is also a process known as **passive eruption** in which the attachment epithelium moves from the crown of the tooth apically. Remember that as the tooth breaks through into the oral cavity the attachment epithelium is formed from the reduced enamel epithelium. This is frequently referred to as the primary attachment epithelium. Later on, the **primary attachment epithelium** is replaced by a **secondary attachment epithelium,** which arises from the gingiva. Passive eruption is generally considered as having the following four stages (Fig. 8-7).

Stage I—The attachment epithelium at the base of the gingival sulcus rests entirely on enamel.

Stage II—The attachment epithelium is primarily on enamel with a bit on cementum.

Stage III—The attachment epithelium extends from the cementoenamel junction (CEJ) onto cementum.

Stage IV—The attachment epithelium is entirely on cementum apical to the CEJ.

There is no specific timing for this process, and it may never reach stage IV, which is considered by some as pathological and is generally referred to as gingival recession.

The attachment of epithelium to tooth is an extremely active process. The cells that provide this attachment are replaced every 3 to 5 days. This rapid turnover aids in the repair of early gingival or periodontal disease.

CHANGES IN ORAL MUCOSA

Sometimes the tissue of the oral cavity deviates from its normal color. It may appear quite reddened or whitish. What causes these changes? Why is the mucosa reddish? Epithelial cells have no color themselves. They may take up pigments produced by the body and carry them to the surface. It is this carried pigment that gives differential colors to the skin. The redness of the mucosa comes from the oxygen-carrying pigment in the blood, known as hemoglobin. These blood vessels are located immediately beneath the mucosa in the connective tissue, and the reflection of the

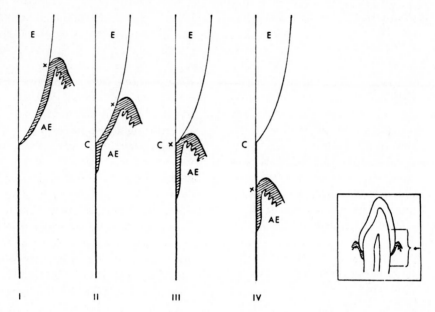

Fig. 8-7 Four stages of passive eruption. X, Base of sulcus; *AE,* attachment epithelium.

blood through the epithelium imparts a red color to the mucosa. What happens when the mucosa is very red? This is caused by inflammation—the blood vessels beneath the mucosa expand and bring more blood to the area to fight the causative irritation. In a pathological condition you will find that redness is one of the primary signs of inflammation. How then can the epithelium appear whitish? Is it because there is less blood beneath the epithelium? It generally is the result of irritation of the mucosa, which causes the cells to multiply faster and the epithelium to become thicker, a condition similar to the development of a callus. When it becomes thicker, the tissue becomes more **opaque,** and the blood does not show through so easily; therefore the tissue is whiter than normal.

It cannot be stressed too strongly that the oral mucosa is a very important indicator for both the oral and general health of the person. The color and tone of the tissue are extremely important health indicators. Study these tissues carefully—they will provide much important information!

REVIEW QUESTIONS

1. What are the three divisions of the oral mucosa, and where are they located?
2. What are the three variations of stratified squamous epithelium, and how are they determined?
3. What determines the mobility of the epithelium?
4. What are the general causes of change in mucosal color?
5. What is the average depth of the gingival sulcus?
6. What is the function of the interdental papilla?
7. What is the descriptive term used for gingival appearance?
8. Describe the relationship of the attachment epithelium to the tooth in the four stages of eruption.

9

The Tongue

OBJECTIVES

- To describe the formation of the tongue as it relates to germ layer and pharyngeal arch origin
- To discuss the difference between extrinsic and intrinsic muscles of the tongue
- To describe briefly how tongue movement is accomplished
- To describe the papillae of the tongue and their function
- To describe the kinds of changes seen on the tongue that indicate health problems

DEVELOPMENT OF THE TONGUE

If you will refer to Chapter 3 on the development of the face, you will recall that there are a number of bars of tissue found on the anterior surface of the developing embryo that are referred to as pharyngeal arches. The first pharyngeal arch is the mandibular arch, the second is the hyoid arch, and the remainder are numbered III, IV, and V (or VI). Just above the first arch and extending down behind all the arches is a hollow tube, the digestive tract. You will also recall that before the third embryonic week this tube is closed off at the upper end by the buccopharyngeal membrane, which separates the upper end, or foregut, from the primitive oral cavity. The epithelium anterior to the buccopharyngeal membrane develops from the outer germ layer, or ectoderm. The tube behind the buccopharyngeal membrane develops from the inner germ layer, or entoderm. At 4 weeks the buccopharyngeal membrane ruptures, but the epithelium in that

area still comes from two distinct germ layers. It is at about this point that the tongue starts to develop, and a swelling begins to arise out of the back part of the pharyngeal arches (Fig. 9-1). This swelling develops from the future floor of the mouth. The covering of the tongue, the epithelium, develops from ectoderm and endoderm— the anterior two thirds from ectoderm and the posterior one third from entoderm. The tongue is a sac of epithelium filled with muscles. These muscles arise from the middle germ layer of the embryo, known as mesoderm; therefore the tongue is unusual, since it originates from all three germ layers. Each one of the pharyngeal arch areas is associated with a particular nerve of the brain, or cranial nerve. In Chapter 19 we discuss the nervous system, and you will discover from which pharyngeal arch the various parts of the tongue develop.

TONGUE MUSCLES

As mentioned before, the tongue is an epithelial sac filled with muscles. These muscles can be controlled willfully and are generally referred to as skeletal muscle. They are divided into two groupings: **intrinsic** and **extrinsic** muscles. Those that start and end wholly within the tongue are referred to as intrinsic muscles, and are the following four groups:

1. Superior longitudinal group—Runs from front to back (anterior to posterior) and lie near the top
2. Inferior longitudinal group—Also runs from front to back but lie near the bottom

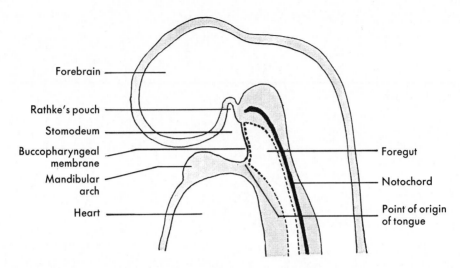

Forebrain

Rathke's pouch

Stomodeum

Buccopharyngeal membrane

Mandibular arch

Heart

Foregut

Notochord

Point of origin of tongue

Fig. 9-1 Section through embryo anteroposteriorly. Mandibular, or first, pharyngeal arch is marked, and others are below it partially covered by the heart. Tongue arises from area at lower end of buccopharyngeal membrane. (Bhaskar: Orban's.)

3. Transverse group—Runs from side to side
4. Vertical group—Runs from top to bottom (dorsal to ventral)

What happens when the muscles in these groups contract? Keep in mind the direction of these fibers and imagine the tongue as an oblong balloon with a constant volume. If the longitudinal group of fibers contracts, the tongue is shortened. Shortening the tongue makes it thicker and wider. If you contract the group that runs transversely, the tongue may get a little thicker and longer. Contract the vertical group, and the tongue may get wider and longer. Try to picture what would happen if you contracted two of these groups at the same time.

Along with the intrinsic muscles in the tongue are groups of muscles that originate outside the tongue and run into it. These are called extrinsic muscles.

The extrinsic muscles of the tongue actually are more directly related to gross anatomy than oral histology, but since they also affect intrinsic muscle action, they should be mentioned here. As we look at origins we might want to study the osteology of the skull in Chapter 11 to be more

familiar with locations. There are four pairs of muscles. The **hyoglossus** muscle runs from the **hyoid** bone upward into the lateral borders of the tongue and pulls the lateral edges down onto the floor of the mouth (see Fig. 13-4). The **styloglossus** runs from the styloid process down and forward into the lateral borders of the tongue and blends in with the hyoglossus muscle. The styloglossus pulls the tongue backwards and upwards. The **palatoglossus** muscle runs from the anterior soft palate downward and a little forward into the lateral borders of the tongue (see Fig. 16-1). It elevates the tongue and pulls it slightly backward. The **genioglossus** muscle originates from the **genial tubercles** on the midline of the mandible and inserts into the midline of the tongue from the tip to the base (see Fig. 13-6). It can aid in protrusion or depression of the tongue.

PAPILLAE

The tongue is covered with stratified squamous epithelium. The undersurface, or ventral surface, of the tongue has very thin epithe-

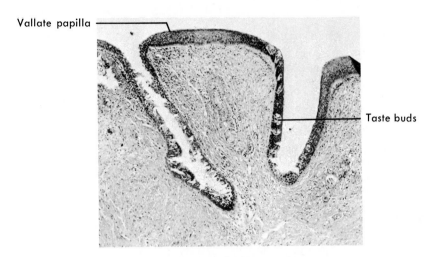

Vallate papilla

Taste buds

Fig. 9-2 Large vallate papilla in trough, with light-colored taste buds along its side. (Bhaskar: Orban's.)

lium, but the upper surface has thick parakeratinized to keratinized epithelium. Scattered throughout this epithelium on the upper surface are four types of elevated structures known as papillae.

Circumvallate or Vallate Papillae

One type is **circumvallate** or **vallate papillae,** a V-shaped row of circular raised papillae. There are about 13 elevations in the V, which is located about two thirds of the way back on the tongue, with the point of the V facing backward. This row divides the anterior two thirds of the tongue from the posterior one third and marks the area that develops from different branchial arches with different nerve supplies. (See also Chapter 19.) If you look at these vallate papillae under a microscope, you will see that they appear to rest in troughs and that they have many tiny **taste buds** all around their lateral surfaces (Fig. 9-2). These taste buds are made up of many cells supporting several little hairlike nerve endings that perceive taste. There are small salivary glands located beneath these papillae, which serve to wash the papillae clean, making them ready to perceive new tastes (Fig. 9-3).

Fungiform Papillae

If you look closely at the tongue, you will see that the anterior two thirds have tiny, round, raised spots. In younger persons they appear redder than the area around them. These are the **fungiform papillae.** There are a few taste buds in these papillae similar to those in the vallates (Fig. 9-4, *A*).

Filiform Papillae

The remainder of the anterior two thirds of the tongue is covered with tiny pointed projections of parakeratinized to keratinized epithelium, known as **filiform papillae** (Fig. 9-4, *B*). They have no taste function and probably only provide tactile sensation, or the ability to know that there is something on the tongue. In the cat, they are well developed, and you can feel the rough surface of these papillae when a cat licks your hand. Sometimes the epithelium on these papillae grows very long and traps food and pigments originating from oral bacteria and food in between them. This is referred to as hairy tongue. There are other times when the epithelium of these papillae are lost and the surface of the epithelium becomes very smooth. This is re-

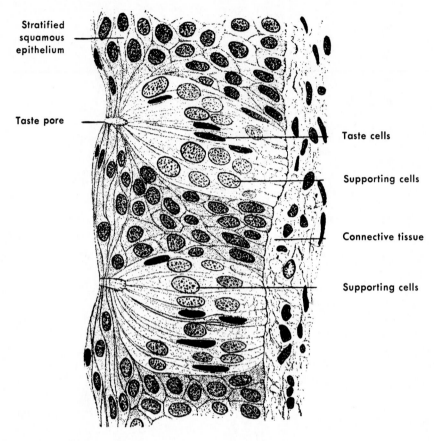

Stratified squamous epithelium

Taste pore

Taste cells

Supporting cells

Connective tissue

Supporting cells

Fig. 9-3   Hairlike receptor of taste bud is located in taste pore. (Bhaskar: Orban's.)

ferred to as glossitis, and it occurs in a number of disease processes, one of which is vitamin deficiencies.

Foliate Papillae

If you grasp the tip of the tongue with a piece of gauze and pull it out and to the side, you will see a roughened lateral surface back in the region of the vallate papillae. In lower forms of animals these are another set of well-developed papillae with many taste buds, known as the **foliate papillae.** In humans these are not so well developed and contain fewer taste buds than those in animals.

The tip of the tongue is an area that can become irritated and reddened. It is also an area where oral cancer can begin but be obscured because of the location and folds of tissue. It is therefore an important area to check in oral examinations (Fig. 9-5).

Another area that should be mentioned is a region near the midline on the dorsum of the tongue just behind the vallate papillae, known as the **lingual tonsils.** This is tissue similar to the palatine tonsil and provides a defense mechanism for infection in that area. Infection in this part of the tongue will involve the lingual tonsils, and they will become reddened and enlarged.

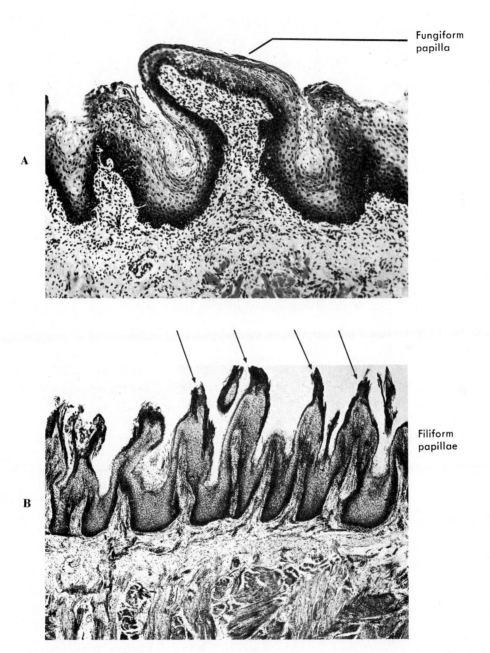

Fungiform
papilla

Filiform
papillae

Fig. 9-4 **A,** Fungiform papillae. Although taste buds are not visible in fungiform papillae, they are present in small numbers. **B,** Filiform papillae. (Bhaskar: Orban's.)

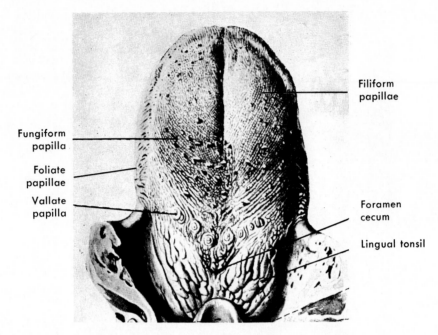

Fungiform
papilla

Foliate
papillae

Vallate
papilla

Filiform
papillae

Foramen
cecum

Lingual tonsil

Fig. 9-5 Overall view of tongue showing large lingual tonsils on posterior and roughened area of foliate papilla on side. (Bhaskar: Orban's.)

Therefore this is an important clinical indicator of potential problems (Fig. 9-5).

The tongue as a whole is a good indicator of the patient's overall health, as is the gingival tissue. These should be carefully studied when a patient is being examined.

REVIEW QUESTIONS

1. How many different germ layers form the entire tongue?

2. What is the difference between extrinsic and intrinsic muscles?
3. How are various tongue movements and shapes accomplished?
4. Name the papillae of the tongue, where they are located, and what their functions might be.
5. What kinds of changes can you see in the tongue that relate to the health of a person?

10

Salivary Glands

OBJECTIVES

- To describe the components of a salivary gland
- To describe the duct system of a salivary gland
- To describe the arrangement of the cells of a mixed salivary gland.

In this chapter we will attempt to describe only the histology of salivary glands. For the description of size, location, and function of these glands, refer to Chapter 18.

COMPONENTS OF A SALIVARY GLAND

In Chapter 2 you learned that salivary glands arise from a tube of epithelium growing into the underlying connective tissue. At the end of this tube a cluster of secretory cells form. This endpiece can be clusters of cells shaped like a grape, or a tube.

Acini

The secretory endpieces are known as **acini**. There are two kinds of acinar cells, **mucous** and **serous**. Because these cells form a circular pattern, they are described as being **pyramidal cells** (Fig. 10-1). The outer edge, or base, of the cells rests on connective tissue. The apex of the cells face the center of the tube or circular structure. The base of the cells are surrounded by connective tissue, and partially surrounding each secretory acinus is a **myoepithelial cell** (Fig. 10-2). This cell has long cellular projections that would make it look like a squid. These projections sur-

round the acinus, and when the myoepithelial cell contracts, it squeezes the acinus and aids in the secretion of saliva into the hollow center of the acinus and out the duct system.

Mucous acini. A **mucous** secretion is a slightly viscous secretion caused by the production of several mucins. Although its product is 99% water, it does have a number of inorganic ions such as Na^+, K^+, and Cl^- and some **amylase** (carbohydrate-splitting) enzymes that begin to break down starches into long-chain sugars. It probably also has some proteins that aid in inhibiting caries and probably periodontal disease. A mucous acinus is more tubular and has a larger **lumen** than a serous acinus and the cell membranes can more easily be seen at adjacent sides of the cells. The nucleus of a mucous cell is usually very flat and lies against the basal part of the cell. The apical end of these cells appear frothy under the light microscope. In the electron microscope one would see a great number of mucus droplets that stain very poorly and so give an empty frothy appearance.

Serous acini. A serous acinus has a fairly similar makeup of secretions without the mucins. The secretory granules stain deeply, the lumen is very small and difficult to see, and the adjacent cell membranes are not easily seen. A serous cell is also pyramidal in shape. The nucleus is round and is close to the base of the cell.

Seromucous acini. In glands that have both mucous and serous components you will see the separate types of acini, and you will also see them joined together as a mixed acinus or **seromucous** acinus. The mucous cells form a tube-

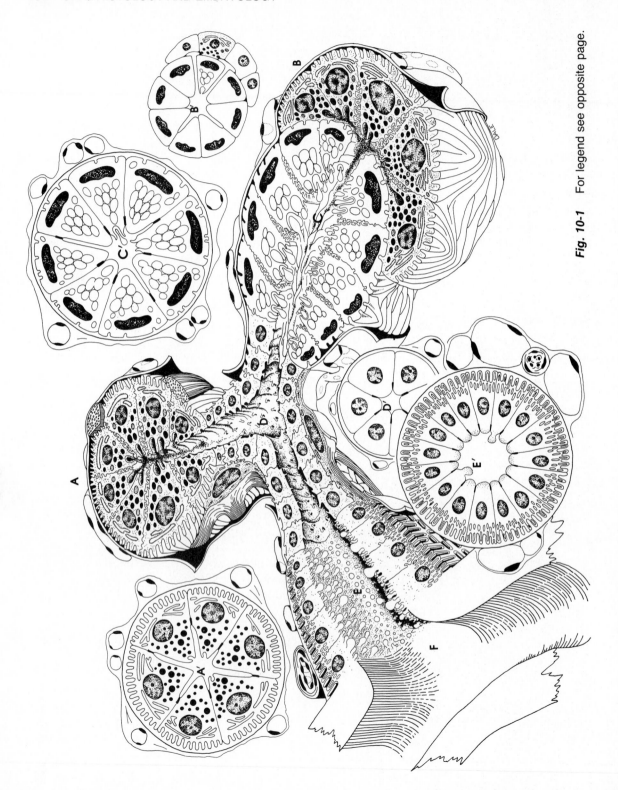

For legend see opposite page.

Fig. 10-1

Fig. 10-1   Schematic diagram of typical salivary gland. **A,** Seromucous endpiece; **A′,** in cross section. **B,** Seromucous demilune; **B′,** in cross section. **C,** Mucous endpiece; **C′,** in cross section. **D,** Intercalated duct; **D′,** in cross section. **E,** Striated duct; **E′,** in cross section. **F,** Terminal excretory duct. (From Ten Cate AR: Oral histology, ed 2, St Louis, 1985, The CV Mosby Co.)

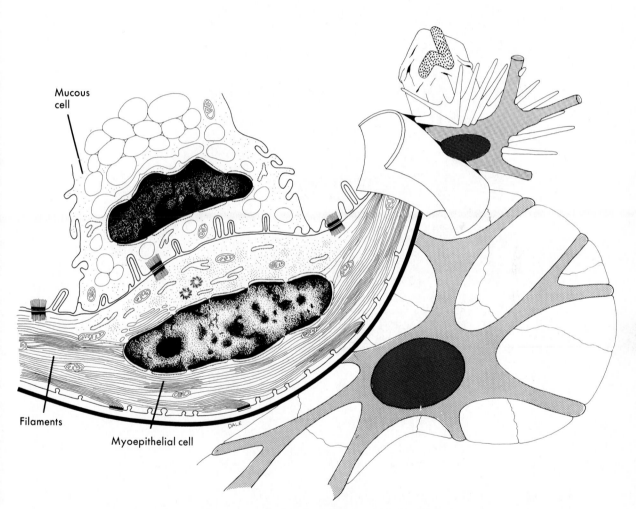

Fig. 10-2   Myoepithelial cell can be seen with its processes surrounding an acinus.

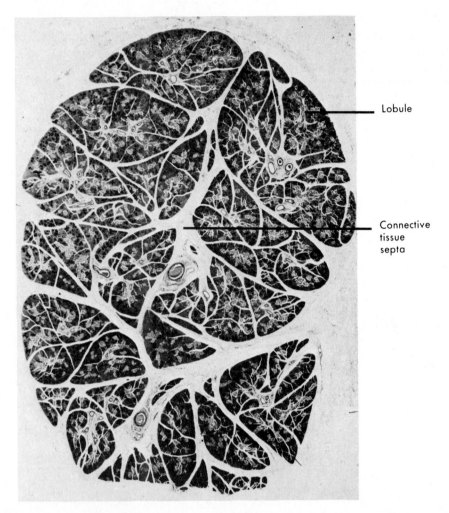

Lobule

Connective tissue septa

Fig. 10-3 Connective tissue surrounds this salivary gland and further subdivides it into lobules.

like structure, and on the end of the tube a group of serous cells are found looking like a half-moon cluster of cells. These are referred to as **serous demilunes.** These acini produce both mucous and serous secretions (Fig. 10-1).

Connective Tissue Capsule

A salivary gland is surrounded by a connective tissue capsule. The connective tissue not only surrounds the gland but also sends partitions into the gland carrying nerves and blood vessels with it, and this connective tissue divides the gland into lobes and smaller units called lobules (Fig. 10-3).

Duct System

Salivary glands have varying numbers of lobules, depending on their size. As just mentioned, each one of these lobules is surrounded by connective tissue. There are a series of different

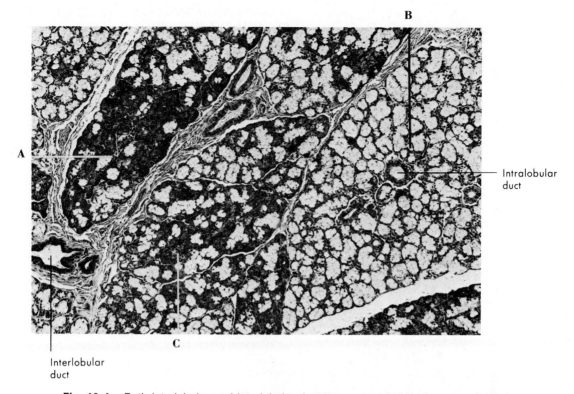

Intralobular
duct

Interlobular
duct

Fig. 10-4   Both intralobular and interlobular ducts are seen. **A,** Mostly serous lobule. **B,**
Mostly mucous lobule. **C,** Lobule fairly even in mucous and serous acini.

kinds of ducts, some of them within the lobule, some between the lobule, and some outside of the gland leading onto the surface of the oral cavity. Within the lobule we can see two kinds of ducts that by location are called **intralobular ducts,** meaning 'within the lobule.'

Intercalated ducts. Intercalated ducts are very small ducts that directly drain the acini. The cells in these ducts are not much higher than their nuclei. In some glands they are longer and can be more easily seen, whereas in others they are so short that they are rarely seen. These intercalated ducts carry the secretions to the next set of ducts within the lobule.

Striated (secretory) ducts. These **striated ducts** are so named because the base of the cell seems to have stripes in it. The reason is that the basal part of the cell membrane is thrown up into long folds with mitochondria trapped between these folds. These mitochondria can be stained, and they look like stripes. These ducts are also called "secretory" because as the salivary fluid passes through them their content is modified. Water and various substances such as sodium, potassium, calcium, and other ions are absorbed into the cell and secreted out of the basal end of the cell where they are picked up again by the bloodstream. This function conserves water and electrolytes and is a very important conservation function (Fig. 10-1).

Interlobular ducts. Interlobular ducts lie within the connective tissue between lobules of the gland. Some of these are striated like the intralobular ducts, but most of them are nonstriated and large. They are generally referred to as **excretory ducts.** They do not modify the salivary secretions but simply carry them out of the gland and to the surface tissues of the oral cavity (Fig. 10-4).

Control of Secretions

Secretory control is from the **autonomic nervous system** (see Chapter 19). The control of secretion is tied to the chewing process, taste, and smell. Each of these is capable of modifying the amount and consistency of the salivary secretions.

REVIEW QUESTIONS

1. What are acini, and what are three types?
2. What is a myoepithelial cell and what is its function?
3. Define the following:
   a. Intercalated duct
   b. Striated duct
   c. Secretory duct
   d. Excretory duct
   e. Intralobular duct
   f. Interlobular duct
4. What are serous demilunes?

TEST

1. Which of the following is *not* a cell organelle?
   a. nucleus
   b. glycogen inclusion
   c. endoplasmic reticulum
   d. Golgi apparatus
   e. all are organelles

2. The skin and mucosa of the oral cavity are an example of _____ epithelium.
   a. simple squamous
   b. simple columnar
   c. transitional
   d. stratified squamous
   e. pseudostratified squamous

3. Which of the following would *not* be classed as connective tissue?
   a. bone
   b. cartilage
   c. collagen
   d. tendon
   e. ligament
   f. all are connective tissue

4. Which of the following is *not* a granulocyte blood cell?
   a. neutrophil
   b. lymphocyte
   c. basophil
   d. eosinophil

e. all are granulocytes

5. Which of the following muscle tissues is classified as striated voluntary muscle?
   a. cardiac
   b. skeletal
   c. smooth
   d. a and b
   e. b and c
   f. a, b, and c

6. The protective sheath around a nerve cell is known as a _____ sheath.
   a. dendrite
   b. axon
   c. myelin
   d. cellulin
   e. none of the above

7. The developmental period of the embryo is:
   a. 0-2 weeks
   b. 3-8 weeks
   c. 8-12 weeks
   d. 12-36 weeks

8. The upper lip develops from the
   a. medial nasal process
   b. lateral nasal process
   c. maxillary process
   d. mandibular process
   e. a and b
   f. b and c
   g. a and c
   h. none of the above

9. The upper lip forms by a process of _____, while the palate forms by a process of _____.
   a. elongation, migration
   b. migration, fusion
   c. fusion, elongation
   d. none of the above

10. The premaxilla comes from the
    a. lateral nasal process
    b. medial nasal process
    c. mandibular process
    d. maxillary process
    e. none of the above

11. The buccopharyngeal membrane breaks down during the _____ embryonic week.
    a. second

b. third

c. fourth

d. fifth

12. The critical time for facial development is _____ weeks.
    a. 2-5
    b. 3-6
    c. 5-9
    d. 7-10

13. The critical time for palatal development is _____ weeks.
    a. 2-6
    b. 3-7
    c. 5-9
    d. 7-11

14. There are _____ pharyngeal arches that develop
    a. two
    b. three
    c. four
    d. five

15. Cleft lips occur about once in every-_____ births.
    a. 300
    b. 800
    c. 1500
    d. 7,000
    e. 10,000

16. Which of the following are *not* a part of an early pharyngeal arch?
    a. cartilage
    b. bone
    c. nerve
    d. blood vessel
    e. mesodermal tissue

17. The first signs of tooth development are seen in the _____ week.
    a. fourth
    b. sixth
    c. tenth
    d. twelfth
    e. none of the above

18. The first stage of the enamel organ is the _____ stage.
    a. cap

b. bell

c. bud

d. incisive

e. none of the above

19. The beginning of the bell stage occurs when the _____ appears.
    a. outer enamel epithelium
    b. stellate reticulum
    c. stratum intermedium
    d. inner enamel epithelium
    e. none of the above

20. Which of the following *does not* arise from the dental sac?
    a. dentin
    b. cementum
    c. periodontal ligament
    d. they all arise from it

21. The ameloblast arises from the
    a. dental papilla
    b. inner enamel epithelium
    c. outer enamel epithelium
    d. stellate reticulum
    e. none of the above

22. Enamel is about _____ hydroxyapatite crystals.
    a. 30%
    b. 70%
    c. 95%
    d. 5%

23. The last thing the ameloblast produces is the
    a. primary enamel cuticle
    b. Nasmyth's membrane
    c. reduced enamel epithelium
    d. secondary enamel cuticle
    e. a and b

24. Cracks in the enamel are known as
    a. enamel spindles
    b. enamel tufts
    c. imbrication lines
    d. enamel lamellae
    e. none of the above

25. Dentin is about _____ crystal in composition.
    a. 10%
    b. 30%

c. 50%

d. 70%

e. none of the above

26. Dentin formed beneath an area of decay is known as _____ dentin.
    a. mantle
    b. circumpulpal
    c. primary
    d. reparative
    e. secondary
    f. none of the above

27. Pulp develops from
    a. dental papilla
    b. mesenchyme
    c. pulp stones
    d. dental sac
    e. a and b
    f. none of the above

28. Cementum is about _____ inorganic crystals.
    a. 10%
    b. 30%
    c. 50%
    d. 70%
    e. 90%

29. Hertwig's root sheath comes from
    a. enamel organ
    b. dental papilla
    c. dentin
    d. dental sac
    e. none of the above

30. At the cementoenamel junction, cementum overlaps enamel about _____ of the time.
    a. 10%
    b. 20%
    c. 30%
    d. 60%
    e. 90%

31. Which of the following is *not* a true statement concerning Sharpey's fibers?
    a. They are found in cementum.
    b. They are found in dentin.
    c. They are found in alveolar bone.
    d. They are the embedded portion of the periodontal ligament.
    e. All of the above are true statements.

32. Cellular cementum is usually found
    a. at the cementoenamel junction
    b. in the cervical third of the root
    c. in the middle third of the root only
    d. in the apical third of the root

33. Which of the following is *not* found originally as alveolar bone is forming?
    a. bundle bone
    b. cribriform plate
    c. spongy bone
    d. cortical plate
    e. they are all an original part of alveolar bone

34. Which of the following alveolodental fibers would resist the forces of mastication?
    a. apical
    b. horizontal
    c. oblique
    d. alveolar crest
    e. none of the above

35. In active tooth eruption, the "eruptive" stage begins when
    a. crown formation begins
    b. root formation begins
    c. tooth erupts into the oral cavity
    d. root formation is completed
    e. none of the above

36. The most probable cause of tooth eruption is
    a. growth of pulpal tissue
    b. root growth
    c. bone growth in socket
    d. changes within periodontal ligament
    e. none of the above

37. The permanent molars develop
    a. between the roots of the primary molars
    b. between the roots of the premolars
    c. apical and lingual to primary molars
    d. lingual to primary molars
    e. none of the above

38. Attached gingiva is an example of
    a. specialized mucosa
    b. lining mucosa
    c. masticatory mucosa
    d. b and c
    e. none of the above

39. Specialized mucosa is found
    a. on the hard palate
    b. on the soft palate
    c. on the dorsum of the tongue
    d. on the mucosa of the cheek
    e. a and b
    f. in none of the above
40. The height of the free gingiva is generally the same height as the
    a. attached gingiva
    b. alveola mucosa
    c. gingival sulcus
    d. interdental papilla
41. Which of the following papillae of the tongue have *no* taste buds on them?
    a. filiform
    b. fungiform
    c. vallate (circumvallate)
    d. foliate
    e. all have taste buds
42. The intrinsic muscles of the tongue run
    a. front to back
    b. top to bottom
    c. side to side
    d. all of the above
    e. none of the above
43. Hairy tongue is an elongation of the
    a. fungiform papillae
    b. filiform papillae
    c. circumvallate papillae
    d. foliate papillae
    e. none of the above
44. The ducts in salivary glands that carry the secretions directly out of the acini are the _____ ducts.
    a. interlobular
    b. excretory
    c. striated
    d. intercalated
    e. none of the above
45. The enzyme found in saliva that splits starches into long-chain sugars is
    a. peptidase
    b. sucrase
    c. amylase
    d. protease
    e. none of the above
46. Intralobular ducts are surrounded by
    a. connective tissue
    b. blood vessels
    c. other ducts
    d. acini
    e. none of the above
47. Striated salivary ducts
    a. aid in conserving water
    b. aid in conserving electrolytes
    c. modify the saliva
    d. all of the above
    e. none of the above

SECTION TWO

REFERENCES

SUGGESTED READINGS

Bevelander G: Outline of histology, ed 8, St Louis, 1979, The CV Mosby Co.

Bevelander G: Atlas of oral histology and embryology, Philadelphia, 1967, Lea & Febiger.

Bhaskar SN: Orban's oral histology and embryology, ed 10, St Louis, 1985, The CV Mosby Co.

Langman J: Medical embryology, ed 5, Baltimore, 1985, The Williams & Wilkins Co.

Melfi R: Permar's oral embryology and microscopic anatomy: a textbook for students in dental hygiene, ed 8, Philadelphia, 1988, Lea & Febiger.

Provenza DV: Fundamentals of oral histology and embryology, ed 2, Philadelphia, 1972, JB Lippincott Co.

Ten Cate AR: Oral histology: development, structure, and function, ed 3, St Louis, 1989, The CV Mosby Co.

ILLUSTRATION SOURCES

Bevelander G: Outline of histology, ed 7, St Louis, 1971, The CV Mosby Co.

Bevelander G: Atlas of oral histology and embryology, Philadelphia, 1967, Lea & Febiger.

Bhaskar SN: Orban's oral histology and embryology, ed 8, St Louis, 1976, The CV Mosby Co.

Bloom W and Fawcett DW: A textbook of histology, ed 10, Philadelphia, 1975, WB Saunders Co.

DuBrul EL: Sicher's oral anatomy, ed 7, St Louis, 1980, The CV Mosby Co.

Elias H et al.: Human microanatomy, ed 4, Philadelphia, 1978, FA Davis Co.

Ham AW and Cormack D: Histology, ed 8, Philadelphia, 1979, JB Lippincott Co.

Langman J: Medical embryology, ed 3, Baltimore, 1975, The Williams & Wilkins Co.

Meckel AH, Griebstein WJ, and Neal RJ: Structure of mature human dental enamel as observed by electron microscopy Arch Oral Biol 10:775, 1965.

Pawlak E and Hoag PM: Essentials of periodontics, ed 2, St Louis, 1980, The CV Mosby Co.

Provenza DV: Fundamentals of oral histology and embryology, ed 2, Philadelphia, 1972, JB Lippincott Co.

Ross RB and Johnston MC: Cleft lip and palate, Baltimore, 1978, The Williams & Wilkins Co.

Ten Cate AR: Oral histology: development, structure, and function, ed 2, St Louis, 1985, The CV Mosby Co.

HEAD AND NECK ANATOMY

11

Osteology of the Skull

OBJECTIVES

- To name the bones of the neurocranium and the viscerocranium
- To label the various bones and sutures as seen from anterior, lateral, posterior, inferior, and interior views of the skull
- To name the openings, foramina, and canals as seen from the aforementioned views
- To describe the pterygoid processes of the sphenoid bone and their components
- To describe in detail the various parts and landmarks of the maxillae
- To describe in detail the various parts and landmarks of the mandible

The bones of the skull play several different roles. They surround the brain and protect it from injury and also form the facial features and participate in the growth process of the jaws, which in turn controls whether a patient has a malocclusion (improper relationship of the teeth and jaws).

In this chapter we discuss the more important bones and their landmarks. The discussion is certainly not all-inclusive.

Excluding the three small **ossicles** (the bones in each ear that aid in hearing), there are 22 bones that make up the skull. Some of these are single and some are paired bones. They are grouped into two categories: one group surrounds the brain and one group forms the face.

Following are the eight bones that make up the **neurocranium,** or the bones surrounding the brain:

frontal bone (single)	**occipital bone** (single)
sphenoid bone (single)	**temporal bones** (paired)
ethmoid bone (single)	**parietal bones** (paired)

Of these eight, the sphenoid and ethmoid are rather difficult to picture because they cannot easily be seen in their entirety on the surface. The ethmoid bone is primarily located in the facial area of the nose, but since a small part of it surrounds the brain, it is classified as part of the neurocranium.

Following are the fourteen bones that make up the **viscerocranium,** or the bones of the face:

mandible (single)
vomer (single)
nasal bones (paired)
lacrimal bones (paired)
zygomatic bones (paired)
inferior nasal conchae (paired, referred to in plural form *-ae*)
palatine bones (paired)
maxillae (paired, referred to in plural form *-ae*)

Some of these bones are extremely small and do not contribute significantly to facial growth and configuration. Most of these bones are discussed as a group and the sphenoid, maxillae, and mandible are studied in more detail.

Instead of considering the bones around the brain and of the face as two completely separate groups, we will explore various views of the skull and study their relationships to one another. In doing this, refer to the groupings just listed.

However, in preparation, several terms that are used in the following chapters should be introduced. Probably one of the first terms you will hear is **suture.** This is a firm joining together of two or more bones. Two other terms are **foramen** and **canal.** A foramen is a *short* tubelike opening through bone, and a canal is a *long* tubelike opening through bone.

VIEWS OF THE SKULL
Anterior View

In Fig. 11-1, an anterior, or frontal, view of an adult skull, you can see that the area from the eyes up to the top of the skull is made up of the frontal bone. The area below the eyes down to

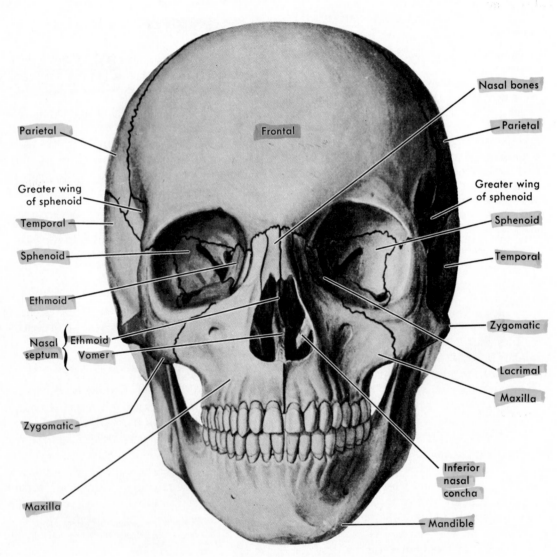

Fig. 11-1   Anterior view of skull. (Sicher and DuBrul.)

the occlusal plane between the upper and lower teeth comprises the paired zygomatic, or cheek, bones and the paired maxillae. The nasal bones form the bridge of the nose, and the lower jaw is formed by the single mandible. Looking more closely, you can see that the inner, or medial, corner of the eye cavity **(orbit)** contains a small lacrimal bone; within the nasal cavity the vertical **nasal septum** is composed of the vomer and ethmoid bones. The inferior nasal conchae are found in the lower, lateral portions of the nasal cavity. If you look back into the orbit, you can see another part of the ethmoid bone and parts of the sphenoid bone. At the lateral edges of the skull some parts of the parietal and temporal bones are visible, as well as another part of the sphenoid bone.

Lateral View

From a side, or lateral, view, parts of many bones can be seen: frontal bone, zygomatic bone, maxilla, mandible, nasal bone, lacrimal bone, a small bit of the ethmoid bone in the medial wall of the orbit, part of the sphenoid bone, temporal

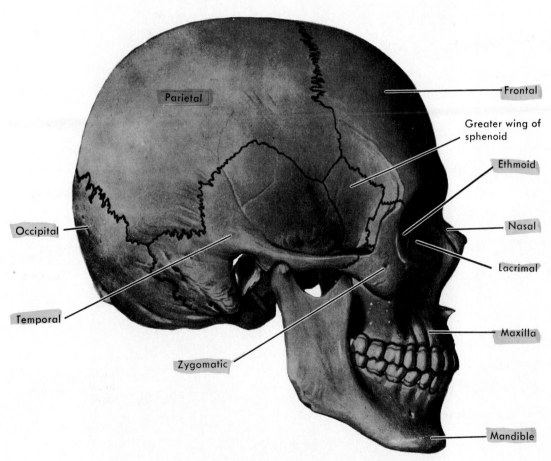

Fig. 11-2   Lateral view of skull. (Sicher and DuBrul.)

bone, parietal bone, and occipital bone. Fig. 11-2 shows jagged suture lines separating one bone from another. It may be difficult to see some of them, but it is probably more important to be able to visualize the relationship of one bone to the other rather than to differentiate every single suture.

Inferior View

The most difficult view of the skull for the beginning student of anatomy is the inferior view. It is difficult for two reasons; there are numerous points of study, or landmarks, and it is difficult to see the suture lines between the bones in many instances. Nevertheless, in the anterior region in

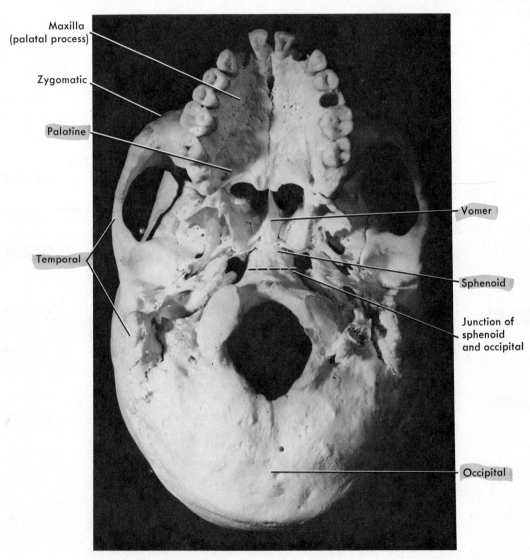

Fig. 11-3   Inferior view of skull.

Fig. 11-3, the hard palate, which is formed by the **palatal processes of the maxillae** and the palatal processes of the palatine bones, is visible. Just behind and above the palate a small portion of the vomer bone can be seen forming the lower part of the nasal septum. Just behind that and running the full width of the skull is the sphenoid bone, which is discussed in greater detail on p. 126. It is difficult to see the suture line between the sphenoid and the occipital bones because it disappears when a person is about 18 years of age. From this view, portions of the zygomatic bones, the temporal bones, and just a tiny portion of the posterior part of the parietal bones can also be seen.

Interior View

There is one other view of the skull that should be considered, and that is a view of the inside of the skull with the top removed (Fig. 11-4). Much of the front of the skull is formed by the frontal bone; however, there is a small area

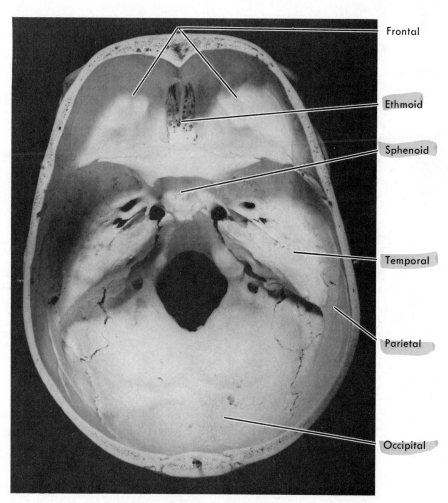

Frontal

Ethmoid

Sphenoid

Temporal

Parietal

Occipital

Fig. 11-4 Floor of cranial cavity with top of skull removed.

near the middle that is part of the ethmoid bone. Immediately behind these bones is the sphenoid bone, and behind it laterally are the temporal, parietal, and occipital bones.

LANDMARKS OF THE SKULL

Now let us reexamine the same views of the skull this time concentrating on the landmarks

rather than on the arrangement of the bones. Again, not every point of study on these views will be named but only those most important for consideration at this stage.

Anterior View

As you look again at the anterior view of the skull in Fig. 11-5, you can see that the rim of the orbit is formed by the frontal, zygomatic, and

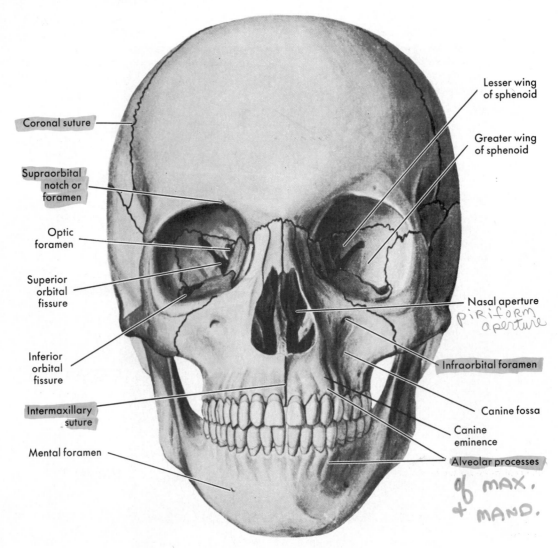

Coronal suture

Supraorbital notch or foramen

Optic foramen

Superior orbital fissure

Inferior orbital fissure

Intermaxillary suture

Mental foramen

Lesser wing of sphenoid

Greater wing of sphenoid

Nasal aperture
PIRIFORM aperture

Infraorbital foramen

Canine fossa

Canine eminence

Alveolar processes
of MAX. + MAND.

Fig. 11-5 Anterior landmarks of skull. (Sicher and DuBrul.)

maxillary bones. The **supraorbital notch, or fora-men,** is seen in the upper rim of the orbit in the frontal bone. Toward either side, at the top, you can see a part of the **coronal suture,** also called the **frontoparietal suture.** A few sutures have special names, such as the coronal, but most of them are named by the two bones they join. You can also see the nasal, or **piriform aperture.** Below the orbit, in the maxillae, are the **infraorbital foramina** and the **intermaxillary suture.** The canine eminence is the ridge of bone over the maxillary canine. The depressions in the maxillae, just above the canine, are the **canine fossae.** The alveolar processes are the areas in the maxillae and the mandible that form the sockets for the teeth. You can also clearly see the **mental foramen** in the mandible. More of the mandible is discussed on pp. 130 to 133 (Fig. 11-5).

Within the orbit are the **superior** and **inferior orbital fissures, optic foramen,** and parts of the **greater** and **lesser wings of the sphenoid.**

Lateral View

We will now reconsider the lateral view of the skull. In Fig. 11-6 you can see the coronal suture, as well as the **lambdoid suture,** or the **parietooc-cipital suture.** The lambdoid suture forms an inverted V, only half of which can be seen from this view. The area outlined by the dotted line is the **temporal fossa** and is made up of areas of the

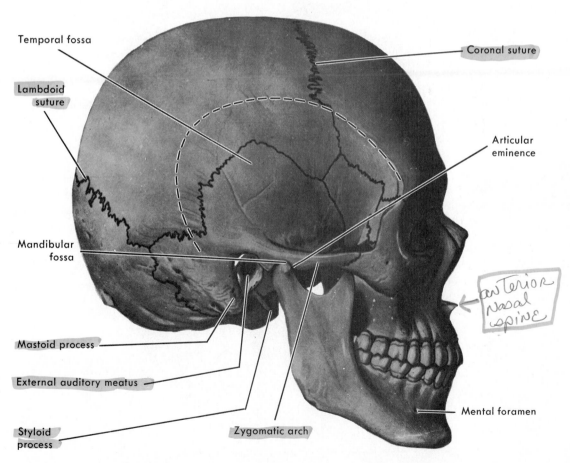

Temporal fossa

Lambdoid suture

Mandibular fossa

Mastoid process

External auditory meatus

Styloid process

Coronal suture

Articular eminence

anterior nasal spine

Zygomatic arch

Mental foramen

Fig. 11-6 Lateral landmarks of skull. (Sicher and DuBrul.)

frontal, parietal, sphenoid, and temporal bones. The **mastoid process** is the projection on the temporal bone just behind the **external auditory meatus,** or outer ear canal. Projecting forward from the temporal bone and joining with the zygomatic bone is the **zygomatic arch.** The **mandibular fossa,** which articulates with the **mandibular condyle,** is found in this area. Just anterior to the mandibular fossa is the **articular eminence** of the temporal bone. Below the ear area is a small projection, the **styloid process,** for the attachment of some muscles of the neck region.

Inferior View

Again, the most difficult of the views is that of the inferior portion of the skull, seen in Fig. 11-7. In the palatal region you can see the **incisive foramen, median palatine suture,** and **transverse palatine,** or **palatomaxillary, suture.** In the posterolateral portion of the hard palate you can also see the **greater palatine foramina,** and just behind that the **pterygoid hamuli,** or **hamular processes.**

You can also see the **pterygoid processes** of the sphenoid bone, which include the **medial** and **lateral pterygoid plates** and the **pterygoid fossa.** Just lateral to that area, still in the sphenoid bone, is the **foramen ovale.** Posterior and slightly lateral are the openings for the internal carotid arteries, the **carotid canals.**

Grouped together are the styloid processes, mastoid processes, and **stylomastoid foramina.** The mandibular fossae of the temporomandibular joint can also be seen, as well as the **jugular**

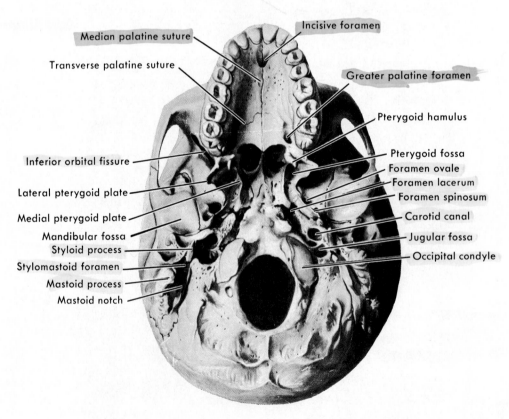

Median palatine suture
Transverse palatine suture
Incisive foramen
Greater palatine foramen
Pterygoid hamulus
Inferior orbital fissure
Lateral pterygoid plate
Medial pterygoid plate
Mandibular fossa
Styloid process
Stylomastoid foramen
Mastoid process
Mastoid notch
Pterygoid fossa
Foramen ovale
Foramen lacerum
Foramen spinosum
Carotid canal
Jugular fossa
Occipital condyle

Fig. 11-7 Inferior landmarks of skull. (Sicher and DuBrul.)

fossae, or **foramina,** and the **occipital condyles.** Although there are many more points of study in this view, it is probably sufficient to be familiar with those mentioned.

Interior View

Internally you can see the **crista galli,** which serves as an attachment for the layers covering the brain, and the **cribriform plate,** which is the passageway for the **olfactory** nerves, or nerves of smell, from the nasal cavity to the brain. Both are parts of the ethmoid bone. Just behind this are the greater and lesser wings of the sphenoid extending from the body of the sphenoid. In the body is a depression called the **hypophyseal fossa,** in which the master control gland of the body, the pituitary gland, lies. Also found in the sphenoid are the **foramen ovale** and **foramen ro-**

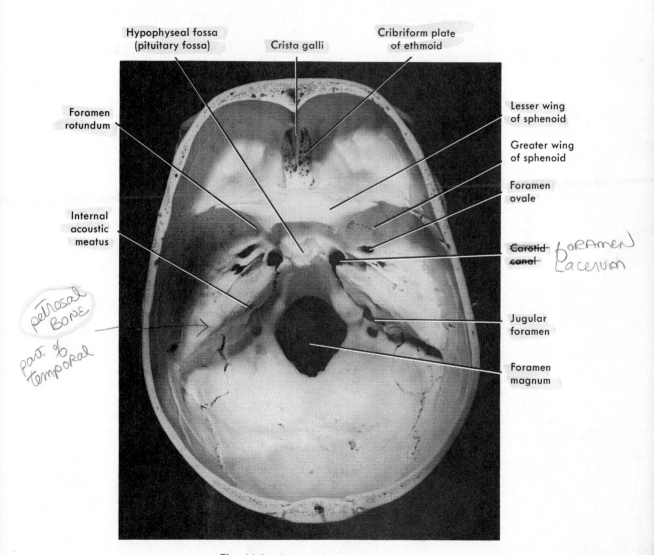

Fig. 11-8   Internal landmarks of skull.

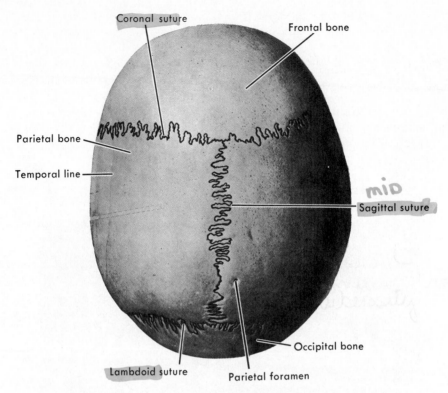

Fig. 11-9   Superior view of skull. (Sicher and DuBrul.)

tundum, where the nerves to the lower and upper teeth leave the skull. The large opening toward the posterior of the skull is the **foramen magnum** of the occipital bone. Just lateral to this the jugular foramen and the **internal acoustic meatus** can be seen (Fig. 11-8).

A brief view of the top of the skull reveals the coronal suture and the lambdoid suture; running between them is the **sagittal,** or **interparietal, suture** (Fig. 11-9).

MAJOR BONES OF THE SKULL
Sphenoid

Now we will examine several of the bones in more detail, beginning with the sphenoid bone. As you have seen, the sphenoid is composed of a body, greater and lesser wings, and paired pterygoid processes. Within the body is one of the pairs of **paranasal sinuses,** the **sphenoid sinuses.** The areas of greatest interest at this time are the pterygoid processes, which project downward from the body of the sphenoid bone, just behind the maxillae. Each has two thin walls of bone that project backward, the medial and lateral pterygoid plates. The area in between these plates is a depression known as a pterygoid fossa. From the fossae and the lateral pterygoid plates originate two pairs of muscles of mastication, which move the jaw (Fig. 11-10). Between the maxillae and the pterygoid processes is an opening into an area at the back of the eye known as the pterygopalatine fossa (Fig. 11-11). Major nerves and blood vessels to the oral and nasal cavity branch in this area.

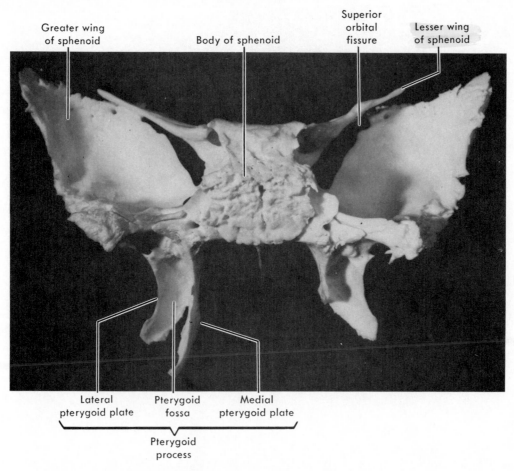

Fig. 11-10   Posterior view of sphenoid bone. Notice pterygoid processes and their components. (Sicher and DuBrul.)

Maxillae

Processes. The maxillae (paired bone) consist of a body and four processes in each bone. Although two of these processes are not particularly important for this discussion, we will mention them all at this time. The frontal process and the zygomatic process are the projections of the maxilla that meet the frontal and zygomatic bones, respectively; between these processes the bone forms about one third of the rim of the orbit. The third process is the alveolar process of the maxilla, which forms the sockets for the up-

per teeth. The fourth is the horizontal palatine process of the maxilla, which, together with its counterpart, forms most of the hard palate.

Maxillary sinuses. Within the bodies of the maxillae are the **maxillary sinuses,** the largest, and possibly the most troublesome, of the paranasal sinuses. As you will study in radiology, the maxillary sinuses are quite large, forming a very thin wall of bone between the roots of the maxillary posterior teeth and the sinus spaces themselves. Infections in the sinuses may affect the

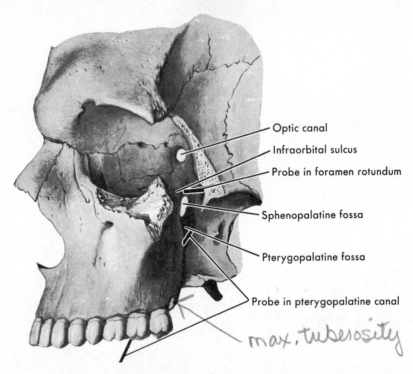

Optic canal
Infraorbital sulcus
Probe in foramen rotundum
Sphenopalatine fossa
Pterygopalatine fossa
Probe in pterygopalatine canal

max. tuberosity

Fig. 11-11 In this lateral view zygomatic bone has been removed to better show opening between maxilla and pterygoid process (pterygomaxillary fissure), which leads into pterygopalatine fossa. (Sicher and DuBrul.)

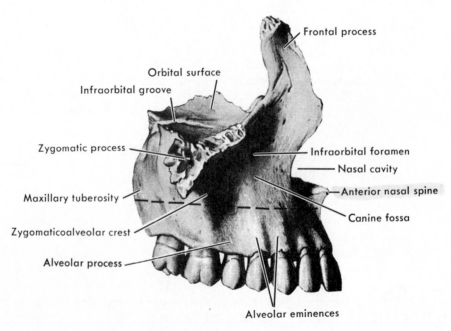

Frontal process
Orbital surface
Infraorbital groove
Zygomatic process
Infraorbital foramen
Nasal cavity
Anterior nasal spine
Maxillary tuberosity
Canine fossa
Zygomaticoalveolar crest
Alveolar process
Alveolar eminences

Fig. 11-12 Lateral view of maxilla. Little room is available for third molars to erupt at this point. *Broken line,* Division between body of maxilla and alveolar process. (Sicher and DuBrul.)

teeth, and, conversely, infections in the teeth may affect the sinuses. (See Chapter 12.)

Lateral view. Fig. 11-12 is a lateral view of the maxilla. Here you can see the body, as well as the alveolar, zygomatic, and frontal processes. You can also see how the maxilla forms half of the opening of the nasal cavity. At the lower end of the nasal cavity, in front, is the **anterior nasal spine.** This is a radiographic landmark frequently used in lateral head films for orthodontics. In the alveolar process you can see how the anterior teeth, and sometimes the premolars, cause bulgings known as **alveolar eminences** in the bone. Above the canine the canine fossa can be seen, and in that fossa area the infraorbital foramen. If you look behind the third molar region, you see the posterior bulging of bone; this is known as the **maxillary tuberosity.** In this area blood vessels and nerves enter the bone to supply the posterior teeth. It is also the area where much of the growth of the maxillae takes place, growth that causes the bones to become longer in an antero-posterior direction. Insufficient growth usually means inadequate room for the third molars to erupt. Growth of these bones and therefore the upper face takes place not only at that point but also between the palatine processes, between the frontal bone and the maxillae, and between the zygomatic bones and the maxillae.

Inferior view. Fig. 11-13 is an inferior or palatal, view of the maxillae. Notice the median palatine suture line, which accounts for lateral palatal growth, and also the incisive foramen in the anterior region. Also visible are the palatine bones that form the posterior part of the hard palate.

Medial view. A medial view of the maxilla from the nasal cavity shows several landmarks seen before, but primarily it shows the opening into the nasal cavity of the maxillary sinus. The opening is known as the **hiatus,** or the **ostium, of the maxillary sinus** and varies considerably in size. The smaller the opening, the more likely the sinus will become clogged from nasal congestion. In this view you can also see the **lacrimal groove,** which runs down from the inner corner of the eye. This is the source from which tears flow into

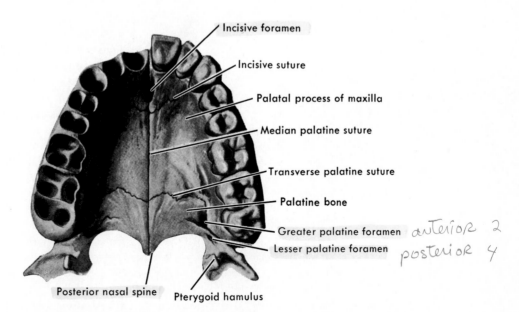

Incisive foramen

Incisive suture

Palatal process of maxilla

Median palatine suture

Transverse palatine suture

Palatine bone

Greater palatine foramen   *anterior 2*

Lesser palatine foramen   *posterior 4*

Posterior nasal spine   Pterygoid hamulus

Fig. 11-13   Inferior, or palatal, view of maxillae and part of palatine bone. Incisive suture tends to disappear in older persons. (Sicher and DuBrul.)

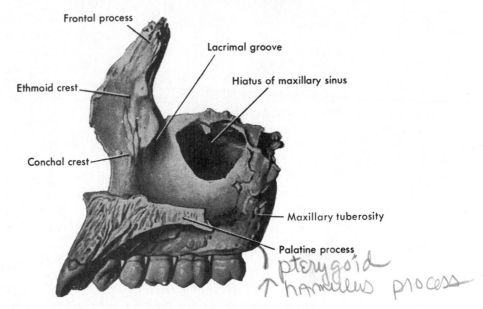

Frontal process

Lacrimal groove

Ethmoid crest

Hiatus of maxillary sinus

Conchal crest

Maxillary tuberosity

Palatine process

pterygoid
↑ hamulus process

Fig. 11-14 Medial view of maxilla. Notice thickness of hard palate separating oral cavity from nasal cavity. Opening in this illustration is exceedingly larger than normal. Many times there are two or more smaller openings. (Sicher and DuBrul.)

the nose, accounting for that runny nose when crying. It is, however, only the filling of the nasal cavity with tears (Fig. 11-14).

Mandible

The mandible is a single bone made up of three parts: the horizontal body, with the alveolar process on top of it, and the vertical portion of bone known as the ramus (Fig. 11-15).

Lateral view. In Fig. 11-16 you can see landmarks of the mandible. The tip of the chin area is referred to as the **mental protuberance.** Just posterior is the mental foramen, from which the blood vessels and nerves for the inside of the lower lip extend. This foramen is just about at a position that divides the body of the mandible below from the alveolar process above it. At the point where the inferior border of the mandible turns upward is the angle of the mandible. This is the dividing line between the body and the ramus. Moving upward along the posterior border

of the ramus, we come to the condyle of the mandible, which articulates with the temporal bone to form the temporomandibular joint. The slightly narrowed area just beneath the condyle is known as the **condylar neck.** In front of the condyle, the depression, or notch, in the ramus is called the **coronoid notch,** or **mandibular notch.** Just anterior to this notch is the **coronoid process,** which is the attachment for one of the muscles of mastication. The anterior border of the ramus ends in the **external oblique line.**

Medial view. In Fig. 11-17 notice many of the landmarks already mentioned and several new ones. About midway up the ramus is the **mandibular foramen,** where the nerves and blood vessels for the lower teeth and lip enter the mandible. Just in front of the foramen and running forward and downward is the **mylohyoid line,** the attachment for the muscle of the same name. Toward the anterior part of that line there are two depressions in the bone, one above the line and

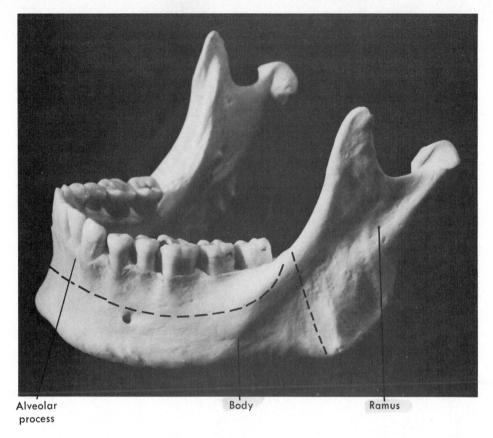

Alveolar
process

Body

Ramus

Fig. 11-15 Lateral view of mandible. Its three components are separated by broken lines.

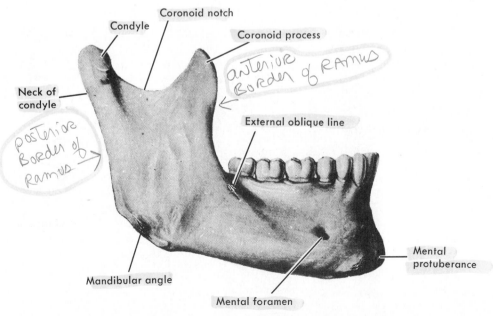

Coronoid notch

Condyle

Coronoid process

anterior Border of RAMUS

Neck of condyle

posterior Border of Ramus

External oblique line

Mental protuberance

Mandibular angle

Mental foramen

Fig. 11-16 Lateral landmarks of mandible. (Sicher and DuBrul.)

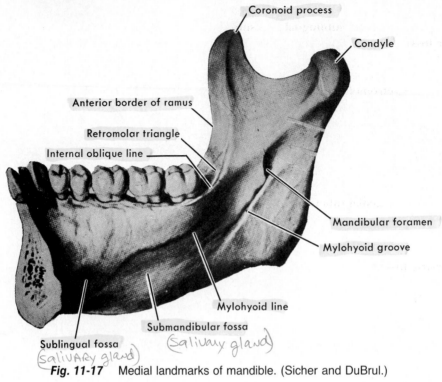

Coronoid process

Condyle

Anterior border of ramus

Retromolar triangle

Internal oblique line

Mandibular foramen

Mylohyoid groove

Mylohyoid line

Submandibular fossa
(Salivary gland)

Sublingual fossa
(salivary gland)

Fig. 11-17 Medial landmarks of mandible. (Sicher and DuBrul.)

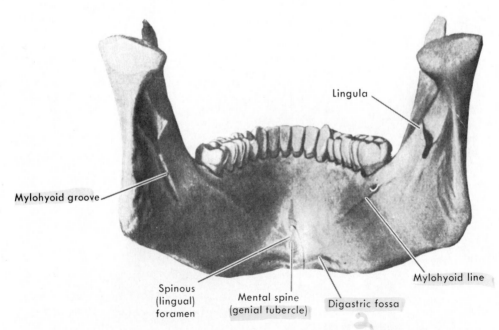

Lingula

Mylohyoid groove

Mylohyoid line

Spinous
(lingual)
foramen

Mental spine
(genial tubercle)

Digastric fossa

Fig. 11-18 Posterior view of mandible. Notice genial tubercles, digastric fossa, and lingula, which could not be easily seen on medial view of mandible. (Sicher and DuBrul.)

one below it. These are the **sublingual** and **submandibular fossae.** The sublingual and submandibular salivary glands lie in these depressions. The area immediately behind the third molars is referred to as the **retromolar triangle.** You may hear more of this in conjunction with denture construction and landmarks.

Posterior view. The last view of the mandible to consider is the posterior, seen in Fig. 11-18. Right at the midline are two small grouped projections, one above and one below. These are the superior and inferior **genial tubercles,** or **mental spines,** muscle attachments that aid in tongue movement and swallowing. Just below these projections at the inferior border of the mandible are the **digastric fossae,** also points of muscle attachment. The last landmark to be mentioned here is the **lingula.** The means 'little tongue'; it is a projection of bone that partially covers the opening of the mandibular foramen. This is a point of attachment for a ligament, and its location, at times, may affect anesthetic solutions injected into the area.

■ ■ ■

From time to time, review this chapter on the osteology of the skull. You will find a great deal of correlation with this material and your radiology studies. A thorough knowledge of osteology will make you a better practitioner of radiological techniques and the subject you are radiographing.

REVIEW QUESTIONS

1. How many bones form the skull? *22*
2. How are they subdivided? *Nuerocranium 8 viscerocranium 14*
3. Define the following:
   a. Suture *JOINING 07 BONES*
   b. Foramen *short tubelike opening*
   c. Canal *LONG tubelike opening*
   d. Fossa *ditch, GULLY,*
   e. Alveolar process
4. Which bones form the hard palate?
5. The pterygoid process is part of what bone?
6. Where is the largest of the paranasal sinuses?
7. Name the area immediately behind the maxillary third molars. *maxillary Tuberosity*
8. What are the divisions of the mandible?
9. Name the major landmarks of the maxillae and mandible.

---

4. palatal processes of maxillae + " " of palatine bones

5. pterygoid process is part of sphenoid bone which includes the lateral & medial pterygoid plates.

6. Largest paranasal sinuses are maxillary & are in the max. bone

8. Mandible consists of horizontal body, vertical ramus, & alveolar process.

12

Nose, Nasal Cavity, and Paranasal Sinuses

OBJECTIVES

- To define the terms nose, nasal cavity, and paranasal sinuses
- To understand the anatomy of the nose, nasal cavity, and paranasal sinuses
- To describe the function of the nasal cavity, nasal epithelium, and paranasal sinuses
- To discuss the anatomical relationship of the maxillary sinus and the maxillary teeth
- To describe the relationship of maxillary teeth to maxillary sinus in infections of either one

NOSE AND NASAL CAVITY
External View

The nose and nasal cavity are a complex arrangement of hard and soft tissues. The nose is that portion of the nasal complex that protrudes outward from the skeletal component. The nose, or more properly external nose, is attached superiorly to the nasal bones and inferiorly to the **anterior nasal spine.** The protruding lateral margins are known as the wing of the nose, or **ala.** The external nose is divided in half by the cartilagenous part of the nasal septum, which is the wall that divides the nasal complex into a right and left half (Fig. 12-1). If you look at a skull, you will see that the nasal aperture, the anteriormost portion of the nasal cavity, is somewhat pear shaped.

Internal View

Peering inside the nasal cavity you see that it has a midline partition, the nasal septum. The lateral walls have three shelves, called nasal conchae, that project inward toward the septum. The superior portion has small holes that open into the anterior cranial fossa through the ethmoid bone to transmit the olfactory nerves for the sense of smell from the nose up to the brain. The septum is formed by the vomer bone and a portion of the ethmoid bone (Fig. 12-2). The inferior portion, or floor, is formed by the bones of the hard palate, which are the palatal processes of the maxillae and the horizontal portion of the palatine bones. The most complicated portion of the nasal cavity is its lateral walls. The upper half to two thirds of the lateral wall of the cavity is formed from more parts of the ethmoid bone. It consists of the wall, which you saw earlier as the part of the ethmoid bone that forms the medial wall of the orbit, and two shelflike structures known as the **superior** and **middle nasal conchae.** The lower part of the lateral walls are formed by portions of the maxillae. Where the maxillae and the ethmoid bone meet in this lateral wall there is a third medial projection, which is a separate bone itself, known as the inferior nasal conchae (Fig. 12-3). As you reach the posterior part of the nasal septum, you come to an area known as the **choana, or posterior nasal aperture.** Posterior to this is the nasal pharynx, which is discussed in a later chapter. The posterosuperior part of the nasal cavity is composed of a portion of the body of the sphenoid bone and is known as the **sphenoethmoidal recess.** If you want to attain an image of this from a sagittal view of a skull, the sphenoidal sinus is below the pituitary fossa.

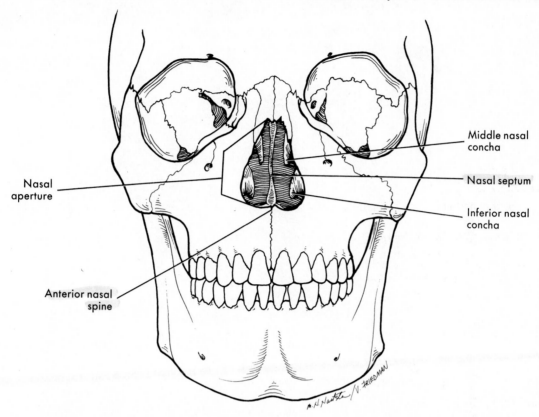

Fig. 12-1   Anterior view of skull showing nasal aperture, nasal septum, and nasal conchae.

Epithelial Lining

Recall from the chapter on epithelial tissues that there was one type of epithelium known as pseudostratified columnar ciliated epithelium with goblet cells. This epithelial type is usually referred to as **respiratory epithelium** because it is primarily found in the respiratory tract, and you should be aware by now that the nasal cavity is the beginning of the respiratory system. The epithelium has many hairlike projections, known as **cilia,** that have the ability to move in a synchronized beating pattern toward the anterior portion of the nasal cavity. The tiny goblet cells secrete a sticky mucous substance onto the cilia, and these trap contaminants as they enter the nasal cavity and move them toward the front where they can be removed by blowing of the nose. For this mechanism to be successful it is important to have as much surface area as possible in the nasal cavity. These conchae accomplish that. The epithelium in the roof, or top, of the nasal cavity and coming down onto the upper surface of the superior concha is modified and has nerve fibers that perceive taste. This is referred to as **olfactory epithelium.**

PARANASAL SINUSES
Location

You now should be having a little better picture in your mind of the nasal cavity. To see it even better, you would be helped by having a

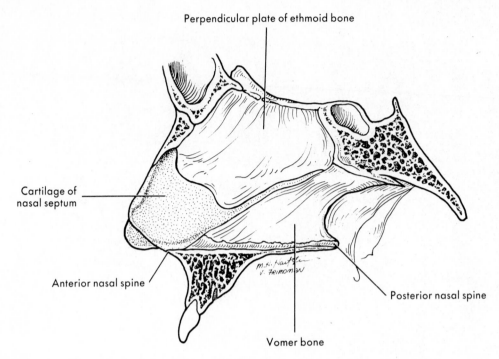

Perpendicular plate of ethmoid bone

Cartilage of nasal septum

Anterior nasal spine

Posterior nasal spine

Vomer bone

Fig. 12-2   Sagittal section showing nasal septum and its components.

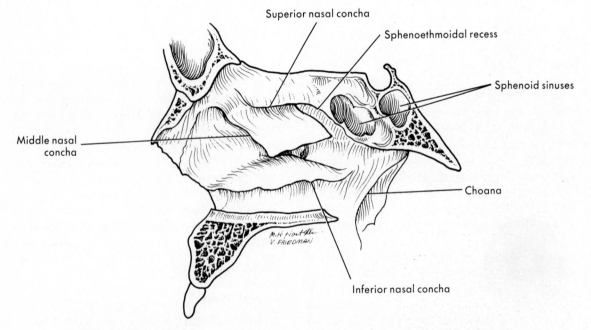

Superior nasal concha

Sphenoethmoidal recess

Sphenoid sinuses

Middle nasal concha

Choana

Inferior nasal concha

Fig. 12-3   Sagittal section as in Fig. 12-2 but with septum removed showing lateral nasal wall and bony conchae.

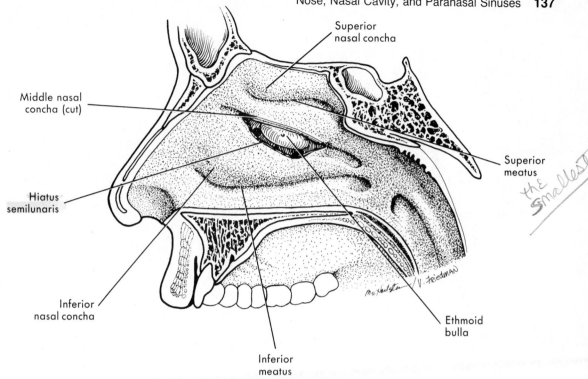

Fig. 12-4   Same view as in Fig. 12-3 but covered with nasal mucosa. Middle concha has been partially removed to show hiatus semilunaris and ethmoid bulla in middle meatus.

skull that has been specially prepared by being split along the midline. This will give you a much better appreciation for the complexity of the structure. When you begin to study this area more closely, you will see that there are a number of openings into this cavity from other areas. Most of these openings are from compartments, or cavities, of various sizes known as the **paranasal sinuses.** There are four pairs of these sinuses, two ethmoids, two frontals, two maxillaries, and two sphenoids. When we first look for these sinuses, they are not easily seen. We must first look at the projections we mentioned earlier, the nasal conchae. These three projections in each half of the nasal cavity are there for several reasons, one of them being to increase the surface area for the respiratory epithelium, which, as we said before, acts as a filter for the incoming air. If you look at the area of the lateral nasal wall sheltered underneath the conchae, you will be look-

ing at what are known as the **meatus.** The **inferior meatus** is beneath the inferior nasal concha and has one small opening in the region, which is the nasolacrimal duct, which carries tears from the corner of the eye into the nasal cavity. The **middle meatus** lies beneath the middle nasal concha. There is a rather crescent-shaped opening here, which is called the **hiatus semilunaris,** which means a half moon-shaped opening. In this area we will find a number of openings, which are to be discussed shortly. There is a bulbous ridge above the hiatus semilunaris, which is known as the **ethmoid bulla.** The **superior meatus** lies beneath the superior concha and is the smallest meatus (Fig. 12-4).

Frontal Sinus

The paired **frontal sinuses** are located in the frontal bone just above the orbital cavity. These vary in size from person to person. They frequently cross the midline and may be partially located on the opposite side. These sinuses drain into the very anterior end of the hiatus semilunaris in the middle meatus beneath the middle nasal concha. Infections in these sinuses cause pressure and pain just above the eye.

Sphenoid Sinus

The paired **sphenoid sinuses** are located in the body of the sphenoid bone just underneath the pituitary fossa, which is located in the middle cranial fossa. These sinuses also cross the midline. They open into the highest and most posterior part of the nasal cavity. This area is referred to as the **sphenoethmoidal recess.** Infections in these sinuses cause a pressure and congested feeling that is hard to localize but is deep in the midline of the head.

Ethmoid Sinuses

The **ethmoid sinuses** are frequently referred to as the **ethmoid air cells** because they are not single-paired sinuses like the other paranasal sinuses but are subdivided into numerous small compartments. These clusters of air cells are further divided into the anterior, middle, and posterior ethmoid air cells.

Anterior ethmoids. The anterior ethmoids are located in the lateral wall of the nasal cavity at the base of the middle nasal concha. These air cells open into the hiatus semilunaris just posteroinferior to the opening for the frontal sinus.

Middle ethmoids. The middle ethmoids are also located in the base of the middle nasal concha just behind the anterior air cells. They are also located within the bulge of bone in the middle meatus that we mentioned, the ethmoid bulla. These may have a couple openings, one on the ethmoid bulla and another possibly in the hiatus semilunaris.

Posterior ethmoids. The posterior ethmoid air cells are located in the base of the superior nasal concha and open into the superior meatus.

These sinus infections are difficult to treat because of all the small compartments. When in-

fected, they give a feeling of congestion and aching within the nasal cavity area.

Maxillary Sinus

The maxillary sinuses are the largest of the paranasal sinuses and open into the posterior end of the hiatus semilunaris through one or more openings. At the time of birth the maxillary sinus in each maxilla is the size of a small pea. As growth takes place, each sinus continues to expand. As it expands, it tends to occupy greater and greater proportions of the body of the maxilla. In young adults we find that the maxillary sinus occupies an area from just posterior to the maxillary canine back to the area of the third molar in an anteroposterior direction. In a superoinferior direction it would extend from the floor of the orbital, or eye, cavity inferiorly to the point where it might extend down around the root tips

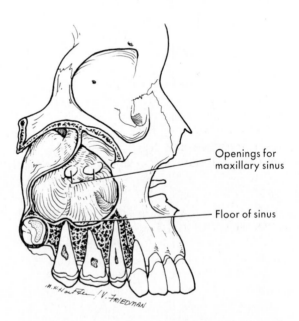

Openings for maxillary sinus

Floor of sinus

Fig. 12-5 Lateral view of facial part of skull with lateral wall of maxillary sinus removed, showing relationship of floor of sinus to maxillary roots of teeth. Opening of maxillary sinus from nasal cavity can be seen two thirds up medial wall of sinus.

of the maxillary posterior teeth (Fig. 12-5). The maxillary sinus may develop compartmental walls, but generally all of them are connected by large openings. If you look at the location of the opening for the maxillary sinuses in the middle meatus region and compare it with its location on the medial wall of the sinus, you will find that this opening is almost two thirds of the way up the medial wall (Fig. 12-5). You can appreciate the significance of trying to drain a cavity through an opening that is near the top of the space. Several things come into play here, the first being that everybody's maxillary sinus is different. Sometimes there is more than one opening in each sinus; sometimes the opening or openings are very small; and sometimes they are very big. If we get a nasal infection, we get a swelling in our nasal mucosa. If our maxillary sinus has a very small opening or openings, the mucosa may swell so much that it closes the openings to the sinus cavity. Since there is already infection in the sinus, it continues to multiply. As it increases in severity, we feel the pressure in the maxillae. If we tilt the head forward, we can frequently feel the pressure seeming to increase as the fluid produced by the infection flows forward against the anterior wall of the sinus. The use of nasal sprays frequently give some relief, but then it clogs right up again and continues. If there is some opening of the sinus, you can tilt your head to one side while laying down, and you may get some drainage from the opposite side. When this clogging happens repeatedly, the ENT (ear, nose, and throat) specialist sometimes punches a hole from the inferior meatus into the medial wall of the maxillary sinus, near its base, and enlarges it until it effects good drainage and a decrease in maxillary sinus infections.

FUNCTION OF SINUSES

There have been several functions discussed in regard to these sinuses. Probably the most popular one was that they warmed the air as it passed into the respiratory system. Later on, studies showed that the flow of air into and out of these sinuses was very minimal. The general belief now is that the probable function of the nasal sinuses is to lighten the overall bone weight by being hollowed-out cavities. They are a constant source of infections caused by organisms getting into them and multiplying rapidly because of the excellent atmosphere of warm and moist mucosa.

CLINICAL PROBLEMS

Aside from the problems mentioned regarding the maxillary sinus, we also have to consider the dental implications of this structure. As you will find later on in the chapter discussing nerves, the same nerves that supply the maxillary posterior teeth also supply the maxillary sinus. These are sensory nerves carrying different types of messages back to the brain. As we go about our everyday lives, we are constantly sending messages back to the brain from the nerves of the maxillary teeth. We bite down on a piece of bone, or maybe a piece of seed from fresh fruits, and a painful stimulus is sent back to the brain. However, under normal circumstances that same nerve to the teeth also has fibers from the maxillary sinus, but the sinus very seldom sends any messages back to the brain. The brain gets used to interpreting everything that travels along that nerve as messages from the tooth because the sinus never sends a message. Now, one day, we get an infection in the maxillary sinus. For the first time the sinus sends a message back along the same nerve from the tooth and the brain correctly interprets this message as pain; however, it incorrectly interprets it as coming from the tooth because that's where all the messages have been coming from in the past. What do you suppose the person does about this? Correct! He or she contacts the family dentist and complains about rather severe toothache. An appointment is set up, and the patient comes in. When that patient is examined, no apparent signs of any caries are found; there are no periodontal pockets; and the tooth is only mildly sensitive to percussion. A **periapical** radiograph shows no periapical lesion and no interproximal caries. Pulp testing appears to be normal. Where do we go from here? There could be things that are many times undetectable, such as a cracked tooth, but we need to cover one other area before we proceed with any other tests or treatment. We need to go back to the medical and dental history form and look for a history of sinus infections. If your history does not have that category, it is then appropriate to question the patient concerning this. If you get a positive response, you should then question the patient concerning recent sinus problems. If this question is positive, the patient should then be referred to the physician for treatment of the sinus infection. This will usually take care of it unless it recurs after medical treatment for the sinus infection. Under those circumstances, further evaluation must be done. Similarly, there may be tooth infections that involve the maxillary sinus.

Another area of concern is the relationship of the floor of the sinus to the teeth. In a number of instances the floor of the sinus dips down around the tip of one or more roots of the posterior teeth. Under some circumstances it is possible that a periapical infection of a tooth may involve the sinus. It is also possible that the sinus may dip between the roots of a maxillary molar. If that molar has roots that are **dilacerated** (curved because of disturbances in development) and needs to be extracted for any reason, one must have good reliable radiographs to assess the situation. It is terribly embarrassing and negligent treatment if one has no radiographs of the region, proceeds to extract that molar tooth,

and finds that besides the extracted tooth a part of the floor of the maxillary sinus was also extracted.

When maxillary teeth are extracted and healing takes place, there is a tendency for the maxillary sinus to enlarge into the area formerly occupied by the posterior maxillary teeth. This means that the thickness of bone in the maxillary tuberosity and alveolar ridge up to and sometimes including the canine region may be very thin and has to be evaluated in deciding what type of treatment to use to replace those teeth with a **prosthetic appliance.**

As you can now understand, our evaluation and treatment needs to go beyond the teeth and involve other areas or systems of the patient. This is just one reason why the members of the dental team need to know more about the total evaluation of the patient.

REVIEW QUESTIONS

1. Which bone or bones form the nasal septum?
2. What is a meatus?
3. What is the function of respiratory epithelium?
4. What opens into the
   a. inferior meatus? *Nasolacrimal canal*
   b. middle meatus? *Frontal sinus, Ant. & mid. ethmoids* [MAX?]
   c. superior meatus? *Posterior ethmoids*
   d. sphenoethmoidal recess? *sphenoid sinus*
5. Where specifically is the olfactory epithelium found?
6. Why may a maxillary sinus infection seem to be coming from the teeth? *they are proximal to max. molar roots*

Handwritten notes:

1. ethmoid (top) + vomer (bottom)
2. meatus = space beneath shelter of each nasal conchae.
3. respiratory epithelium is made of pseudostratified columnar ciliated epi. which contain goblet cells.
5. olfactory epithelium is located on roof of nasal cavity + extends down to top surface of superior conchae.

13

Muscles of Mastication, Hyoid Muscles, and Sternocleidomastoid Muscle

OBJECTIVES

- To describe the origin, insertion, action, and nerve and blood supply of the muscles of mastication
- To categorize the muscles according to their roles in elevation, depression, protrusion, retrusion, and lateral excursion
- To name the suprahyoid and infrahyoid muscles and their role in mandibular movement, as well as swallowing and phonation

Since this is the first of three chapters dealing with muscles and their functions, it seems appropriate to mention briefly some relative terms. In general, as one reads about muscles, there are five terms that are constantly seen-origin, insertion, action, nerve supply, and blood supply. Because nerve and blood supply are self-explanatory, we will be primarily concerned with the first three. The **origin** of a muscle is the end of the muscle that is attached to the least movable structure. The **insertion** of a muscle is the other end of the muscle that is attached to the more movable structure. The **action** is the work that is accomplished when the muscle fibers contract. If you are familiar with the action of a muscle but are not sure which end is the origin or the insertion, keep in mind that, in general, the insertion moves toward the origin when the muscle is contracted. Likewise, if you know the direction of the muscle fibers, you can usually deduce the action by imagining the insertion moving toward the origin and picturing what happens.

MUSCLES OF MASTICATION

The muscles of **mastication** are four pairs of muscles attached to the mandible and primarily responsible for elevating, protruding, retruding, or causing the mandible to move laterally. They develop from the first (mandibular) pharyngeal arch, which is also responsible for the development of some of the bony facial structures. Since they develop from this arch, they are innervated by the nerve of the first arch, the fifth (V) cranial nerve (trigeminal nerve). More specifically, the muscles are innervated by the third part of the fifth nerve, which is called the mandibular division, or V_3. The blood supply to these muscles comes from the maxillary artery, which is a branch of the external carotid artery. Blood vessels and nerves are further discussed in Chapters 17 and 19.

Masseter Muscle

The **masseter muscle** is probably the most powerful of the muscles of mastication. It takes its origin from two areas on the zygomatic arch. Part of it attaches to the inferior border of the zygomatic arch and the remainder is from the medial side. The fibers run downward and slightly backward to be inserted into the angle of the mandible on the lateral side. When the muscle contracts, it elevates the mandible, closing the mouth (Fig. 13-1).

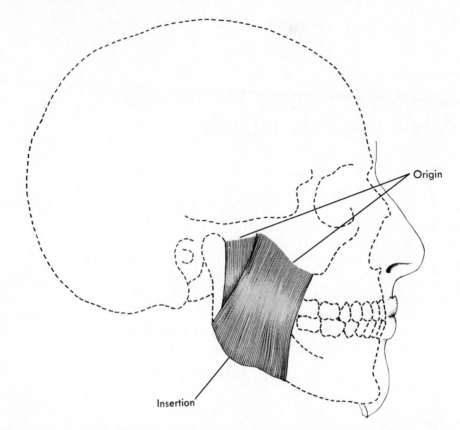

Fig. 13-1 Lateral view of skull showing origin of masseter muscle from zygomatic arch. Fibers run downward and slightly backward to insert into angle of mandible.

Temporal Muscle

The **temporal muscle** has a very wide origin from the entire temporal fossa and fascia covering the muscle. The anterior fibers run almost vertically, but the posterior fibers run in a more horizontal direction over the ear. All these fibers insert into the coronoid process of the mandible and sometimes run down the anterior border of the ramus of the mandible as far as the third molar. If the entire muscle contracts, the overall action is to pull upward on the coronoid process and elevate the mandible, closing the mouth. If only the posterior fibers are contracted, the result is a horizontal pulling action in a posterior direction. This tends to pull the mandible backward, which is referred to as retruding the mandible (Fig. 13-2).

Medial Pterygoid Muscle

In studying the origin of the **medial pterygoid muscle**, it is probably best to examine the skull while reading the description. The muscle has two origins. The larger and major origin is from the medial side of the lateral pterygoid plate and the pterygoid fossa. The smaller origin is just anterior to that area, coming from the maxillary tuberosity just behind the third molar. All the fibers run downward and slightly laterally to be in-

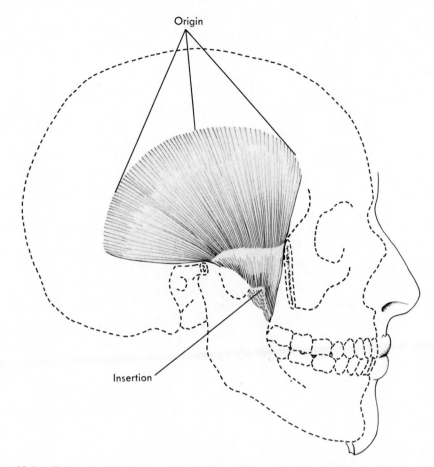

Fig. 13-2   Temporal muscle has wide origin from temporal fossa. Notice vertical, inclined, and horizontal muscle fibers, which insert primarily on medial side and tip of coronoid process.

serted into the angle of the mandible on the medial side. This is just opposite the masseter insertion on the lateral side. When the muscle contracts, the resultant action is to elevate the mandible and close the mouth (Fig. 13-3).

Lateral Pterygoid Muscle

The **lateral pterygoid muscle** has two separate origins. The smaller, superior origin arises from the area referred to as the infratemporal crest of the greater wing of the sphenoid bone. The larger, inferior origin arises from the lateral side

of the lateral pterygoid plate. Notice that this is just opposite the origin of the medial pterygoid muscle. The fibers from both origins run rather horizontally in a posterior direction. Some of the fibers from the superior head penetrate the capsule of the temporomandibular joint and insert into the anterior border of the disc of the joint. The remainder of the fibers from that origin and the fibers of the inferior head insert into the neck of the condyle. The action of the muscle is twofold. The inferior head pulls the condyle forward, and the disc is also brought forward be-

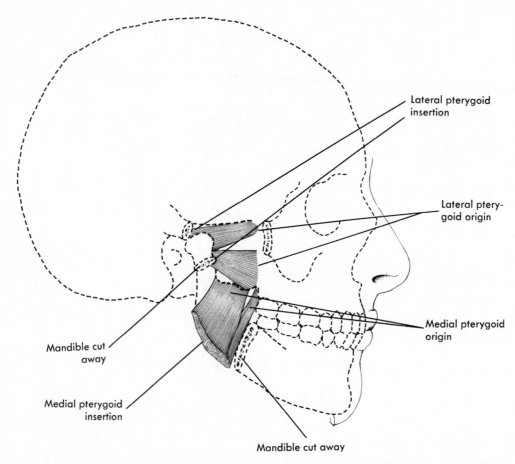

Fig. 13-3 Lateral view of skull showing origins of lateral pterygoid muscle from infratemporal crest and pterygoid plate with fibers inserting into disc and neck of condyle. Notice medial pterygoid muscle originating from pterygoid area, as well as small origin from maxillary tuberosity. Insertion onto medial side of angle of mandible is also visible.

cause of its attachment to the condyle. When both left and right inferior heads function, the mandible is protruded. If only one lateral pterygoid is contracted, there will be lateral excursion to the opposite side of the contracted muscle. The superior head of the lateral pterygoid functions only in the action of biting, or what is referred to, at times, as the power stroke. It functions to guide the posterior movement of the disc and condyle as it goes back to a centric position (Fig. 13-3).

HYOID MUSCLES

We have just discussed the muscles that accomplish virtually all jaw movements except depression of the mandible, or opening the mouth. This is accomplished by muscles in the neck referred to as the **hyoid muscles.**

The hyoid muscles are so named because they attach to or are associated with the hyoid bone in the neck. The hyoid is a horseshoe-shaped bone suspended beneath the mandible, with the open end of the horseshoe pointed posteriorly. It is

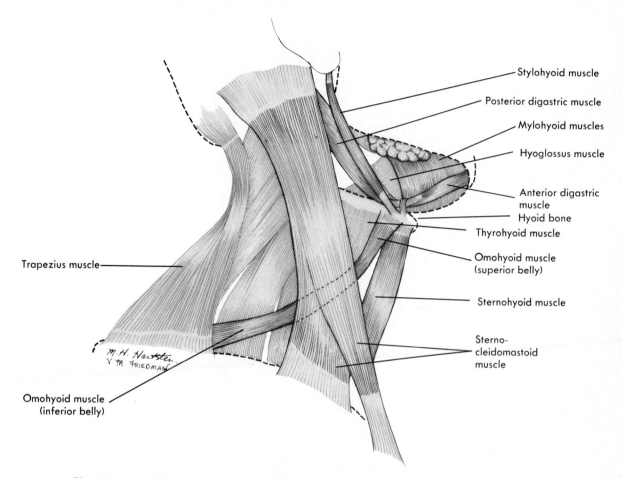

Fig. 13-4   Lateral view of neck showing digastric muscle suspended above hyoid bone and attaching to it by ligamentous loop. Mylohyoid and stylohyoid muscles are also visible above hyoid bone, and omohyoid, thyrohyoid, and sternohyoid muscles are visible below hyoid bone. Also, large sternocleidomastoid muscle covers large area on side of neck.

unusual in that it articulates with no other bone. Its only connection with other bones is by muscles. These muscles are divided into two groups. Those above the hyoid are referred to as **suprahyoid muscles;** those below the hyoid are referred to as **infrahyoid muscles.**

Suprahyoid Group

Digastric muscle. The **digastric muscle** has a relatively unusual arrangement of fibers. There are muscle fibers at either end with a collage-nous tendon in the middle. Classically, it has been described as having an origin at either end with an insertion in the middle. For the sake of clearer understanding, it might be best to say that its origin is at the digastric notch just medial to the mastoid process behind the ear. The fibers run forward and downward to the area of the intermediate tendon, which attaches to the hyoid bone by a tendinous loop through which it can slide. From here the muscle fibers extend forward, to be inserted into the digastric fossa on

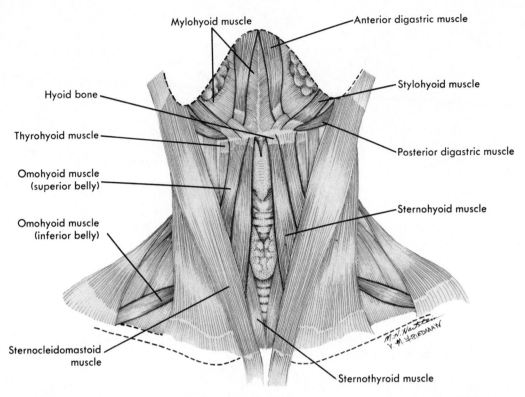

Mylohyoid muscle

Anterior digastric muscle

Hyoid bone

Stylohyoid muscle

Thyrohyoid muscle

Posterior digastric muscle

Omohyoid muscle
(superior belly)

Omohyoid muscle
(inferior belly)

Sternohyoid muscle

Sternocleidomastoid
muscle

Sternothyroid muscle

Fig. 13-5 Anterior and inferior view of mylohyoid muscle. Left and right muscles fuse in midline and form slinglike arrangement that forms mouth floor. You can also see anterior view of digastric, stylohyoid, sternohyoid, sternothyroid, and sternocleidomastoid muscles.

the inferior surface of the mandible at the midline (Figs. 13-4 and 13-5).

The action of this muscle is twofold. By contracting, it can create a backward pull on the mandible, thus retruding it. If the jaw is clenched, contraction of the muscle elevates the hyoid bone and lifts up on the larynx, or voice box. It can also aid in pulling the mandible downward.

The digastric is also an unusual muscle in that it has two nerves supplying it. The anterior part of the muscle is supplied by the third part of the trigeminal nerve (V_3), and the posterior part is supplied by the facial nerve (VII).

Mylohyoid muscle. The **mylohyoid muscle** forms what is referred to as the floor of the mouth. The muscle originates from the mylohyoid line on the medial surface of the mandible, running downward and inserting into the hyoid bone. The left and right muscles also fuse together in the midline of the neck. The action is related to the depression of the mandible or the elevation of the hyoid bone. The nerve supply is the mylohyoid branch of V_3 (trigeminal). The bloody supply is a branch of the inferior alveolar artery (Figs. 13-4 and 13-5).

Geniohyoid muscle. The **geniohyoid muscle** originates from the inferior genial tubercle, or mental spine. It lies deep to the mylohyoid, running downward and backward to insert into the hyoid bone. It also acts as a depressor of the mandible or elevator of the hyoid bone. Its nerve

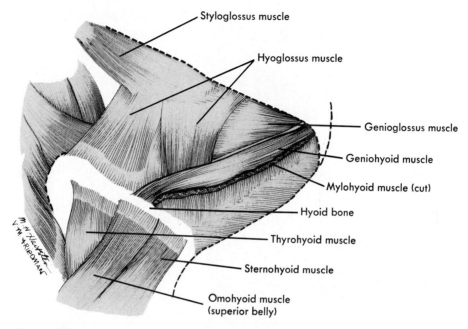

Fig. 13-6 With mylohyoid muscle cut away, geniohyoid muscle extends from genial tubercles of mandible downward to hyoid bone.

supply comes from the first cervical nerve in the neck. The blood supply is a branch of the lingual artery (Fig. 13-6).

Stylohyoid muscle. The **stylohyoid muscle** takes its origin from the styloid process of the skull. The muscle runs downward and forward to insert into the posterior part of the hyoid bone. At its insertion on the hyoid bone the muscle splits, and part of the posterior portion of the digastric passes through it. The action of the muscle is to pull the hyoid bone backward and upward. The nerve supply is a branch of the facial nerve (VII), which also supplies the posterior part of the digastric muscle. The facial and occipital arteries provide its blood supply (Figs. 13-4 and 13-5).

Infrahyoid Group

Omohyoid muscle. The two muscular bellies of the **omohyoid muscle** are separated by an intermediate tendon. One of the bellies arises from the upper border of the scapula (shoulder blade) and the other from the hyoid bone. Two bellies are joined by an intermediate tendon beneath the **sternomastoid (sternocleidomastoid)** muscle in the side of the neck. When the muscle contracts, it pulls the hyoid bone downward. The nerve supply comes from the second and third cervical nerves and the blood supply from the lingual and superior thyroid arteries (Figs. 13-4 and 13-5).

Sternohyoid muscle. The **sternohyoid muscle** takes its origin from the upper border of the sternum. It runs upward to be inserted into the front part of the hyoid bone. When the muscle contracts, it pulls the hyoid bone downward. Its nerve supply is from the second and third cervical nerves. Its blood supply is the lingual and superior thyroid arteries (Figs. 13-4 and 13-5).

Sternothyroid muscle. The **sternothyroid**

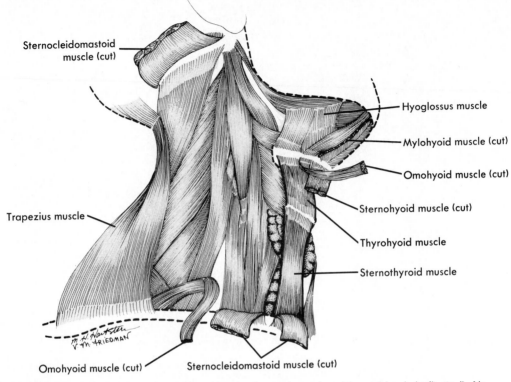

Sternocleidomastoid muscle (cut)

Hyoglossus muscle

Mylohyoid muscle (cut)

Omohyoid muscle (cut)

Sternohyoid muscle (cut)

Thyrohyoid muscle

Sternothyroid muscle

Trapezius muscle

Omohyoid muscle (cut)

Sternocleidomastoid muscle (cut)

Fig. 13-7 Lateral view of neck with several muscles cut and turned back (reflected). Notice extent of sternothyroid and thyrohyoid muscles.

muscle arises from the upper part of the sternum, running upward to be inserted onto an oblique line on the side of the thyroid cartilage of the larynx. When the muscle contracts, it pulls the larynx downward. The nerve supply comes from the second and third cervical nerves. The blood supply is from the superior thyroid artery. (Figs. 13-5 and 13-7).

Thyrohyoid muscle. The **thyrohyoid muscle** originates from the oblique line on the lateral side of the thyroid cartilage, which serves as the insertion of the sternothyroid muscle. The fibers run upward to be inserted into the hyoid bone. When the muscle contracts, it either lifts the thyroid cartilage and raises the **larynx** or helps depress the hyoid bone. The first cervical nerve provides the nerve supply, and the superior thyroid artery is the blood supply (Figs. 13-4 and 13-7).

MOVEMENTS OF THE JAW AND LARYNX

Following is a brief description of the movements accomplished by the muscles of mastication and the hyoid muscles.

Mandibular Protrusion

Lateral pterygoid muscles acting together produce mandibular **protrusion.**

Mandibular Retrusion

The posterior or horizontal fibers of the temporal muscle, as well as the digastric muscle, accomplish **retrusion** of the mandible.

Lateral Excursion of the Mandible

One of the lateral pterygoid muscles, acting by itself, accomplishes **lateral excursion.** If the left lateral pterygoid muscle contracts, the left condyle is pulled forward, and the mandible will

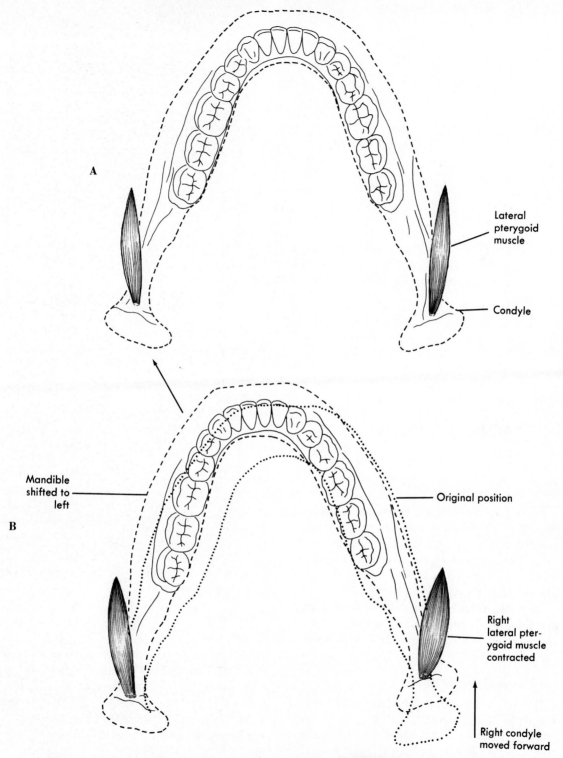

Fig. 13-8 **A,** Superior view of mandible in rest position showing condyles and lateral pterygoid muscles. **B,** Right lateral pterygoid muscle has contracted, pulling condyle on that side forward. Mandible swings to opposite side, as shown by dashed line and arrow.

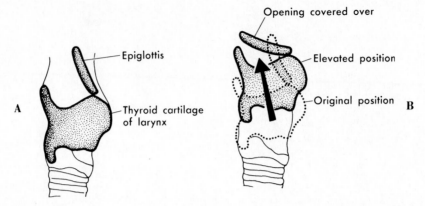

Fig. 13-9 **A,** Thyroid cartilage of larynx and epiglottis are suspended, in part, from hyoid bone. **B,** As suprahyoid muscles are contracted along with thyrohyoid muscle, larynx is elevated, and epiglottis moves back and down to cover laryngeal opening.

move to the right. Contraction of the right lateral pterygoid accomplishes the opposite movement. While the one lateral pterygoid is contracting, the opposite elevators of the mandible hold the other condyle in place (Fig. 13-8).

Elevation of the Mandible

The medial pterygoid, masseter, and temporal muscles accomplish **elevation.**

Depression of the Mandible

The **depression** of the mandible is accomplished by the hyoid muscles. It is important to know that this includes the suprahyoid and infrahyoid muscles. If the mandible is to be depressed, or lowered, it is important that the infrahyoid muscles contract and pull down on the hyoid bone. Once the hyoid bone is stabilized, or held down from below, contraction of the suprahyoid muscles can aid in pulling the mandible downward.

Laryngeal Movements

The larynx moves upward and downward in swallowing and phonation. For this to be accomplished, certain muscles must contract. Before continuing, try this demonstration. Place your fingers lightly on the larynx and swallow. What happened? The upward movement of the larynx helped to pull the **epiglottis** over the laryngeal opening so that anything being swallowed would pass over the laryngeal opening and enter the esophagus. If this elevation did not take place, you could choke when trying to swallow food. How is this accomplished? The hyoid bone is pulled upward slightly by the contraction of the suprahyoid muscles. The thyrohyoid muscle then contracts, elevating the thyroid cartilage of the larynx and, along with the contraction of the muscles attached to the epiglottis and the backward movement of the tongue, moves the epiglottis over the opening of the larynx, allowing the swallowed material to enter the esophagus (Fig. 13-9).

■ ■ ■

This by no means covers all the muscles in the neck area, but it does include those most intimately involved in mandibular and laryngeal movements, providing a better understanding of some of the controls of mastication and swallowing **(deglutition).**

STERNOCLEIDOMASTOID MUSCLE

The sternocleidomastoid muscle of the neck should be mentioned at this time, even though it does not fit the subject areas already mentioned. In an extraoral examination of a patient, it will be necessary to press, or palpate, beneath the anterior border of the muscle to check for enlargement of the lymph nodes lying against the jugular vein in the neck.

The sternocleidomastoid muscle, sometimes referred to simply as the sternomastoid muscle, has its origin in the upper border of the sternum and the medial one third of the clavicle, or collarbone. The muscle runs upward and backward on the side of the neck to insert into the mastoid process of the temporal bone. The action of the muscle is involved in tilting and rotating the head. It is innervated by the eleventh (XI) cranial nerve (accessory nerve), and its blood supply is a branch of the external carotid artery (Figs. 13-4 and 13-5).

REVIEW QUESTIONS

1. How can you distinguish the origin from the insertion of a muscle?
2. Describe the action of a muscle.
3. Define or describe the following terms:
   a. Elevation   *closing the mand.*
   b. Protrusion   *pulls mand, forward.*
   c. Retrusion   *pulls mand. backward*
   d. Depression   *opens mand.*
   e. Lateral excursion of the mandible   *sideway movement*
4. Name the muscles involved in creating the actions mentioned in Question 3.
5. Which muscles or general groups of muscles affect the movements of the larynx?
6. What is found beneath the sternomastoid muscle?   *Lymph nodes*
7. Name or point out the origins and insertions of the muscles of mastication.

1. origin is the part of muscle that's attached to the least movable structure.

2. the action is the work accomplished when muscle fibers contract.

4. elevation — masseter, temporal, medial pterygoid

protrusion — lateral pterygoid, medial pterygoid

lateral excursion — lateral pterygoid

retrusion — temporal

depression — digastric, mylohyoid, geniohyoid, stylohyoid,

5. Affects movements of larynx — omohyoid, sternothyroid, thyrohyoid

14

Temporomandibular Joint

OBJECTIVES

- To diagram and label a sagittal section of the temporomandibular joint (TMJ)
- To define the role of a synovial cavity
- To describe the two movements of the TMJ as the mouth opens and know where these movements take place
- To describe the role of the superior posterior elastic lamina, the inferior posterior collagenous lamina, and the superior and inferior heads of the lateral pterygoid muscle as the jaw goes through the various functions
- To define disc derangement, subluxation, bruxism, and TMJ sounds
- To discuss probable causes of TMJ pain

STRUCTURE

As the name indicates, the **temporomandibular joint** (TMJ) is the articulation between the temporal bone and the mandible. A joint is a joining together of two bones. There are a number of types of joints. A suture of the skull is one type of joint that we have already studied, and now the TMJ is another type, since it is a joint in which the surface of one bone moves over the surface of another.

Actually the TMJ is two joints that move and function as one. It is also a bilateral, or two-sided, joint in that the mandible is fused at the symphysis, so the left and right joints are interrelated. In Chapter 11 you learned the osteology, or the system of bony parts, of this joint. Fig. 14-1 shows the fossa, posterior tubercle, and articular eminence and tubercle of the temporal bone, as well as the condyle and its neck of the mandible. Between these two bones you can see a small fibrous pad of dense collagen tissue called the **articular disc.** The upper surface of the disc is concavo-convex to match the contours of the mandibular fossa and articular eminence, whereas the lower surface of the disc is concave to match the contour of the condyle. Looking at Fig. 14-1 you will see that the articular disc is thickest at the posterior end; As you get to the middle, it is thinnest; and then there is a slight increase in thickness at the anterior end. The thick posterior area is called the posterior band, the thin middle area is called the intermediate zone, and the slightly thicker anterior area is called the anterior band. Above and below this disc are small saclike compartments called **synovial cavities.** Part of the tissue lining these cavities is an epithelium that secretes a few drops of lubricating liquid, called **synovial fluid,** which allows the surfaces to rub over one another without any irritation.

The entire joint is surrounded by a thick fibrous capsule. The lateral side of this **capsule** is thickened between the articular tubercle and the lateral pole of the condyle. This thickened area is known as the **temporomandibular ligament.** This ligament prevents the condyle from being displaced too far inferiorly and posteriorly and provides some resistance to lateral displacement (Fig. 14-2).

The disc is attached both medially and laterally to the poles of the condyle (Fig. 14-3). Anteriorly the disc is attached to fibers of the superior head of the lateral pterygoid muscle. These fibers pen-

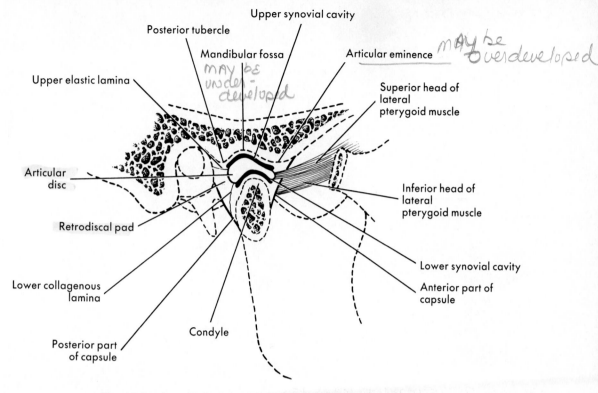

Posterior tubercle

Upper synovial cavity

Mandibular fossa

may be under-developed

Articular eminence *may be overdeveloped*

Upper elastic lamina

Superior head of lateral pterygoid muscle

Articular disc

Inferior head of lateral pterygoid muscle

Retrodiscal pad

Lower synovial cavity

Anterior part of capsule

Lower collagenous lamina

Condyle

Posterior part of capsule

Fig. 14-1   Longitudinal section through temporomandibular joint.

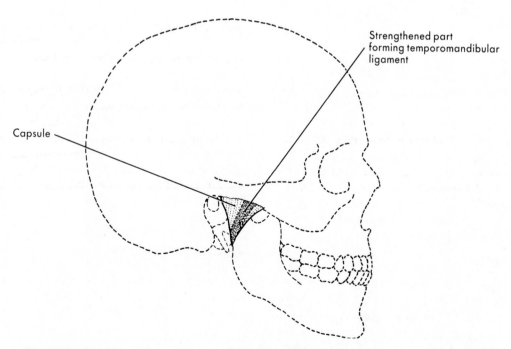

Strengthened part forming temporomandibular ligament

Capsule

Fig. 14-2   Capsule surrounding entire temporomandibular joint. Capsule is strengthened on the deep side of lateral surface by temporomandibular ligament, which helps prevent lateral, posterior, and inferior movement of condyle out of fossa.

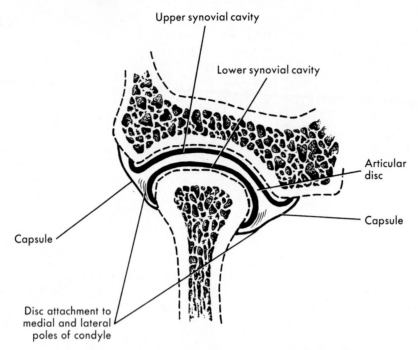

Upper synovial cavity

Lower synovial cavity

Articular disc

Capsule

Capsule

Disc attachment to medial and lateral poles of condyle

Fig. 14-3 *Left to right,* Frontal section through condyle, disc, capsule, and fossa. Disc fibers curve down to insert into poles of condyle.

etrate the capsule and insert into the disc. The area posterior to the disc is known as the **retrodiscal pad.** Running from the posterior upper part of the disc is an elastic lamina, or layer of tissue, that lies above the retrodiscal pad and inserts into the posterior upper end of the TMJ capsule where it attaches in the area of the tympanic plate of the temporal bone. Running from the posterior lower border of the disc is a collagenous lamina that lies below the retrodiscal pad and attaches into the posterior neck of the condyle where the capsule attaches to it.

MOVEMENT

What kind of movement is this joint capable of creating, and how does it do it? There are two distinct types of movement that can be accom-

plished: a rotational movement and a gliding movement along an inclined plane. As the teeth begin to separate (the first few millimeters), there is a rotational movement in the lower synovial cavity between the condyle and the disc. The reason for the rotational movement is the posterior elastic lamina. As the condyle begins rotating, the disc wants to move anteriorly with it, since it is attached to the poles of the condyle. However, the elastic lamina pulls posteriorly on it, and the disc and condyle rotate on one another. As the jaw opens further, the rotational movement continues, but now there is also an anterior gliding movement along the posterior slope of the articular eminence. This gliding movement takes place between the disc and the temporal bone. The forward movement is caused by contraction of the inferior head of the lateral pterygoid muscle (Chapter 13). The condyle and disc move forward until they reach just slightly anterior to the crest of the articular eminence.

If you now slowly move the jaw back into a centric relation, the superior head of the lateral pterygoid controls the posterior movement of the disc by controlling the release of its contraction and balancing the posterior pull exerted by the elastic lamina. The lower posterior collagenous lamina prevents the elastic lamina and disc from being pulled too far forward and injured.

Let us consider what happens in the power stroke when you chew on something from the protruded, open position of the mandible. As you begin and continue to bite down on a thick piece of meat placed between the teeth on the right side, the right condyle will be in a position where the condyle, disc, and temporal bone are in contact with each other. However, on the left side, as you continue to bite down, the condyle, disc, and temporal surfaces will be pulled slightly apart. This would make the left side of the joint somewhat wobbly. This wobble could cause the surfaces to bounce against one another and possibly injure the structures. This does not happen because the superior head of the lateral pterygoid contracts, pulling the disc forward. In doing so it moves the thicker posterior part of the disc forward and this thicker part fills the space created by the surfaces moving slightly apart and so balances and stabilizes the joint on that side. As continued contraction takes place, the upper head of the lateral pterygoid again controls the posterior movement of the disc with a posterior pull from the superior elastic lamina, and a smooth movement takes place.

PROBLEMS ASSOCIATED WITH THE TMJ

There are a myriad of problems associated with the TMJ, and in many cases there is disagreement over how these problems should be treated. Our job will be to present some of these problems and their possible causes. It is quite likely that you will see many of these cases in the office where they will either be treated or referred elsewhere for treatment.

Pain in the TMJ Area

Many patients come into the office complaining of pain in the region of the TMJ. If radiographic studies seem to show a normal TMJ and there does not seem to be any pain on palpation of the area, one might consider the possibility of **referred pain.** This is a condition in which sensory messages, apparently coming from the area of the TMJ, are actually traveling to the brain from other regions of the body. Many of these pains come from spasms in neck muscles and from the muscles of mastication. Many times muscle relaxants or physical therapy allow these muscles to relax and subsequently relieve pain. In Chapter 19 you will study the cranial nerves. Four of these nerves, the V, VII, IX, and X, have sensory areas around the ear that they supply. Involvement with these nerves may cause pain that seems to come from the TMJ.

Internal Problems of the TMJ

TMJ sounds. Many patients complain of a popping, clicking, or grinding in the TMJ yet have no other symptoms, such as pain. The popping or clicking noise may occur when the disc is pulled too far forward in the opening movement. The thick posterior band of the disc gets caught between the head of the condyle and the articular eminence. It then pops forward and is displaced too far anteriorly. Many times the dentist is not able to hear the clicking or popping but may do so with the aid of a stethoscope. Sometimes by palpating the joint as the popping occurs, you can feel the jumping movement of the condyle as the disc pops forward. If it only happens on one side, you can frequently see the movement by standing in front of the patient as they open seeing if the mandible moves in a straight downward movement or if it shifts to one side as it opens and then moves back to the midline. Many times these problems can be treated with ultrasound, physical therapy, or a plastic splint, similar to a nightguard; the disc may return to its normal position. The grinding sound may come from adhesions in the synovial membranes of the joint. It may also be treated by ultrasound, although it may recur.

Disc derangement. The cause of TMJ sounds may be considered a type of disc derangement, but here we will discuss additional problems. In constant anterior displacement of the disc, there possibly may be permanent damage to the components of the disc. In anterior displacement the posterior laminae possibly may be torn and the disc permanently displaced anteriorly. Also, the medial or lateral attachments of the disc to the poles of the condyle possibly may be torn. If this happens, it tends to be a tear to the lateral pole attachment. Both of these require surgery, and the surgery tends to be fairly successful.

Subluxation. The student should understand how some other clinical problems occur. A person may open the mouth too wide and not be able to close it again. This happens when the condyle glides too far forward and moves too far anterior to the height of the articular eminence (Fig. 14-4). When the patient tries to close, the condyle cannot move posteriorly because the muscles are trying to pull upward and posteriorly, and the articular eminence does not allow it to move back. You can remedy this in the dental office by placing the thumbs on the occlusal surface of the mandibular posterior teeth, with the index fingers beneath the inferior border of the mandible, and pushing downward while at the same time guiding the jaw slowly back into its posterior position. It is advisable to wrap the thumbs in gauze so that they are protected in case the patient closes down on them. In general, there are several reasons for this condition,

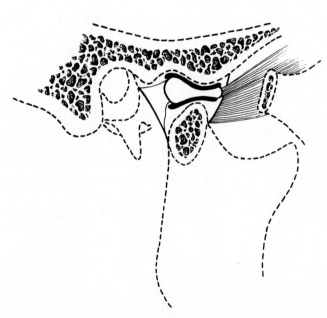

Fig. 14-4 Condyle has ridden forward to height of eminence. If it moves further forward, it may become trapped and unable to move backward because of contour. It therefore has to be pushed downward, or depressed, before it can be eased back into its normal position.

which is called **subluxation.** One is the shape of the influential condylar fossa and articular eminence. Another is the position of the capsule around the joint, a factor that controls the amount of contraction of the lateral pterygoid muscle. This can be treated by surgically decreasing the height of the articular eminence.

Bruxism. Many people grind their teeth. Most of the time this is done during sleep, though some of the time it occurs during waking hours. This is referred to as **bruxism.** Over a long period of time it may tend to wear down the teeth faster, but the immediate result is that the TMJ becomes very tired and sore. Much of this tenderness has to do with the muscles of mastication tiring, yet it is the joint that seems to ache. One of the methods of treatment is to make a plastic nightguard to cover the patient's teeth. To a great extent this eliminates the excessive wear on the teeth and tenderness of the teeth from stress on the periodontal ligament. Others might be treated with tranquilizers to relieve the tension that may contribute to the bruxism.

Arthritis and other pain in the TMJ. The TMJ is also subject to such conditions as **arthritis** and the pain that results from it. **Cortisone** may relieve it, but the pain can still be a major problem. Other patients have a grinding sensation in the joint. Authorities contend that this is caused by excessive wear of the disc in the joint so that there is no longer a smooth gliding movement within the snyovial cavities. This seems very reasonable, since we tend to think of the TMJ as a stress-bearing joint and believe that too much stress will cause it to wear out early in life and cause problems. However, there are reports of people who have had both condyles fractured so severely that they had to be removed surgically, and the patients have continued to function well without a real joint. This points out that not enough is known about the TMJ and that it is more complicated than was formerly believed.

Over the years a patient may wear away some of the occlusal surfaces of teeth and begin to experience pain in the TMJ. Many times, simply rebuilding the teeth to their original height with crowns and onlays eases the pain. Most authorities would now agree that most of the problems in these cases rest not in the joint itself but in the muscles of mastication, other head and neck muscles, and the occlusion of the teeth. With changes in the relationship of the jaws caused by tooth wear, the muscles of mastication are no longer in their normal relaxed position. Therefore they might tend to go into **spasm** and cause pain.

REVIEW QUESTIONS

1. What is a synovial cavity, and what is its function?
2. Describe the TMJ capsule and ligament.
3. What are the two TMJ movements, and when do they occur? ROTATIONAL + gliding
4. Describe the roles of the posterior laminae and the lateral pterygoid muscle in mastication.
5. What are some of the causes of TMJ pain? referred pain
6. What may cause TMJ sounds?
7. What is a disc derangement?

1. synovial cavity - epithelium-lined space that secretes tiny amounts of fluids, synovia, + is found in free-moving joints.
2. capsule covers the entire TMJ joint. Lateral side of capsule is thicker + is the TMJ ligament.
6. TMJ sounds may be from disc pulling too far forward in opening movement.
7. disc derangement possibly from torn post. laminae OR medial OR lateral attachments torn.

15

Muscles of Facial Expression

OBJECTIVES

- To name the various groupings, or locations, of the muscles of facial expression and their nerve supply
- To name all the muscles surrounding the mouth, with their origin, insertion, and action
- To discuss the role of the buccinator muscle in mastication

The term "facial expression" may be a bit misleading, since the muscles included in this chapter are located around the ears, scalp, neck, eyes, nose, and mouth. Although some of them are not located in an area normally thought of as the face, they are located in areas that can physically display some kind of emotion or attentiveness. All these muscles are innervated by the seventh (VII) cranial nerve (facial). Although most of the muscles are mentioned, only the muscles around the oral cavity are discussed in greater detail. These are the muscles you will be most concerned with, and they are responsible for some functions related to speech and mastication.

EARS

The muscles around the ears are not well developed. In lower forms of animals, however, they are better developed, and the ears can be easily moved and repositioned to better catch sounds. There are three pairs of ear muscles (Fig. 15-1).

Anterior Auricular Muscle

The **anterior auricular muscle** arises from connective tissue of the scalp in front of the ear and runs posteriorly into the anterior part of the ear. The action of this muscle pulls the ear slightly forward.

Superior Auricular Muscle

The **superior auricular muscle** arises from connective tissue of the scalp above the ear, and the fibers run downward to be inserted into the upper part of the ear. The action of this muscle raises the ear.

Posterior Auricular Muscle

The **posterior auricular muscle** arises from the **superior nuchal line** of the occipital bone and the mastoid area. The fibers run forward to insert into the posterior part of the ear. The action of this muscle is to pull the ear backward. This is probably the best developed of the ear muscles.

SCALP

The muscles of the scalp allow for its mobility—the ability to move it forward and backward.

Occipitofrontalis (Epicranius)

The **occipitofrontalis (epicranius)** is a paired muscle having groups of fibers in front and back connected by a broad flat band of **fascia.** The anterior and posterior groups of muscle fibers take their origin from connective tissue of the scalp. This kind of attachment allows for either forward or backward movement of the scalp (Fig. 15-1).

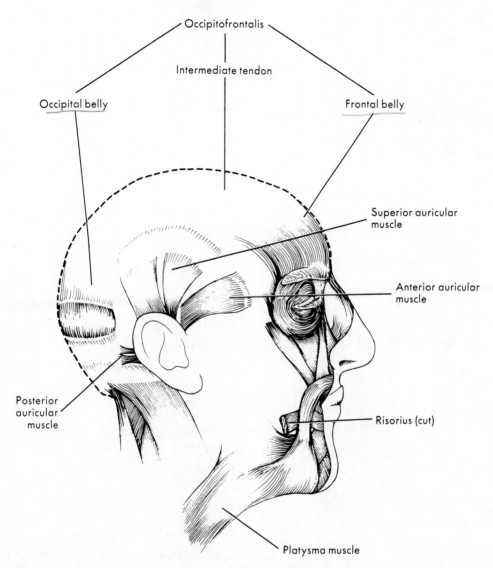

Occipitofrontalis

Intermediate tendon

Occipital belly

Frontal belly

Superior auricular muscle

Anterior auricular muscle

Posterior auricular muscle

Risorius (cut)

Platysma muscle

Fig. 15-1   Three groups of auricular muscles around ear. There are two bellies of occip-itofrontalis with intermediate tendon.

NECK

You may wonder how a muscle in the neck can show facial expression. However, pulling down the corners of the mouth, as in a grimace, is partly accomplished by this muscle.

Platysma

There is some disagreement as to which end of the **platysma** is the origin and which is the insertion. The upper end of the fibers attaches to the inferior border of the mandible, near the angles of the mouth and back along the mandible. They pass downward in a broad flat sheet to end in the skin of the chest area just below the clavicle. The muscle lies just below the skin of the neck; thus it moves the skin over the neck quite noticeably when it contracts.

EYES

Several muscles located around the eyes close the eyes and move the eyebrows (Fig. 15-2).

Orbicularis Oculi

Although the long Latin names may prove a problem for some, by studying the words care-

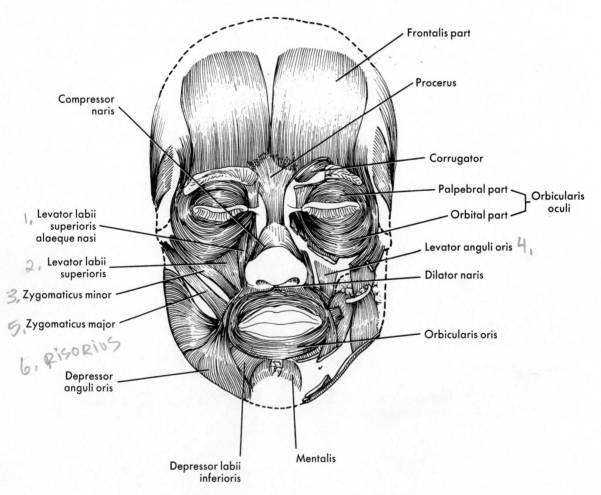

Fig. 15-2   Muscles of eye, nose, and mouth.

fully you can infer their meaning. The term "orbicularis" relates to the word "circular." In this age of astronauts, space shuttles, and orbits, it is easy to understand how this circles the eye.

There are two parts to the **orbicularis oculi.** The part that encircles the eye is called the orbital part. It attaches to the skull at the medial and lateral edges of the orbit. The muscle fibers in the eyelid are called the palpebral part. The fibers also attach at the medial and lateral corners of the orbit. The action of the muscle involves closing the eyelids and contracting the skin around the eye.

Corrugator

The **corrugator** runs from the bridge of the nose upward and lateral to the lateral part of the eyebrow. It pulls the eyebrow medially and downward, as in a frown.

Procerus

From the nose the fibers of the **procerus** extend upward into the medial end of the eyebrow. They pull the eyebrow at the medial end downward.

NOSE

The muscles of the nose primarily circle the opening of the nostrils (Fig. 15-2). The **nasalis** is the muscle that opens and closes the nostrils. It is composed of two parts.

Dilator Naris

The **dilator naris** pulls downward on the nostrils, causing them to flare or dilate.

Compressor Naris

The **compressor naris** causes the nostrils to close or compress.

MOUTH

The muscles grouped around the mouth influence expression and speech and aid in mastication. The pressure of these muscles on the teeth

helps to hold them in alignment if the pressures are normal. Abnormal pressures caused by cheek biting, lip biting, and lip compression may cause them to move out of alignment (Fig. 15-2).

Orbicularis Oris

The **orbicularis oris** circles the oral cavity in the tissue of the lip. It has some bony attachment at the anterior nasal spine and at the midline above the chin. The fibers circle the lip like a purse string, and all the muscles surrounding the lips interlace with them. The action of the muscle is to close and compress the lips.

Levator Labii Superioris   ALAQUE NASi

As its name indicates, the **levator labii superioris** elevates the upper lip. It has its origin just beneath the lower rim of the orbit. The fibers run downward to be inserted into the fibers of the orbicularis oris of the upper lip, midway between the center of the lip and the corner of the mouth. O → frontal process of max.
I → medial - ala of nose, lateral - upper lip

Zygomaticus Minor Between CORNER & middle

The **zygomaticus minor** is a smaller muscle coming from the area of the zygomatic bone. The fibers run downward and forward to be inserted into the orbicularis oris just lateral to the levator labii superioris. It also raises the upper lip, though it is usually a very poorly developed muscle and therefore does not exert great influence in this function.

Zygomaticus Major

The **zygomaticus major** is the larger muscle originating from the zygomatic bone. Its origin is lateral to the zygomaticus minor and runs downward and forward to insert into the orbicularis oris at the angle of the mouth. Its action is to elevate the corners of the mouth, as in a smile.

Levator Anguli Oris

The **levator anguli oris** lies deep to the levator labii superioris and the zygomaticus major and zygomaticus minor. It originates from the maxilla, just below the infraorbital foramen. The fibers run downward and laterally to blend into the orbicularis oris at the corners of the mouth. As the name indicates, this muscle pulls the angles of the mouth upward and somewhat toward the midline.

Depressor Labii Inferioris

The origin of the **depressor labii inferioris** is the area beneath the angles of the mouth and just above the inferior border of the mandible. The fibers run upward and medially to insert into the

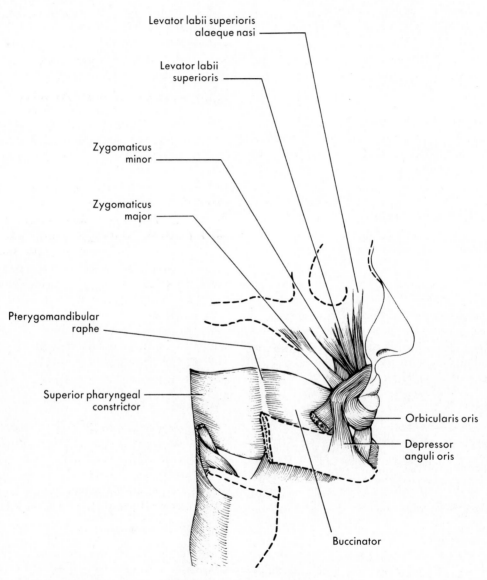

Fig. 15-3 Muscles of mouth.

fibers of the orbicularis oris toward the middle of the lower lip. The name indicates that this muscle functions by pulling down the lower lip. This kind of action is accentuated in a pout.

Depressor Anguli Oris

The origin of the **depressor anguli oris** is from the same general area as that of the depressor labii inferioris, and the fibers partly overlap it. From the origin the fibers run upward and converge to blend into the orbicularis oris at the angle of the mouth. As the name indicates, this muscle pulls the corners of the mouth downward.

Mentalis

The **mentalis** originates on the anterior surface of the mandible just beneath the lateral incisors. The fibers run downward and toward the midline, where some even cross to meet the muscle on the opposite side, terminating with insertion into the skin of the chin. When the muscle contracts, it pulls this skin upward.

Buccinator

The **buccinator** is probably the most important muscle in this group. Although it is a muscle of facial expression, it plays a role in mastication. The muscle originates from a fibrous band (the **pterygomandibular raphe**) that runs from the pterygoid hamulus down to the medial surface of the mandible, near the posterior part of the mylohyoid line. This pterygomandibular raphe connects the anterior part of the **superior constrictor muscle** of the pharynx with the posterior part of the buccinator.

The buccinator also originates from the buccal alveolar bone of the maxillary molars, as well as the corresponding area of the mandibular molars. From these two bony origins and from the raphe the fibers of the buccinator run anteriorly, making up the musculature of the cheek. The fibers insert into the orbicularis oris at the corners of the mouth. When the muscle contracts, it pulls the corners of the mouth backward and compresses the cheek. When one chews, the food is crushed and ground between the molars. As it is squeezed out from the occlusal surfaces, some of the food is pushed onto the tongue and the remainder is deposited into the buccal vestibule. The food on the tongue can be pushed back up onto the occlusal surface by the action of the tongue. The food that is forced out into the vestibule is pushed back up onto the occlusal surfaces, in part, by the contraction of the buccinator muscle.

The buccinator muscle has frequently been referred to as an accessory muscle of mastication because of the help it provides in chewing food. A person with facial muscle paralysis would have difficulty chewing food. It would pile up in the buccal vestibule because the buccinator muscle could not force it back up on the occlusal surfaces (Fig. 15-3).

Risorius

The **risorius** is a small muscle that arises from the soft tissue near the angle of the mandible. It runs forward on the surface of the buccinator and inserts into the corner of the mouth. It also aids in smiling but is usually very poorly developed (Fig. 15-1).

REVIEW QUESTIONS

1. Describe or name the head and neck locations of muscles of facial expression.
2. Which nerve innervates the muscles of facial expression? FACIAL (VII)
3. Of all the muscles of facial expression, which one do you believe to be the most important for mastication? Why? Orbicularis oris encircle the mouth
4. List the muscles around the oral cavity and diagram where they enter the orbicularis oris muscle and the direction from which they enter.

---

3. <u>Buccinator</u> — has major role in mastication.

16

Soft Palate and Pharynx

OBJECTIVES

- To describe the origins, insertions, actions, and nerve supplies of the muscles of the soft palate and pharynx.
- To describe the interrelationship of all of these muscles in chewing, swallowing, and speech

The muscles of the soft palate and **pharynx** are rather intricate in their arrangement and interrelationship. They share some common boundaries between the upper end of the digestive and respiratory systems and are also important in the production of the sounds that we call speech. The soft palate forms the posterior end of the roof of the mouth. The pharynx has three components: the upper part, known as the nasal pharynx, is located at the posterior end of the nasal cavity; the middle part, the oral pharynx, is the back throat wall; and the lower end, the laryngeal pharynx, is below the tongue where the digestive and respiratory systems branch into their respective parts, the esophagus and larynx.

SOFT PALATE

There are five pairs of muscles in the soft palate. These muscles help to move the soft palate up and back to contact the posterior throat wall and seal off the nasal cavity from the oral cavity and also to narrow the space between the two palatine tonsils. This space is referred to as the fauces and is used in swallowing.

Palatoglossal Muscle

If you open the mouth and look at the tonsils on the side of the throat wall, you will see that there is a vertical fold of tissue in front of and behind the tonsil. These are known as the anterior and posterior faucial pillars, or the palatoglossal and palatopharyngeal folds. Beneath the palatoglossal fold is the **palatoglossal muscle.** It originates from the posterior end of the hard palate and the anterior part of the soft palate. The fibers run downward, laterally, and forward to insert into the posterior and lateral part of the tongue. When the palatoglossal muscle contracts, it pulls the sides of the tongue upward and back, pulls the soft palate downward on the lateral edges, and narrows the space between the left and right faucial pillars. The nerve that supplies this muscle is a part of the eleventh (XI) cranial nerve (Figs. 16-1 and 16-3).

Palatopharyngeal Muscle

The posterior faucial pillar is formed by the **palatopharyngeal muscle.** It originates from the posterolateral part of the soft palate and runs downward and laterally to insert into the pharyngeal constrictor muscle and the thyroid cartilage of the larynx. When it contracts, it narrows the fauces and elevates and dilates the pharynx, or throat area, behind the tongue. The nerve supply is also the eleventh cranial nerve (Figs. 16-1 to 16-3).

Muscles of Uvula

The uvula is that small fold of tissue that hangs down in the throat from the posterior part of the

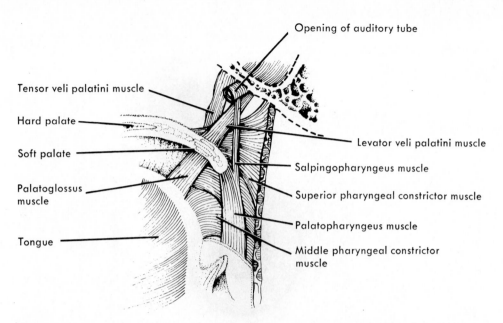

Opening of auditory tube

Tensor veli palatini muscle

Hard palate

Soft palate

Palatoglossus muscle

Tongue

Levator veli palatini muscle

Salpingopharyngeus muscle

Superior pharyngeal constrictor muscle

Palatopharyngeus muscle

Middle pharyngeal constrictor muscle

Fig. 16-1 View of lateral throat wall looking from midline. Mucosa has been removed and various muscles can be seen. Palatoglossal and palatopharyngeal muscles form anterior and posterior pillars, respectively; palatine tonsil would lie between them. (Redrawn after Snell.)

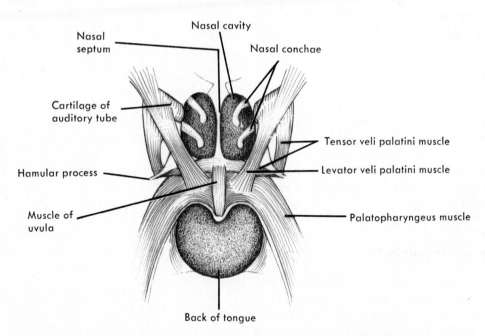

Nasal septum

Nasal cavity

Nasal conchae

Cartilage of auditory tube

Hamular process

Muscle of uvula

Tensor veli palatini muscle

Levator veli palatini muscle

Palatopharyngeus muscle

Back of tongue

Fig. 16-2 Posterior view of muscles of soft palate. Pharyngeal constrictor muscles have been removed, and view is from behind throat. Notice especially how levator veli palatini runs directly downward into soft palate, whereas tensor veli palatini runs downward and forward around lateral side of hamular process and then turns medially into soft palate. You can see how shortening of this muscle would tense soft palate. (Redrawn after Snell.)

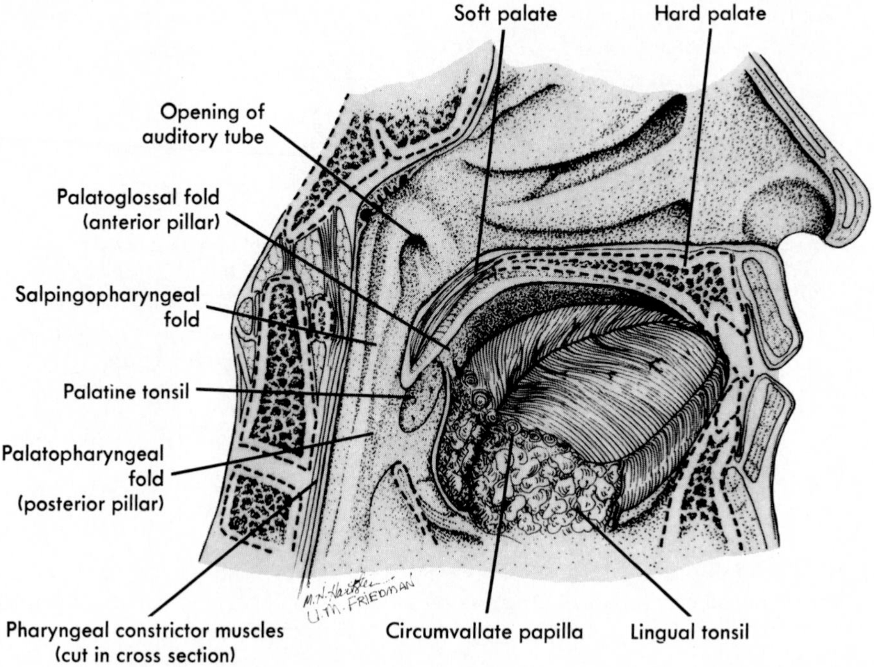

Fig. 16-3 View of lateral throat wall similar to Fig. 16-1 but with mucosa in place. Anterior and posterior pillars can be seen, as can opening of auditory tube in nasal pharynx; fold caused by salpingopharyngeal muscle runs downward from it. (Redrawn after Snell.)

soft palate. It is formed by two small bands of muscle that originate from the posterior end of the hard palate and run backward and downward in the soft palate to form that structure. When the **muscle of the uvula** contracts, it shortens and broadens the uvula and changes the contour of the posterior end of the soft palate so that it adapts to the posterior throat wall when it is moved up against it. This muscle is also innervated by the eleventh cranial nerve (Fig. 16-2).

Levator Veli Palatini

The **levator veli palatini,** as the name indicates, elevates the posterior end of the soft palate. It originates from the petrous part of the temporal bone just anterior to the carotid canal and from the medial wall of the cartilagenous part of the auditory canal, or tube, which lies in the lateral wall of the nasal pharynx. The fibers run down-

ward and slightly medially into the posterior part of the soft palate. When the muscle contracts, it pulls the posterior end of the soft palate upward and backward to contact the posterior pharyngeal (throat) wall. The nerve supply to this muscle is also the eleventh cranial nerve (Figs. 16-1, 16-2, and 16-5).

Tensor Veli Palatini

The last of the muscles of the soft palate is the **tensor veli palatini.** This muscle takes its origin from an area near the base of the medial pterygoid plate, where it meets the body of the sphenoid bone, as well as from the lateral wall of the cartilage of the auditory tube. The fibers run downward and forward to pass around the lateral side of the hamular process on the medial pterygoid plate; as they pass around the hamular process, they turn medially and insert into the posterior edge of the hard palate and the anterior portion of the soft palate. As the name indicates, contraction of the muscle slightly tenses the anterior portion of the soft palate. The nerve supply to this muscle is the third part of the fifth (V) cranial nerve and is usually denoted V_3 (Figs. 16-1, 16-2, and 16- 5).

PHARYNX
Pharyngeal Constrictors

The pharynx has two groups of muscles associated with it, one group that constricts the pharynx and another group that elevates and dilates the pharynx. There are three pairs of pharyngeal constrictors, all of which insert into a midline tendon in the posterior throat wall known as the **median raphe.** These three muscles also overlap one another in their insertion into this raphe.

Superior pharyngeal constrictor muscle. The **superior pharyngeal constrictor muscle** takes its origin from the lower part of the medial pterygoid plate and its hamular process, from the mandibular alveolar process on the lingual side just above the mylohyoid line, and from a tendinous band that runs between these two areas and is known as the pterygomandibular raphe. These points are also the origin of the buccinator muscle discussed previously. The buccinator muscle runs forward, whereas the superior pharyngeal constrictor runs backward to insert into the base of the skull just in front of the foramen magnum and into the midline raphe mentioned earlier. When the muscle contracts, it constricts the upper part of the pharynx and is able to force the

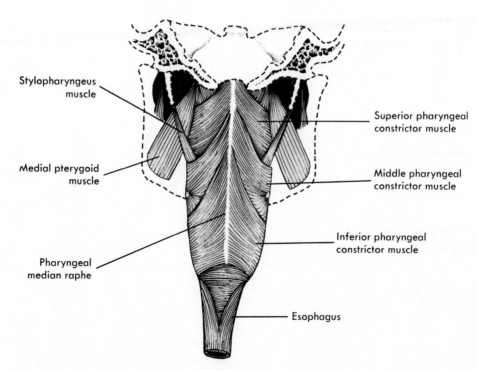

Fig. 16-4   Posterior view of pharyngeal wall. You can see overlapping of pharyngeal constrictor muscles and position of stylopharyngeal muscle running down into them. (Redrawn after Snell.)

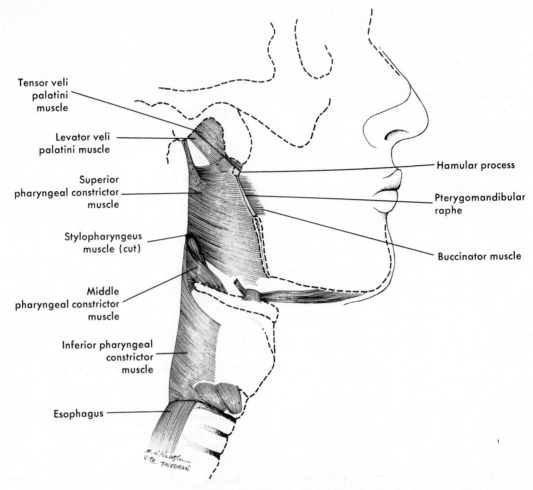

Fig. 16-5   Lateral view of pharyngeal constrictor muscles. Above them you can see tensor and levator veli palatini running downward into soft palate.

contents of the pharynx downward. The muscle is supplied by the ninth, tenth and eleventh cranial nerves (Figs. 16-4 and 16-5).

Middle pharyngeal constrictor muscle. The **middle pharyngeal constrictor muscle** takes its origin from the posterior part (greater and lesser cornua) of the hyoid bone and from the stylohyoid ligament. The fibers run backward, overlapping the superior constrictor muscle above and underlying the inferior constrictor below. When the muscle contracts, it also constricts the pha-

ryngeal opening and forces the food downward toward the esophagus. This is also supplied by the ninth, tenth, and eleventh cranial nerves, which make up what is known for most of these muscles as the **pharyngeal plexus of nerves** (Figs. 16-4 and 16-5).

Inferior pharyngeal constrictor muscle. The **inferior pharyngeal constrictor muscle** takes its origin from the posterior part of the thyroid cartilage of the larynx. The fibers run backward, overlying the middle pharyngeal constrictor, and insert into the midline raphe. The lowest of these fibers blend in with the upper part of the wall of the esophagus so that contraction of this muscle also constricts the lower end of the pharynx and forces the food into the esophagus, which then continues the movement of the food toward the stomach. The nerve supply to this muscle is also the ninth, tenth, and eleventh cranial nerves (Figs. 16-4 and 16-5).

Pharyngeal Elevators and Dilators

The second group of muscles in the pharynx aids in elevating and dilating the pharynx.

Palatopharyngeal muscle. Although the palatopharyngeal muscle has already been listed as a muscle of the soft palate, you can see from its action that it also has the ability to elevate and slightly dilate the pharynx. This action is necessary to receive the food that is to be swallowed.

Stylopharyngeal muscle. The **stylopharyngeal muscle** takes its origin from the base of the styloid process on the medial side and runs downward and medially to blend in with some fibers of the palatopharyngeal muscle, which then insert into the lateral pharyngeal wall and the thyroid cartilage of the larynx. Contraction of the muscle causes dilation and elevation of the pharynx. The nerve supply to this muscle is the ninth cranial nerve (Fig. 16-4).

Salpingopharyngeal muscle. The **salpingopharyngeal muscle** takes its origin from the end of the auditory tube in the lateral wall of the nasal pharynx. The fibers run downward to blend in also with the palatopharyngeal muscle and the lateral pharyngeal wall. Contraction of the muscle primarily lifts the pharyngeal wall in the act of swallowing as does contraction of the other muscles just listed. The nerve supply to this muscle is also the ninth, tenth, and eleventh cranial nerves (Figs. 16-1 and 16-3).

ACTIONS

Let us first consider the action of the muscles of the soft palate as they relate to speech and then compare that with their actions in swallowing. When we speak, we pull the soft palate upward and backward to contact the posterior pharyngeal wall. This is accomplished primarily by the tensor and levator veli palatini, and the muscle of the uvula.

If the soft palate is unable to adapt well to the posterior pharyngeal wall, the speech will have a nasal sound. A common example of this occurs when a person has enlarged adenoids (pharyngeal tonsils) that are in the posterior pharyngeal wall just where the soft palate contacts it. These enlarged adenoids give the voice a definite nasal tone. As another example, if there is a large open contact region, as occurs in a cleft palate, the voice may be unintelligible.

While we are considering the act of swallowing, let us look at what precedes it and follow it through to completion using the example of meat. The meat is incised by the anterior teeth and ground up by the posterior teeth. While this is going on, the meat is also being mixed with saliva. When it reaches the proper consistency, it is shaped into a ball of food by the teeth, cheeks, and tongue; this ball is referred to as a **bolus of food.** The bolus is placed on the tongue, the tongue is moved upward and backward, and the bolus is shifted onto the posterior part of the tongue and moved back into the oral pharyngeal area. As the tongue moves upward and backward, the muscles of the soft palate raise the posterior end of the soft palate to contact the posterior pharyngeal wall and narrow the fauces so that it presses tightly to the sides of the tongue, sealing off the back part of the tongue and the oral pharynx from the front part of the tongue and the oral cavity.

If we look at the action of the pharyngeal muscles in this swallowing process, we see that the elevators and dilators of the pharynx lift it up and widen it to accommodate the bolus of food that has just been moved back into the oral pharynx. Next the constrictors compress the upper part of the oral pharynx and push the food down into the laryngeal pharynx. As this happens, some of the pharyngeal muscles elevate the thyroid cartilage of the larynx with assistance from the thyrohyoid muscle and a number of others. This allows the epiglottis to help shelter the laryngeal opening from food moving into it, and the food moves down into the upper end of the esophagus. The upper half of the esophagus is also a voluntary skeletal muscle, and a person can willfully move the food about halfway down the esophagus before the further movement is taken over by involuntary smooth muscle, which creates wavelike constrictions of the digestive tube known as **peristaltic contractions.** At one time or another we have all moved too much food into the esophagus too quickly and have felt like it was stuck halfway down. In essence this is true because we can move the food only that far; then it has to stop and wait for the involuntary peristaltic waves to take it the rest of the way; these waves proceed at a much slower rate than the voluntary waves of contraction that we can create.

REVIEW QUESTIONS

1. What are the muscles of the soft palate that narrow the fauces and what other actions can they accomplish? Describe their origins and insertions.
2. Which muscles of the pharynx aid in elevation and dilatation of the pharynx? Which nerves supply them?
3. Name the origins and insertions of the pharyngeal constrictors as well as their nerve supply.
4. What creates nasal sounds in a person's speech?
5. Try to make a list of the sequences of events that take place when food is masticated and swallowed.
6. Why do we sometimes feel like food is caught halfway down our throats?

1. muscles that narrow the fauces - palatoglossal, palatalpharyngeal, uvula, levator veli palatini, tensor veli palatini

2. pharyngeal elevators & dilators - palatopharyngeal, stylopharyngeal, salpingopharyngeal

3. pharyngeal constrictors - Superior, middle, & inferior pharyngeal constrictor muscles.

4. Nasal sound is when soft palate is unable to adapt well to the posterior pharyngeal wall.

17

Arterial Supply and Venous Drainage

OBJECTIVES

- To trace the blood supply from the heart to all areas of the oral cavity, including all the teeth
- To trace the venous drainage from the teeth and oral cavity back to the heart
- To define hematoma
- To discuss the possible problems associated with a posterior superior alveolar injection

Within the head and neck are many blood vessels, each with numerous branches. In this chapter we concentrate on those vessels that supply and drain the teeth and oral cavity. We start with the heart and trace the blood up into the head and neck and then back down to the heart again.

ARTERIAL SUPPLY

Blood leaves the heart through the **pulmonary artery** and travels to the lungs to pick up fresh oxygen. It returns to the heart through the **pulmonary veins** and then leaves the heart again by way of the **aorta.** The pathways to the right and left sides of the head and neck are slightly different. On the right side the **brachiocephalic artery** (*brachio-*, 'arm'; *cephalic,* 'head') branches off the aorta.

Common Carotid Artery

Coming off the brachiocephalic is the **common carotid artery.** On the left side the common carotid artery branches directly off the aorta. In the neck, on both sides, this artery lies beneath the sternomastoid muscle, which runs along the side of the neck. At about the level of the larynx, the common carotid divides into the **external carotid** and the **internal carotid arteries.**

The internal carotid artery has no branches in the neck region but goes upward to enter the skull. Only when inside the skull does it branch to supply the eye, the brain, and the coverings of the brain (Fig. 17-1).

The external carotid artery has a number of branches in the neck, as shown in Figs. 17-1 and 17-2, but we will consider only the **facial, lingual,** and **maxillary arteries.**

Facial artery. The facial artery ascends the side of the neck, runs deep to the submandibular gland, and crosses the lower border of the mandible just in front of the angle of the mandible. (You can feel a small depression on the lower border of the mandible at this point.) After crossing the mandible, the artery travels across the face, ending near the inner corner of the eye. On its way it supplies the skin and muscles of facial expression.

Lingual artery. The lingual artery branches off the external carotid artery below the facial artery. The lingual artery then travels forward and deeper, going beneath some of the extrinsic, or external, muscles of the tongue and ending as it enters the tongue on its inferior surface. It supplies the tongue and the tissue in the floor of the oral cavity. If you have ever cut your tongue, you realize that there is an extremely well-developed blood supply within this tissue. This is completely supplied by the lingual artery (Fig. 17-3).

Maxillary artery. The maxillary artery is also a

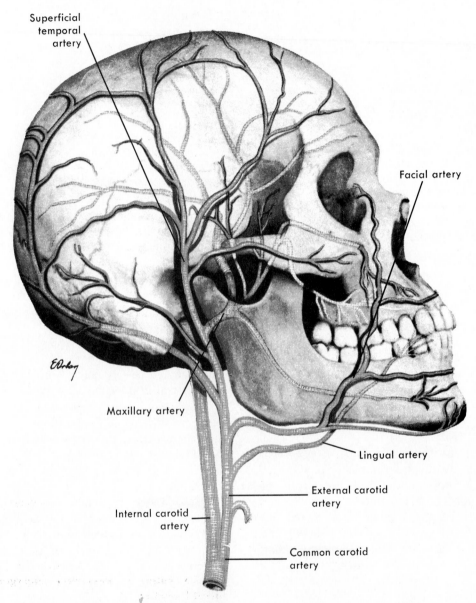

Fig. 17-1 General distribution of arteries from lower part of neck up through skull area. (DuBrul.)

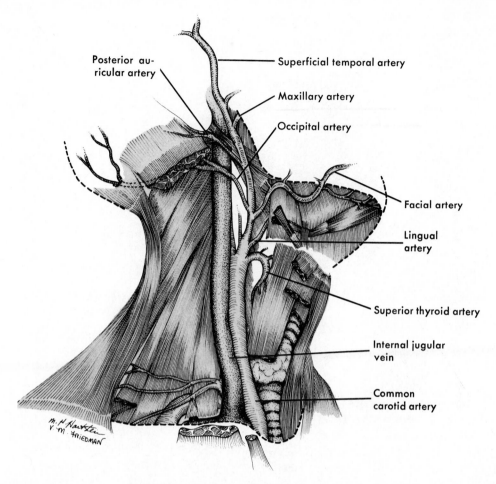

Posterior au-
ricular artery

Superficial temporal artery

Maxillary artery

Occipital artery

Facial artery

Lingual
artery

Superior thyroid artery

Internal jugular
vein

Common
carotid artery

m. H. Hawlstin
v. m. Friedman

Fig. 17-2   Branches of external carotid artery.

branch of the external carotid artery. It diverges from the vessel at the level of the neck of the condyle on its deep surface. There are about 15 branches of this artery; we will be concerned with a little more than half of them. In general, this artery supplies the muscles of mastication, the teeth, the oral and nasal cavities, and several smaller areas.

From its beginning, where it branches off the external carotid artery, the maxillary artery runs forward in an area known as the **infratemporal fossa,** where it crosses the surface of the lateral

pterygoid muscle to enter the **pterygopalatine fossa,** behind and below the eye.

INFRATEMPORAL FOSSA BRANCHES. The more important branches of the maxillary artery in the infratemporal fossa are the **inferior alveolar, mental, temporal, masseteric, pterygoid** and **buccal branches** (Fig. 17-4).

Inferior alveolar branch. The inferior alveolar branch runs downward to enter the mandibular foramen and run into the mandibular canal. It sends off branches into each of the mandibular teeth and into the bone. In the premolar region

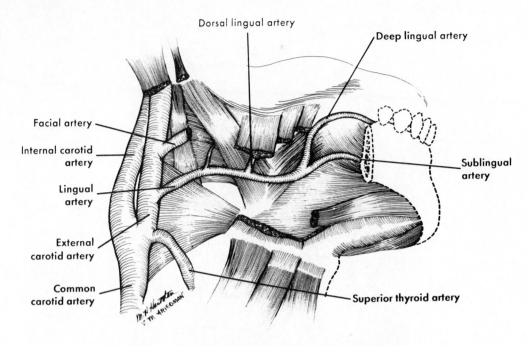

Fig. 17-3 Branches of lingual artery that supply tongue.

the inferior alveolar artery sends off a small branch called the **mental artery,** which exits from the mandible through the mental foramen. It supplies the buccal gingiva and mucosa from the premolars to the incisors and also supplies the mucosa of the lower lip.

Temporal branches. Two temporal branches arise from the maxillary artery to supply the temporal muscle. There is an anterior and a posterior deep temporal artery.

Masseteric branch. The masseteric branch comes off the maxillary artery and runs laterally through the coronoid notch, entering the deep surface of the masseter muscle to supply it with blood.

Pterygoid branches. There may be one or more pterygoid branches, which extend to the medial and lateral pterygoid muscles. Their course and direction vary.

Buccal branch. The buccal branch runs downward and forward to supply the mucosa of the cheek and the buccal mucosa and gingiva of maxillary and mandibular posterior teeth (Fig. 17-4).

PTERYGOPALATINE FOSSA BRANCHES. At this point the maxillary artery reaches the pterygopalatine fossa, at the back of and slightly below the orbital cavity. From here branches divide into five general directions: backward to the nasal pharynx, down to the palate, medially into the nasal cavity and eventually to the anterior palatal area, laterally to the maxillary tuberosity, and forward onto the infraorbital area of the face (Figs. 17-4 and 17-5).

Descending palatine artery. The **descending palatine artery** extends downward from the maxillary artery to the posterior hard palate through the pterygopalatine canal. There it splits into two branches: the **lesser palatine artery,** which supplies the soft palate, and the **greater palatine artery,** which travels forward along the lateral part of the hard palate to supply the palatal mucosa

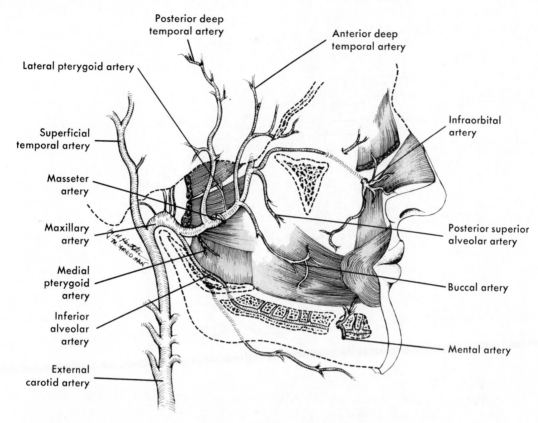

Fig. 17-4   Cutaway section showing origin of maxillary artery from external carotid artery just medial to what would be neck of condyle. Most branches of maxillary artery can be seen.

and maxillary lingual gingiva. These vessels emerge onto the palatal area through the lesser and greater palatine foramina (Fig. 17-5).

Posterior superior alveolar artery. The **posterior superior alveolar artery** comes out of the pterygopalatine fossa through the pterygomaxillary fissure, descends onto the maxillary tuberosity, and enters the bone behind the third molar. From there it supplies blood to all the maxillary posterior teeth (Figs. 17-4 and 17-6).

Pterygopalatine (sphenopalatine) artery. The **pterygopalatine (sphenopalatine) artery** comes off the maxillary artery and runs medially

through the pterygopalatine foramen into the nasal cavity, supplying most parts of the nasal cavity. It finally emerges from the incisive foramen to anastomose (join) with the greater palatine artery (Fig. 17-5).

Infraorbital artery. The **infraorbital artery** is the end part of the maxillary artery. From its location in the floor of the orbital cavity it sends a branch, the **anterior superior alveolar artery,** downward into the wall of the maxillary sinus, supplying the maxillary anterior teeth. It also anastomoses with the posterior superior alveolar artery in the wall of the sinus. The remainder of the infraorbital ar-

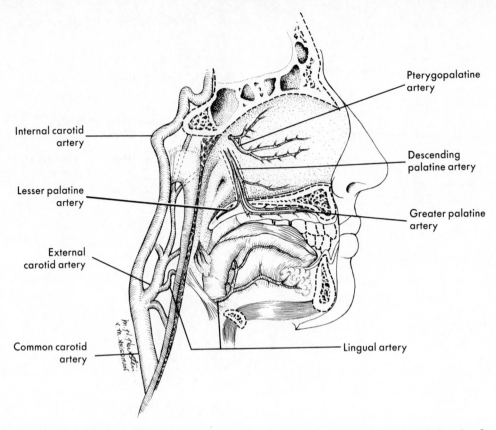

Fig. 17-5 Section of lateral part of hard palate, showing blood supply to hard and soft palates and nasal cavity area.

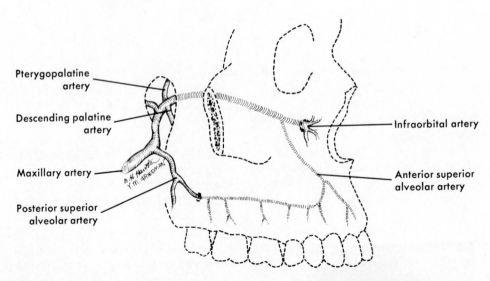

Fig. 17-6 Infraorbital artery extending across floor of orbit, with anterior superior alveolar artery branching off and supplying anterior teeth and possibly premolars. Anterior and posterior superior alveolar arteries join, or anastomose, with one another.

tery emerges through the infraorbital foramen onto the face and supplies the upper lip and its mucosa, labial gingiva, lower eyelid, and side of the nose (Figs. 17-4 and 17-6).

■ ■ ■

You should at this time be able to name the blood supply sources for all teeth and all tissues of the oral cavity. The supply to the teeth is easy,

but the maxillary and mandibular buccal and lingual gingivae, the palate, the floor of mouth, and the cheek may be more difficult.

VENOUS DRAINAGE

Now that we have considered how blood reaches the head and neck, and in particular the oral cavity, we will examine the return of the blood to the heart. In general, it can be said that

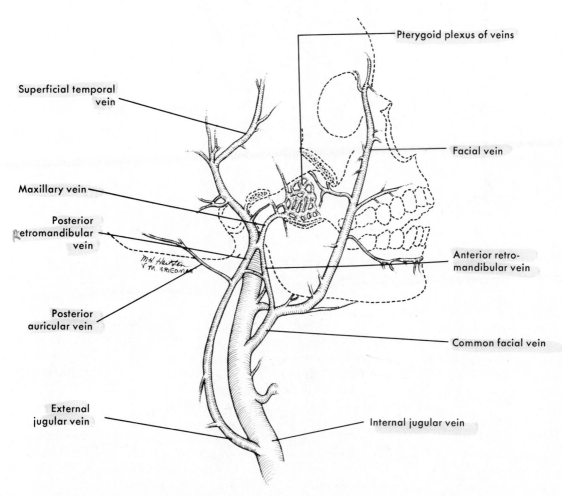

Fig. 17-7 General drainage areas of internal and external jugular veins. Retromandibular vein connects internal and external jugular veins and distributes blood between them.

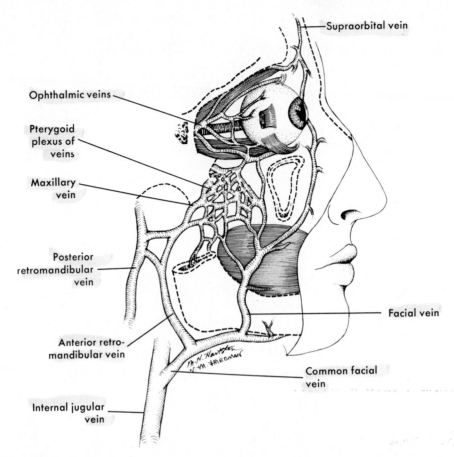

Fig. 17-8 Pterygoid plexus of veins just behind maxillary tuberosity. It may be injured during injection of that area of maxillary molars.

veins follow the same pathways as arteries do and that in most instances they have the same names. For this reason the majority of anatomical texts devote most of the discussion to the blood supply, or arteries, and spend less time on the veins.

Jugular Veins

In the head and neck the names of the veins vary little from those of the arteries. Instead of internal and external carotid veins, they are designated the **internal** and **external jugular veins.** The internal jugular vein drains the entire brain area and passes out of the skull through the jugular foramen. The internal jugular, in general, drains much of the area in front of the ear to the front of the face through veins that correspond to arteries, for example, the facial, lingual, and superficial temporal. The external jugular vein drains the area behind the ear, as well as some flow from the posterior **retromandibular vein** (*retro*, 'behind'). The anterior retromandibular vein joins with the facial vein forming the common facial vein, which enters the internal jugular vein (Figs. 17-7 and 17-8).

One other structure is seen in the area of the

maxillary vein just posterior to the tuberosity of the maxilla. There is an intertwining network of veins known as the **pterygoid plexus of veins.** These veins are so close to the maxillary tuberosity that there is the possibility of piercing them while performing a posterior superior alveolar nerve block if the angulation of the needle is not correct. When this happens, blood escapes into the tissue spaces and a **hematoma** occurs. This is a swelling and discoloration of the area and tends to upset the patient (Figs. 17-7 and 17-8).

Another point of interest is the area at the bridge of the nose, near the inner corner of the eye. Untreated infections in this area may tend to spread through the veins, into a venous sinus, or space, near the base of the brain where the infection may remain and stagnate. This can cause serious damage if left untreated and may even cause death.

The internal jugular and external jugular veins join together and eventually merge with the **subclavian vein** from the arm to form the **brachiocephalic vein.** This vein flows into the **superior vena cava** and on into the heart. The circle for the head and neck is then complete, and the blood can flow out to the lungs again.

REVIEW QUESTIONS

1. How does blood get from the heart into the head and neck? *Brachio cephalic + carotid art.*
2. What are the two divisions of the common carotid artery? *internal + external*
3. Which two branches of the external carotid artery supply all the teeth and oral cavity?
4. Where does the blood supply to the muscles of mastication originate?
5. Name the individual vessels that supply all areas of the oral cavity.
6. What is the major vein that drains most of the head and neck? *internal juglar vein*
7. What is the pterygoid plexus of veins and what is its significance?
8. Trace the blood from the neck to the heart by way of the veins.

3. *lingual + maxillary art. supplies the teeth + oral cavity*

4. *muscles of mastication are supplied by the max. branch of the external carotid artery.*

7. *pterygoid plexus is an intertwining network of veins near the max. tuberosity.*

5. *vessels that supply all areas of oral cavity - lingual, maxillary, inferior alveolar branch, mental, buccal, descending palatine, posterior superior alveolar, pterygoid palatine, anterior superior alveolar,*

8. *internal + external juglar veins merge w/ subclavian vein to form the brachiocephalic vein which flows into superior vena cava + into the heart*

18

Salivary Glands

OBJECTIVES

- To describe the difference between major and minor salivary glands
- To name and locate each of the major and minor glands
- To classify each of the glands according to its type of secretion

As you may recall from Chapter 2, the glands of the body are classified in a number of ways. Salivary glands are classed as exocrine, merocrine, compound tubuloalveolar, serous, mixed, or mucous. They are also divided into major salivary glands, which are the three pairs of large glands, and minor salivary glands, which are found throughout the oral cavity.

MAJOR SALIVARY GLANDS

The major salivary glands are three pairs of glands that produce the bulk of the fluid in the mouth. This is saliva, which is mixed with food to make it easy to swallow. It should be pointed out that this saliva begins to break down starches into smaller carbohydrate units. Further food breakdown takes place in the stomach. The three gland pairs are the parotid, the submandibular, and the sublingual.

Parotid Gland

The **parotid gland** is located on the side of the face near the ear and behind the ramus of the mandible (Chapter 11). It is composed of many grapelike clusters of cells, which secrete into a system of tubes leading to the oral cavity. If you look at the cells of the secretory part of the gland through a microscope, you will see that the cells are all of the same type. They produce a very thin watery secretion referred to as serous secretion. Although these glands are quite large, the pair of them produce only about 25% of the total resting salivary volume. Fig. 18-1 shows the location of the gland. You can see that the duct leading from the gland travels anteriorly across the masseter muscle (Chapter 13) and pierces the buccinator muscle (Chapter 15) to open into the oral cavity opposite the maxillary second molar. Mumps is a virus infection of the parotid gland, causing pain when the gland secretes. Thus eating at this time is sometimes quite painful because it causes stimulation of the gland. Stenson's Duct

Submandibular (Submaxillary) Gland

The **submandibular gland** provides about 60% to 65% of the total resting salivary volume. It is called a mixed gland, since it has serous and mucous cells in it. Mucous secretion is thicker and stickier than is serous, and although almost two thirds of the cells are serous, the mucus component makes it a slightly more viscous secretion. The gland is located below and toward the posterior part of the **body of the mandible** (Chapter 11). Place your finger on the **inferior border of the mandible** and run it back toward the **angle of the mandible** (Chapter 11). As you near the angle, you will feel a slight depression in the inferior border. If you move your finger medially from that point, you will feel a lump in the neck.

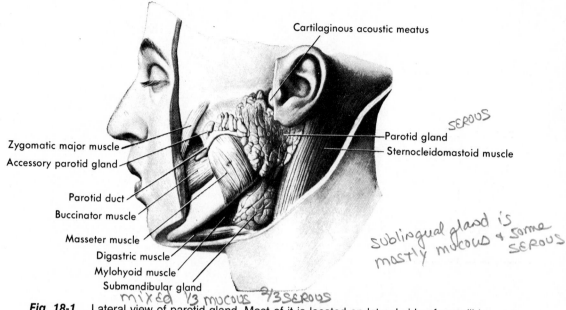

Handwritten annotations: SEROUS (pointing to Parotid gland); sublingual gland is mostly mucous & some SEROUS; mixed 1/3 mucous 2/3 SEROUS

Fig. 18-1   Lateral view of parotid gland. Most of it is located on lateral side of mandible and masseter muscle, wrapping around back of mandible also. Duct pierces buccinator muscle as it opens into oral cavity. (Sicher and DuBrul.)

That is the submandibular gland. The gland is wrapped around a muscle in the neck, known as the mylohyoid muscle (Chapter 13). Part of the gland lies on the more superficial side, and part of it lies on the deep side of the muscle in the posterior and lateral floor of the mouth. The duct extends from the deep part of the gland and runs forward in the floor of the mouth to open onto a small elevation called the sublingual caruncle. This is located at the base of the lingual frenum, the fold of tissue that attaches the tongue to the floor of the mouth (Figs. 18-2 and 18-3).

Sublingual Gland

The **sublingual gland** is the smallest of the three pairs of glands and contributes only 10% of total salivary volume. It is composed of mostly mucous cells with some serous cells; therefore the secretion of this gland tends to be slightly

Handwritten annotation: wharton's duct

more viscous than that of the submandibular gland. It is located in the anterior floor of the mouth next to the mandibular canines. It has one major duct which opens with the submandibular duct, and several smaller ducts, which open in a line along the fold of tissue beneath the tongue, known as the sublingual fold (Figs. 18-2 and 18-3).

All of these glands should be palpated in intraoral and extraoral examinations of the patient. Any enlargement of these glands should be further investigated. Sometimes, when a patient has lost all the teeth and there has been a loss of most of the mandibular ridge of bone, the sublingual gland will appear to bulge up into the floor of the mouth when the mouth is opened wide. This is not too unusual and is no cause for alarm, as long as the new denture replacing those teeth does not press on the gland.

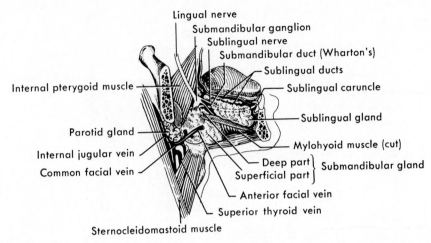

Fig. 18-2 Submandibular gland has superficial part that can be palpated and deep part from which duct runs forward to sublingual caruncle. *Dotted line,* Path of duct. (Pansky and House.)

MINOR SALIVARY GLANDS

The minor salivary glands have a similar structure but are much smaller. One could compare the major and minor glands to a very large bunch of grapes and a much smaller bunch of grapes. The primary differences are size, the number of secretory units or acini, and the number of ducts. The function of the minor glands is not really to produce saliva for mixing with food in the beginning digestive process, but to secrete minor amounts of saliva onto the surface to keep the mucosa moist. Some of these glands are pure serous cells, most are pure mucous cells, and the rest of them are mixed but mostly mucous. They do not have a long duct system; thus there are many clusters of these throughout the mouth, each with its own duct opening. They are located labially, buccally, palatally, glossopalatally, and lingually.

Labial Glands

In the upper and lower lips, opening onto the inner surface, are the **labial glands.** These are mixed glands, mostly mucous. You can see them in a mirror by pulling the lip outward and looking at its inner surface, where they are present beneath the epithelium. This is also a good place to see the distribution of duct openings. Try the following: gently pull your lower lip outward while standing in front of a mirror. Dry off the inner surface with a tissue. Now pull the lip tight and watch for tiny drops of moisture to appear on the lip surface. These drops indicate the location of the labial gland ducts.

Buccal Glands

On the inner cheek region are the **buccal glands.** They are generally considered to be similar to the labial glands, differing only in location.

Palatine Glands

Located in the soft palate and in the posterior and lateral parts of the hard palate are the **palatine glands.** They are pure mucous glands in nature. Since there are no minor salivary glands in the anterior part of the hard palate to keep it moist, it might be assumed that the drying effect tends to cause the epithelium to be more kerati-

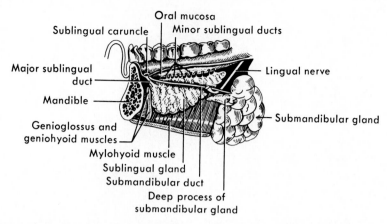

Fig. 18-3 Sublingual gland is just lingual to mandibular canine. Also major duct joins with submandibular and many minor ducts open into sublingual fold. (Pansky and House.)

nized, and this is generally the case. The anterior portion of the hard palate tends to be more keratinized.

Glossopalatine Glands

Continuing from the posterior lateral parts of the palate down into the anterior fold of tissue in front of the palatine tonsil, you will find the **glossopalatine glands.** These are also pure mucous glands.

Lingual Glands

The **lingual glands** are divided into several groups.

Anterior lingual glands. These glands are found near the tip of the tongue and open onto the under, or ventral, surface. They are mostly mucous in nature.

Lingual glands of von Ebner. Lingual **glands of von Ebner** are pure serous glands located beneath the vallate papillae and open into the trough around the gland. These glands function to wash off the taste buds so that they can perceive new tastes.

Posterior lingual glands. These glands are located around the lingual tonsils on the posterior third of the tongue. They are pure mucous glands in nature.

■　■　■

All these glands, whether major or minor, are controlled by the **autonomic,** or automatic, **nervous system.** To be specific the **parasympathetic** part of this system is the main stimulus for salivation. The smell of food or the presence of something in the mouth will start the glands secreting. It does not necessarily have to be a pleasant taste to do this. You can chew on plain paraffin and cause secretion. There are a number of medications that can cause overstimulation or understimulation of these glands, and a history of the patient's medications will help you understand why there may be more or less saliva in the mouth. You should also realize that "normal" amounts of saliva vary considerably from one person to another.

REVIEW QUESTIONS

1. What are the major salivary glands, and where do their ducts open? What is their function?
2. What are the minor salivary glands, and where do their ducts open? What is their function?

19

Nervous System

OBJECTIVES

- To name the basic components of the nervous system
- To describe how a sensory impulse causes a motor response
- To name the twelve cranial nerves and their general function
- To describe the components and general function of the autonomic nervous system
- To name the specific branches of the trigeminal nerve and which areas of the teeth and oral cavity each supplies
- To describe the nerves and areas involved in general and special sensation of the tongue
- To discuss the nerves and pathways involved in the parasympathetic supply to major salivary glands

The nervous system has many functions that it performs routinely. It relays messages from distant parts of the body, which let the brain know exactly what is happening in each part. The brain may file the information in its memory for future reference. The brain coordinates and sends out messages that cause muscles to contract, stimulates glands to secrete, regulates numerous functions, and performs many of these tasks without true consciousness on our part. To accomplish all this, the nervous system has to have tremendous organization and potential. It has both. Some authorities have theorized that we normally use only 10% of our mental capacity. There are clearly more cells in the brain than we could ever use, and sometimes when there is brain damage these unused cells can be called on to replace the damaged ones.

The nervous system is divided into two major categories: the **central nervous system,** consisting of the brain and spinal cord, and the **peripheral nervous system,** which comprises all nerves that extend outward from the brain or spinal cord (Fig. 19-1).

Remember from Chapter 2 that a neuron or group of neurons transmits a message or impulse in only one direction. It is necessary to have both sensory and motor nerves, or more accurately, both sensory and motor neurons. In most instances, whenever you see a nerve or a drawing of a nerve, it represents a bundle of neurons, some of which are sensory and some motor. These are what enable a nerve to carry messages to and from the brain.

CENTRAL NERVOUS SYSTEM

The brain and spinal cord are made up of neurons that are either motor or sensory, but they are only part of the chain. Imagine you have caught your finger in a desk drawer. You feel pain and quickly pull your finger out of the drawer, probably shaking it. This is what has happened neurologically. A pain receptor, or free nerve ending, in the finger picks up the message and carries it back to the spinal cord. A second neuron carries the message up the spinal cord to the lower parts of the brain, and a third neuron takes it to the surface of the brain, where it is recognized as pain. The pain is interpreted by the brain, and past experience tells the brain to

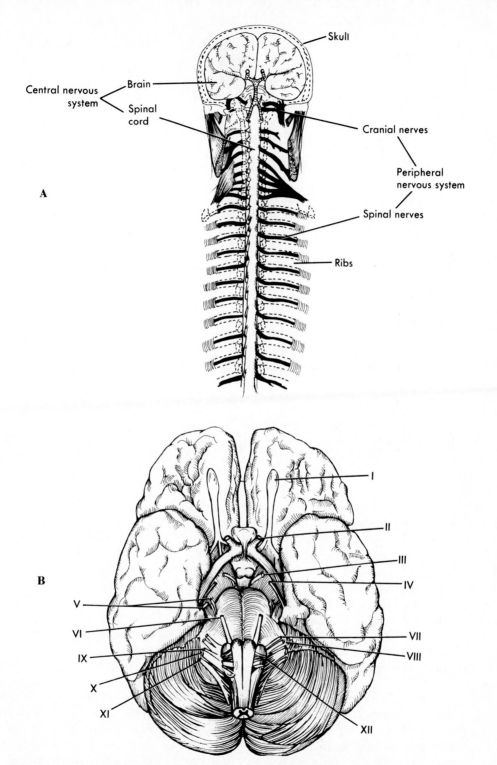

Fig. 19-1 **A,** Central nervous system (brain and spinal cord) and spinal segments and a few cranial nerves of peripheral nervous system. **B,** Inferior view of brain showing origin of 12 pairs of cranial nerves. (Redrawn after Goss.)

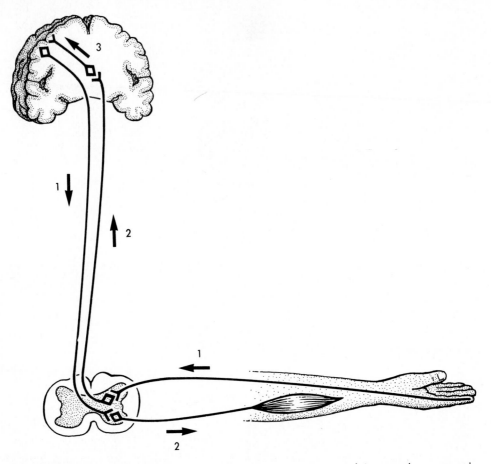

Fig. 19-2 Multiple neurons at various levels necessary to complete conscious sensori-motor reaction.

remove the finger from the drawer so that it will no longer be crushed. A motor message then leaves the brain and goes down the spinal cord; a second motor neuron will carry the message out of the spinal cord along a peripheral nerve to muscles that cause the finger to be pulled out of the drawer (Fig. 19-2).

The nervous system also builds in a shortcut to this system known as a **reflex arc.** This shortcut takes place in the spinal cord between the sensory nerve as it enters the spinal cord. This neuron has a shorter neuron that runs between it and the motor nerve leaving the spinal cord, and

it can actually accomplish the action without the person thinking about it, or more properly, before thinking about it. Touch a hot stove and what happens? You pull your hand away before you actually realize it is hot or before you consciously tell yourself to remove your hand from the stove (Fig. 19-3).

As you can see from this discussion, the brain and spinal cord are only a part of this chain. The spinal cord and brain are the center of nervous activity, but they cannot perform alone. They need the contributions of the peripheral nervous system.

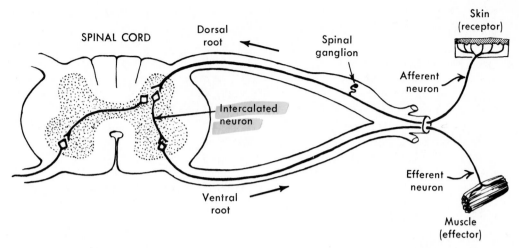

Fig. 19-3   Reflex arc. Message travels into spinal cord and out again without reaching brain. (Chusid and McDonald.)

PERIPHERAL NERVOUS SYSTEM

The peripheral nervous system is traditionally grouped into three components: **spinal nerves, cranial nerves,** and the **autonomic nervous system.** These will be examined individually.

Spinal Nerves

The spinal nerves extend from the spinal cord to distant parts of the body. These nerves generally have both motor and sensory neurons in them. There are 31 pairs of spinal nerves: 8 in the **cervical,** or neck, region; 12 in the **thorax,** or chest, region; 5 in the **lumbar,** or lower back, region; 5 in the **sacral,** or hip, region; and 1 in the **coccygeal,** or tailbone, region (Fig. 19- 4). These nerves are distributed by region from the neck to the toes. Several of the cervical nerves innervate some of the hyoid muscles that depress the mandible and raise the larynx.

Cranial Nerves

The cranial nerves attach directly to the brain. There are 12 pairs of these nerves, and we begin by listing them and briefly describing their general function. A later discussion centers on sev-

eral of these nerves. When referring to these nerves, it is proper to use roman numerals.

I, olfactory nerve. Sensory: provides special sense of smell from the nose to the brain.

II, optic nerve. Sensory: provides special sense of sight from the eye to the brain.

III, oculomotor nerve. Motor: supplies some of the muscles that move the eye in different directions.

IV, trochlear nerve. Motor: supplies one of the muscles that moves the eye.

V, trigeminal nerve. Motor and sensory: sensory from all the teeth and oral cavity, as well as most of the skin of the front part of the face and head; also motor to the muscles of mastication and part of soft-palate muscles; the most important nerve for our consideration and to be covered in greater detail later.

VI, abducens nerve. Motor: supplies one of the muscles that moves the eye.

VII, facial nerve. Motor and sensory: motor to the muscles of facial expression and salivary glands (autonomic); sensory from some areas behind the ear, and taste from the anterior two thirds of the tongue.

VIII, statoacoustic nerve. Sensory: for hearing and balance **(equilibrium).**

IX, glossopharyngeal nerve. Motor and sensory: motor to one of the muscles of the soft palate and the **pharynx** (throat), as well as salivary glands; sensory to the posterior one third of tongue for taste, as well as general sensation such as pain, pressure, heat, cold.

X, vagus nerve. Motor and sensory: motor to the muscles of the pharynx and **larynx,** most of the muscles of the soft palate, most of the smooth muscle of the body, cardiac muscle, and many of the glands; sensory from the skin around the ear and taste sensation from the root of the tongue.

XI, accessory nerve. Motor: supplies the **trapezius muscle** and sternomastoid muscle in the neck; some parts of this nerve run with the vagus nerve and supply most of the soft palate, larynx, and pharynx muscles.

XII, hypoglossal nerve. Motor: supplies most of the muscles of the tongue.

Before we continue with a more detailed description of some of these cranial nerves, a brief discussion of the autonomic nervous system and its function is necessary. This system is also called the automatic nervous system because it is not willfully controlled. The system has motor and sensory fibers. The motor fibers supply smooth and cardiac muscle and glands, and the sensory part carries what is called **visceral** sensation. This is sensation from the various viscera, or organs, of the body.

Autonomic Nervous System

The autonomic system has two parts: the **sympathetic system,** also known as the **thoracolumbar outflow,** and the parasympathetic system, also known as the **craniosacral outflow.** Each of these components innervates all parts of the body, and therefore each organ generally has a sympathetic and a parasympathetic nerve supply. These are **antagonistic** systems, which means they tend to have opposite actions.

Consider the action of the heart. If someone frightens you, the sympathetic nervous system is stimulated and you would find that the following things happen: your heart beats very fast and strong; you become pale and your skin feels cold and "clammy" from shutdown of the surface capillaries; and you feel a "knot" in your stomach from the shutdown of the blood supply to the digestive tract. All of this blood is being shunted to the skeletal muscles of the body; the heart is beating faster and pushing more blood to the lungs for oxygenation and then to the muscles for additional energy. Your body is also releasing a drug called epinephrine (adrenaline), which creates all these actions to help the body meet a stressful situation. You will also find that your mouth becomes dry from shutdown of salivary glands. This is referred to as the "fight or flight" mechanism.

Stimulation of the parasympathetic nervous system and the resultant actions tends to be the opposite of those of the sympathetic nervous system. It is referred to as the "vegetative system" because it relates to the process of digestion. Stimulation of this system slows down the heart and respiration, increases blood to the digestive system, and stimulates secretion of the glands of the body, including the salivary glands.

Where do the terms "craniosacral" and "thoracolumbar" come from? Parasympathetic fibers come off the brain with nerves III, VII, IX, and X and off the spinal cord at the sacral levels (S2 to S4), therefore the name "craniosacral." The sympathetic system comes off the spinal cord at the 12 thoracic levels (T1 to T12) and the first 2 lumbar levels (L1 and L2), therefore the name "thoracolumbar outflow." No attempt will be made to describe how they distribute their fibers to various parts of the body, except to the salivary gland supply (Fig. 19-5).

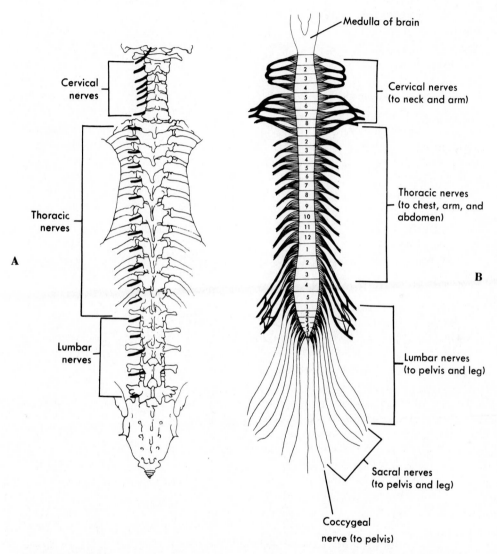

- Medulla of brain

Cervical nerves

Cervical nerves (to neck and arm)

Thoracic nerves

Thoracic nerves (to chest, arm, and abdomen)

Lumbar nerves

Lumbar nerves (to pelvis and leg)

Sacral nerves (to pelvis and leg)

Coccygeal nerve (to pelvis)

A

B

Fig. 19-4   **A,** Some spinal nerves as they emerge from vertebral column. **B,** General arrangement of spinal nerves as they are grouped by regions. (Redrawn after Chusid and McDonald.)

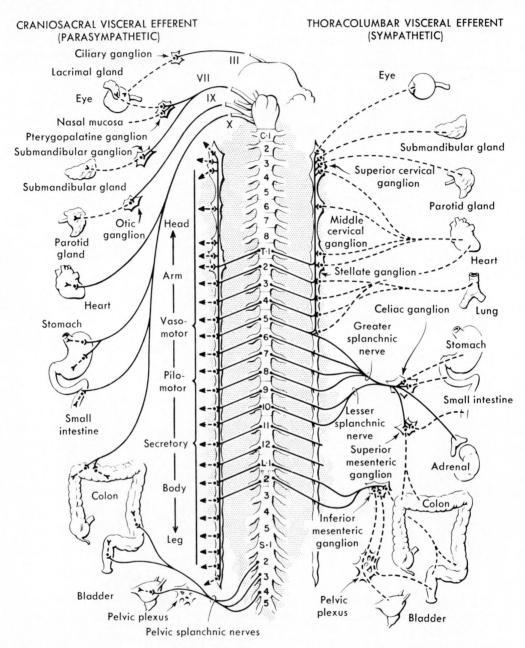

CRANIOSACRAL VISCERAL EFFERENT
(PARASYMPATHETIC)

THORACOLUMBAR VISCERAL EFFERENT
(SYMPATHETIC)

Ciliary ganglion
III
Lacrimal gland
VII
Eye
IX
Nasal mucosa
Pterygopalatine ganglion
X
Submandibular ganglion
Submandibular gland
Otic ganglion
Parotid gland
Heart
Stomach
Small intestine
Secretory
Colon
Bladder
Pelvic plexus
Pelvic splanchnic nerves

Head
Arm
Vaso-motor
Pilo-motor
Body
Leg

Eye
Submandibular gland
Superior cervical ganglion
Parotid gland
Middle cervical ganglion
Heart
Stellate ganglion
Celiac ganglion
Lung
Greater splanchnic nerve
Stomach
Lesser splanchnic nerve
Small intestine
Superior mesenteric ganglion
Adrenal
Inferior mesenteric ganglion
Colon
Pelvic plexus
Bladder

Fig. 19-5 Various levels of origin of autonomic nervous system and some of areas it supplies. (Sections of Neurology.)

NERVES TO ORAL CAVITY AND ASSOCIATED STRUCTURES

Now we consider in greater detail several of the cranial nerves and the parasympathetic functions for those that have them.

Trigeminal Nerve (Cranial Nerve V)

The trigeminal nerve has three separate main branches, or divisions, usually denoted as the **ophthalmic division (V_1), maxillary division (V_2),** and **mandibular division (V_3).** One of the overall functions of these three divisions is the innervation of the skin of the anterior face and head region. Fig. 19-6 shows where each of these three divisions supplies the face.

Ophthalmic division (V_1). The ophthalmic division leaves the skull through the superior orbital fissure and enters the orbital cavity. One of the major branches is the supraorbital nerve, which emerges through the supraorbital notch, or foramen, and supplies the skin above the eye and up into the forehead (Fig. 19-7).

Maxillary division (V_2). The maxillary division exits from the skull through the foramen rotundum and lies in the pterygopalatine fossa behind and below the eye. The branches follow the same kind of distribution pattern as the maxillary artery does, that is, to the upper teeth and oral cavity. They have basically the same names and pathways as the arterial supply to that area does. Thus you have some idea of their distribution. In the pterygopalatine fossa the maxillary division divides into the following four larger branches. It should also be pointed out that the first two divisions of the trigeminal nerve are purely sensory and not motor.

POSTERIOR SUPERIOR ALVEOLAR NERVE. The **posterior superior alveolar nerve** emerges from the pterygopalatine fossa and travels along the posterior portion of the maxillary tuberosity. It supplies the maxillary buccal gingiva of premolars and molars. It then enters the bone to supply the second and third maxillary molars and usually the distobuccal and lingual roots of the first

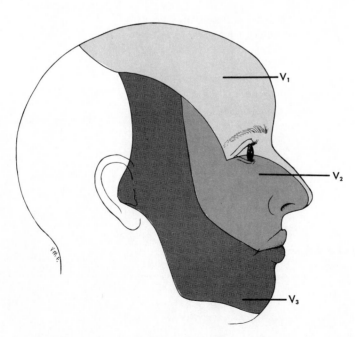

Fig. 19-6   Areas of distribution on facial skin of three divisions of trigeminal nerve.

Nerve supply of oral cavity

Nerve	Mucosa	Teeth	Sinus
Maxillary division (V$_2$)			
Posterior superior alveolar	Buccal; maxillary gingiva	Maxillary molars	Maxillary sinus
Middle superior alveolar	—	Maxillary premolars and mesiobuccal root of first molar	Maxillary sinus
Anterior superior alveolar	Labial gingiva of maxilla	Maxillary anteriors	—
Infraorbital (superior labial)	Labial gingiva of maxilla	—	—
Nasopalatine	Lingual gingiva of maxillary incisors	—	—
Descending palatine			
Greater palatine	All hard palate except lingual gingiva of maxillary incisors	—	—
Lesser palatine	Soft palate	—	—
Mandibular division (V$_3$)			
Inferior alveolar	—	All mandibular teeth	—
Mental	Facial gingivae from mandibular premolar to central incisor, mucosa and skin of lower lip	—	—
Lingual	All mandibular lingual gingivae, floor of mouth, and anterior two thirds of tongue	—	—
Buccal	Cheek and mandibular buccal gingivae from first premolar on back	—	—
Facial nerve (VII)			
Chorda tympani	Taste in anterior two thirds of tongue	—	—
Glossopharyngeal nerve (IX)	Taste and sensation to posterior third of tongue	—	—

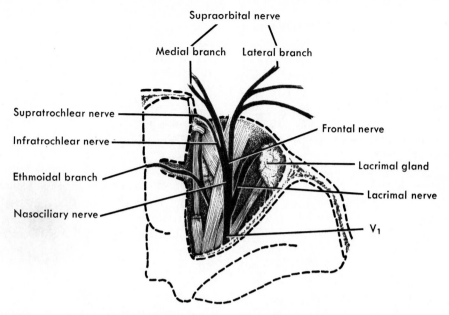

Fig. 19-7 Supraorbital nerve of first division of trigeminal nerve as it comes out through supraorbital notch to supply skin of forehead.

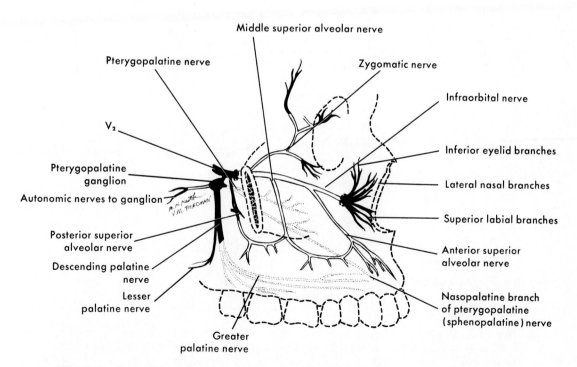

Fig. 19-8 General distribution of maxillary division of trigeminal nerve. Posterior superior alveolar nerve can be seen coming off main trunk of V_2, and middle and anterior superior alveolar nerves can be seen coming off infraorbital nerve.

maxillary molar. It also supplies part of the maxillary sinus (Fig. 19-8).

PTERYGOPALATINE (SPHENOPALATINE) NERVE. The **pterygopalatine (sphenopalatine) nerve** branch comes off the maxillary division, goes through the pterygopalatine foramen, and supplies the nasal cavity. It leaves that cavity through the incisive foramen as the **nasopalatine nerve** in the anterior palate, where it supplies the lingual gingiva just adjacent to the maxillary central and lateral incisors (Fig. 19-9).

DESCENDING PALATINE NERVE. The **descending palatine nerve** runs off the maxillary division straight downward to the posterior part of the hard palate. There it separates into two branches: the **lesser palatine nerve,** which supplies the soft palate, and the **greater palatine nerve,** which supplies all the mucosa of the hard palate except the small area supplied by the nasopalatine branch of the pterygopalatine nerve. The greater palatine nerve extends along the lateral portion of the hard palate; the greater and lesser palatine nerves enter the palatal areas through the greater and lesser palatine foramina (Figs. 19-8 and 19-10).

INFRAORBITAL NERVE. The **infraorbital nerve** runs forward in the floor of the orbit to exit onto the face through the infraorbital foramen. It supplies the skin of the nose, lower eyelid, skin and mucosa of the upper lip, and the maxillary labial gingiva. While in the floor of the orbit, it sends two branches downward to supply the rest of the maxillary teeth. The first branch to come off as the nerve travels forward is the **middle superior alveolar nerve,** which lies in the wall of the sinus to supply the premolars and usually the mesiobuccal root of the maxillary first molar. This nerve also supplies part of the maxillary sinus. The **anterior superior alveolar nerve** extends downward anterior to the wall of the sinus to supply the maxillary anterior teeth (Fig. 19-8).

There are other branches of the maxillary division, but none that supplies the oral cavity.

Mandibular division (V$_3$). The mandibular division, or nerve, leaves the skull through the foramen ovale, traveling downward. As it leaves the skull, it is located in the area known as the infratemporal fossa, adjacent to the pterygoid muscles of mastication. It then breaks up into a number of branches. There are about five motor

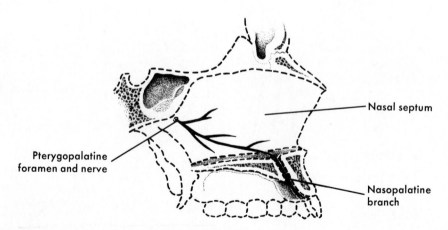

Nasal septum

Pterygopalatine foramen and nerve

Nasopalatine branch

Fig. 19-9 Pterygopalatine (sphenopalatine) nerve enters nasal cavity and one branch, nasopalatine, goes down nasal septum and out through incisive foramen to anterior palatal mucosa.

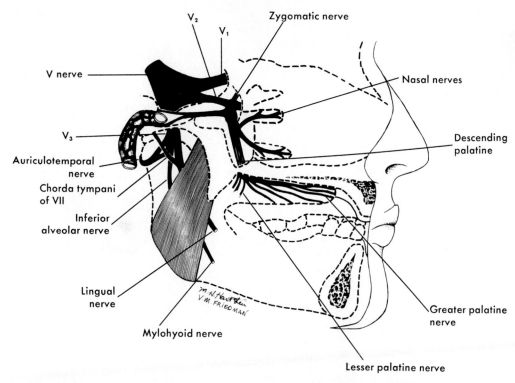

Fig. 19-10   Partial diagram of V₂ and V₃. Notice descending palatine nerve and its greater and lesser palatine branches going to hard and soft palates, respectively.

nerves for the muscles of mastication: two to the temporal and one each to the masseter, medial, and lateral pterygoids. There is a sensory nerve that runs backward to supply the area above and in front of the ear. This is called the **auriculotemporal nerve** (Figs. 19-10 and 19-11). There are also the buccal, lingual, and inferior alveolar nerves.

BUCCAL NERVE. The **buccal nerve** spreads out on the surface of the buccinator muscle and then penetrates the muscle. The lowest of its branches is frequently referred to as the **long buccal nerve** and lies in the posterior portion of the mandibular mucobuccal fold. There it supplies the buccal mandibular gingivae up to the mental foramen. The remainder of the buccal nerve supplies the

skin and mucosa of the cheek and most of the maxillary buccal gingivae (Fig. 19-11).

LINGUAL NERVE. The **lingual nerve** is one of the largest branches of the mandibular division. It supplies sensation to the floor of the mouth, lingual mandibular gingivae, and the anterior two thirds of the tongue. Not too far below the foramen ovale the lingual nerve is joined by a branch from the seventh cranial nerve (facial), known as the **chorda tympani.** This small branch of nerve VII has parasympathetic (secretomotor) fibers to supply the submandibular and sublingual salivary glands and also carries special fibers of taste perception from the anterior two thirds of the tongue. Thus in the floor of the mouth where the lingual nerve is located, there are ac-

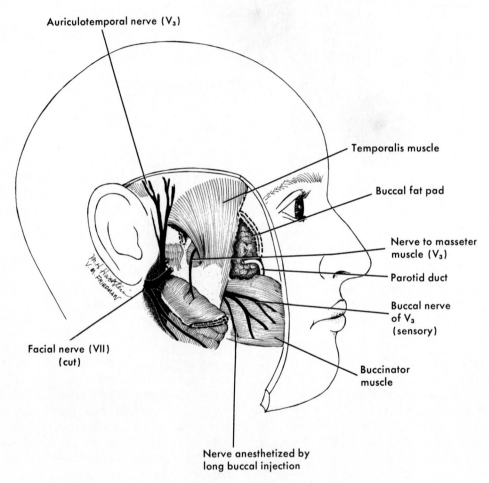

Fig. 19-11   Buccal and auriculotemporal nerves are sensory branches of V₃.

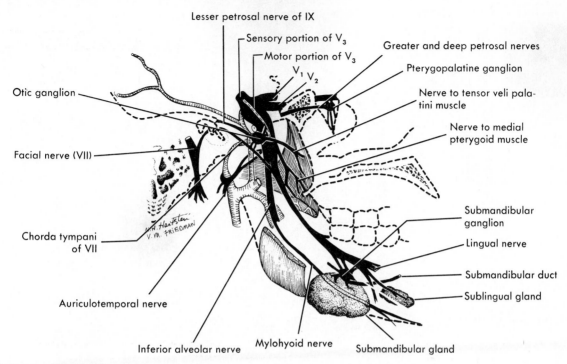

Fig. 19-12 Third (mandibular) division of trigeminal nerve and facial nerve. Notice especially chorda tympani connecting facial nerve to V_3. (This is medial view.)

tually fibers from nerve V and fibers from nerve VII, all wrapped together looking like one nerve. This also means that when the lingual nerve is inadvertently anesthetized during an injection of the lower teeth, the patient not only feels no sensation from the anterior two thirds of the tongue but also loses taste sensation from the same region (Fig. 19-12).

INFERIOR ALVEOLAR NERVE. The last large branch of the mandibular division that should be discussed is the **inferior alveolar nerve.** This nerve primarily serves the lower teeth, though it has a small motor branch called the **mylohyoid nerve** that supplies the mylohyoid muscle and the anterior belly of the digastric muscle. Just after the mylohyoid nerve diverges, the inferior alveolar nerve enters the mandible through the mandibular foramen and supplies all the lower teeth (Fig. 19-13). Between the mandibular premolars a small branch known as the **mental nerve** comes out through the mental foramen to supply the labial mucosa and labial gingiva in the anterior mandible area. This accounts for numbing of the lower lip during anesthetization of the lower teeth, since they are all part of the same nerve.

Facial Nerve (Cranial Nerve VII)

Most of the facial nerve exits the brain through the stylomastoid foramen behind the ear. It comes forward and is found within the substance of the parotid gland. Inside the gland it separates into a number of branches to provide motor supply to the muscles of facial expression. The distri-

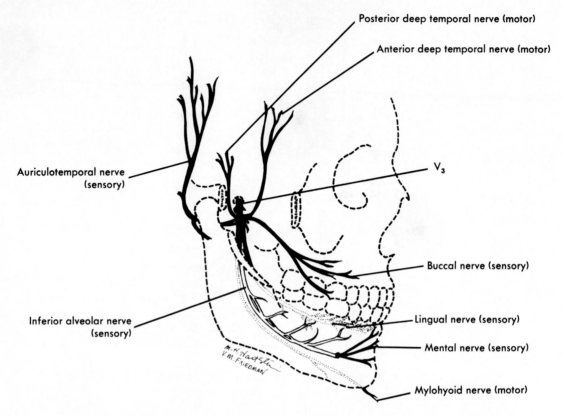

Posterior deep temporal nerve (motor)

Anterior deep temporal nerve (motor)

Auriculotemporal nerve (sensory)

V₃

Buccal nerve (sensory)

Inferior alveolar nerve (sensory)

Lingual nerve (sensory)

Mental nerve (sensory)

Mylohyoid nerve (motor)

Fig. 19-13 Inferior alveolar nerve (V₃) enters mandible through mandibular foramen, and mental nerve branches off it in premolar region. Auriculotemporal nerve extends back over ear.

bution of these branches varies from person to person, but a sample can be seen in Fig. 19-14. There is even one branch that supplies the platysma muscle in the neck. Before the nerve enters the parotid gland, a small section branches to the skin behind the ear and the stylohyoid and posterior digastric muscles. While the facial nerve is still inside the skull, a branch extends through the middle ear and out of the skull as the chorda tympani. As mentioned earlier, this nerve carries parasympathetic (secretomotor) fibers to the submandibular and sublingual glands and special taste fibers from the anterior two thirds of the tongue. These fibers run in

the same bundle with the lingual nerve. There is also another branch of the facial nerve, known as the greater petrosal nerve, that joins up with the maxillary division of the trigeminal nerve to carry some parasympathetic fibers to the minor salivary glands of the hard and soft palate (Fig. 19-12).

Glossopharyngeal Nerve (Cranial Nerve IX)

The glossopharyngeal nerve exits the skull along with the vagus and accessory nerves through the jugular foramen. It then sends one branch to a soft-palate muscle and one to the constrictor muscles of the pharynx, which ac-

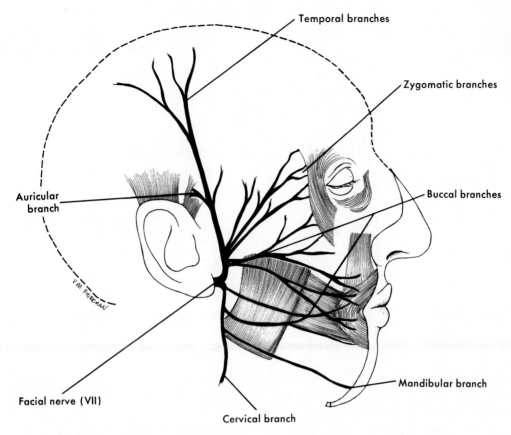

Temporal branches

Zygomatic branches

Auricular branch

Buccal branches

V.M. Freeman

Mandibular branch

Facial nerve (VII)

Cervical branch

Fig. 19-14 Branches of facial nerve that supply muscles of facial expression.

complish swallowing. There is also a branch that goes to the posterior one third of the tongue to supply *both* general sensation and taste to that region.

Another very small branch of this nerve does not exit the skull along with the rest of the nerve but sends a small branch down through the foramen ovale along with the mandibular division of the trigeminal nerve. This branch of nerve IX is known as the **lesser petrosal nerve,** and it joins the auriculotemporal nerve of V_3 as it goes back near the ear. This nerve continues past the parotid gland, and as it does, the lesser petrosal branch of nerve IX, which runs with it, comes off

the nerve and enters the gland to provide parasympathetic fibers for the gland (Figs. 19-12, 19-13, and 19-15).

Vagus Nerve (Cranial Nerve X)

The vagus nerve has the greatest extent of any of the cranial nerves. It sends fibers down to the heart, lungs, kidneys, and most of the digestive tract. The branches in the head and neck area of importance to our discussion are the branches to the larynx and tongue. The vagus sends a small branch to the base of the tongue, where it innervates the base of the tongue and the epiglottis. This branch carries general sensation and has a

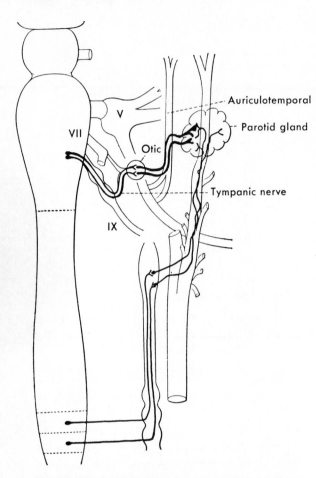

- - - Auriculotemporal

- - Parotid gland

V

VII

Otic

IX

- - - Tympanic nerve

Fig. 19-15 Lesser petrosal nerve of ninth cranial nerve joins auriculotemporal nerve just below foramen ovale and travels with it back to parotid gland. Notice how branch of ninth cranial nerve joins otic ganglion. (Goss.)

few taste fibers. There are two branches that go to the larynx—the superior and inferior laryngeal nerves. These provide general sensation and motor activity to the muscles of the larynx. There is also a motor branch to the muscles of the soft palate and pharynx.

REVIEW QUESTIONS

1. What are the subdivisions of the nervous system? *central nervous system / peripheral nervous system*
2. What happens when the sympathetic nervous system is stimulated? *fight or flight*
3. What happens when the parasympathetic nervous system is stimulated? *relaxation, "veg."*
4. Name the twelve cranial nerves and their general functions.
5. Which nerves carry parasympathetic fibers?
6. Which nerves supply each of the teeth in the mouth?
7. Name the nerves supplying each area of oral mucosa.
8. Name the nerve supply to the major salivary glands and describe their pathway to the glands. *facial*
9. Which nerve is responsible for the sensation of <u>taste</u> to the anterior two thirds of the tongue? *chorda tympani (branch of facial N.)*

peripheral nervous system — spinal, cranial, + autonomic nervous systems.

autonomic system consists of sympathetic + parasympathetic systems
sympathetic A.K.A. thoracolumbar outflow
parasympathetic A.K.A cranial sacral outflow
5. parasympathetic fibers come from III, VII, IX, X at sacral levels S2-S4
sympathetic fibers come from thoracic levels T1 – T12 + lumbar levels L1-L2

20

Lymphatics and Spread of Dental Infection

OBJECTIVES

- To discuss briefly the function of the lymphatic system
- To diagram and label the major groups of lymph nodes that drain the teeth and oral cavity
- To define the following terms as they relate to lymph drainage: primary, secondary, and tertiary
- To name the primary lymph drainage of all the teeth
- To discuss briefly the concept of fascial space infection
- To discuss briefly how a fascial space infection may spread from the oral cavity to the chest
- To define Ludwig's angina

LYMPHATIC SYSTEM

The lymphatic system is an accumulation of tiny channels, or tubules, with small **nodular** structures called **lymph nodes** interconnecting them. The system functions by returning fluids to the bloodstream from the various tissues of the body. Blood plasma is forced out of the capillaries into the surrounding tissues, where it is eventually picked up by the lymphatic vessels. The plasma, now referred to as lymphatic fluid, flows through vessels, then through nodes, back through vessels, and possibly through some more nodes. It finally empties into the venous system of the body and travels back to the heart. This kind of fluid circulation repeats itself continually. The lymph nodes act as filters for the fluids, and the lymphocytes produced within the lymph nodes combat infections that might spread

through the lymphatic channels. Most tissues, including the pulp of the teeth, have lymph vessels in them. The distribution of these vessels has been well determined, and this information can be used as a diagnostic tool in the study of oral infections.

Distribution Pattern

We will now examine the distribution pattern of these channels and nodes and discover how they relate to the head and neck area. Fig. 20-1 shows some of the major groups of nodes in the head and neck. As you can see, the nodes are grouped together into small clusters, which are all interconnected by channels. Each of these groups drains fluids from certain structures or tissue areas. If you are familiar with these areas, you can understand what happens when lymph nodes are involved in spreading infections from an area. A sore throat, for example, can be followed by tender areas in the neck and finally a tender lump in that area. In such an instance the infection from the throat spreads through the lymph channels until it reaches the first lymph node or group of lymph nodes. The lymphocytes in the node begin to combat the infection and also start to multiply, causing the node to become enlarged and tender. If the infection is successfully combated in that node, it will subside; however, if the infection is great, it may spread through that lymph node and on to the next node or group of nodes.

Submental. A very small accumulation of nodes, the **submental nodes,** is found beneath the chin. The lymphatic channels from the man-

primary

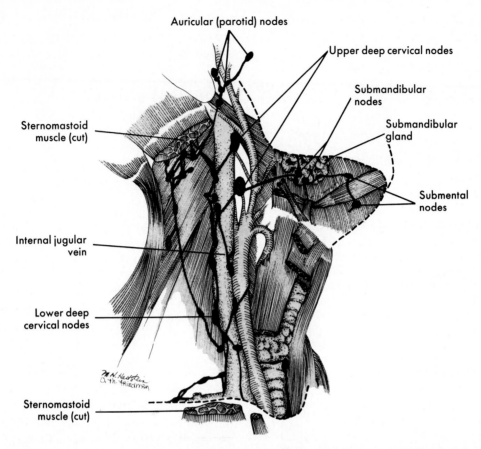

Auricular (parotid) nodes

Upper deep cervical nodes

Submandibular nodes

Submandibular gland

Sternomastoid muscle (cut)

Submental nodes

Internal jugular vein

Lower deep cervical nodes

Sternomastoid muscle (cut)

Fig. 20-1 Locations of some of major groups of lymph nodes that drain head and neck. Retropharyngeal group is not visible because of its location behind throat. Deep cervical chain lies on internal jugular vein beneath sternomastoid muscle, which has been removed in this view.

dibular incisors, the tip of the tongue, and the midline of the lower lip and chin drain into these nodes. Any infection in these areas would generally cause some tenderness and enlargement of the nodes.

Submandibular. The **submandibular nodes** are found grouped around the submandibular gland near the angle of the mandible. The easiest way to locate the gland and the nodes is to place a finger on the inferior border of the mandible near the angle. Run the finger back and forth until you feel a slight depression in the inferior

border. This is the point at which the facial artery and vein cross the inferior border. Just medial to this depression is the submandibular gland, and the submandibular lymph nodes are grouped around it.

Following are the areas draining into these nodes: all maxillary teeth, with the exception of the third molars; the mandibular canines and all mandibular posterior teeth, with the possibility that the third molars may not drain here; the floor of the mouth and most of the tongue; the cheek area; the hard palate; and the anterior nasal cavity. Any infections in these areas tend to cause enlargement and tenderness of the submandibular nodes. This condition may be referred to as **lymphadenopathy.** Another important point is that any lymphatic drainage starting at or near the midline may spread to either side of the face.

Upper deep cervical. The **upper deep cervical nodes** are located on the lateral surface of the internal jugular vein and lie just beneath the anterior border of the sternomastoid muscle, about 2 inches below the ear. A number of other nodes drain into this group—the submandibular nodes, the nodes behind the back throat wall, known as the **retropharyngeal nodes,** the parotid nodes in front of the ear and the parotid gland, as well as others. This is the group affected when you have a particularly sore throat. In addition, the upper deep cervical group drains the third molar regions, the base of the tongue, the tonsillar area, the soft palate, and the posterior nasal cavity region.

Lower deep cervical. The **lower deep cervical nodes** are also found on the lateral surface of the internal jugular vein and beneath the anterior border of the sternomastoid muscle. These nodes are located about 2 inches above the clavicle. They drain the upper deep cervical nodes and many of the nodes at the back of the neck. From here the fluids drain into the junction of the subclavian and internal jugular veins.

NODE GROUPS AFFECTED BY DISEASE

You will hear the terms **primary nodes, secondary nodes,** and **tertiary nodes** used in discussions about infections and cancer, both of which spread through lymphatic channels. These terms refer to the groups of nodes that would be affected in a disease process. If an infection is not stopped by the first (primary) group of nodes, it will spread to the second (secondary) group. If it is not stopped there, it may spread to the third (tertiary) group. If you refer to Fig. 20-1, you will see that one node or group of nodes may be primarily involved in one source of infection

whereas a second group of nodes is involved in another source of infection and even a third group in another area. Look at the upper deep cervical nodes. An infection of the third molars may involve these nodes first—they would be the primary group involved. If the infection were in a first molar, the initial sign of infection would be in the submandibular nodes; if it were not successfully combated there, it would spread secondarily to the upper deep cervical group. Infections originating in the middle of the lower lip would spread first to the submental nodes, secondarily to the submandibular nodes, and then to the upper deep cervical nodes, which in this instance would be tertiary nodes of infection.

An understanding of this concept is necessary to comprehend the spread of oral cancer. Each group of nodes acts as a resistance barrier against the spread of cancer. The nodes slow the spread, and if the cancer is detected early enough, it can be treated more successfully. Once the infection or the cancer reaches the lower deep cervical nodes and passes through them, it enters the bloodstream, moving directly into the heart and then throughout the body. With this in mind, it is easy to understand why cancer on the tip of the tongue does not result in as high a **mortality rate** as cancer does further back on the tongue. The tip of the tongue generally drains through four groups of nodes before it enters the bloodstream and spreads throughout the body, whereas cancer in the posterior portion of the tongue travels to the upper deep cervical nodes, on to the lower deep cervical nodes, and into the bloodstream. In that area there are only two groups to stop the spread of the disease. This knowledge is useful as background information for your involvement in intraoral and extraoral examinations.

SPREAD OF INFECTION IN FASCIAL SPACES

So far the discussion has centered on one manner of the spread of infection, that is, through lymphatic channels. There is another way in which infections may spread—in **fascial spaces**—and although it is much less common, it displays much more dramatic clinical symptoms. The spaces between muscle and tissue layers are referred to as fascial layers or planes, and infections may spread here. You may have seen a cartoon of, or an actual patient with, a large swollen jaw or an area beneath the eye that is also swollen. In this situation the infection of dental origin is not spreading through small lymphatic channels but has broken out of the bone around the tooth and is spreading beneath the tissue. This kind of infection spread will follow certain predictable pathways, depending on its location.

In general, dental infections start in the maxillae or mandible at the apex of a tooth or in the periodontal space around a tooth. Most periodontal space infections cause a swelling of the gingival or mucosal tissue within the oral cavity. Infections at the apices of the teeth cause swelling in one of two directions: buccal or lingual. Most buccal swellings also lead to a swelling in the vestibule of the oral cavity. Many patients will refer to this swelling as a "gumboil," since the infection comes to a pointed head, breaks through the mucosa, and drains into the oral cavity. If a mandibular infection spreads not to the buccal but to the lingual side, it will travel to the tissue spaces in two specific areas, depending on its point of origin—above the mylohyoid muscle in the floor of the mouth or beneath the mylohyoid muscle in the tissue beneath the chin. How can one predict where the infection will go? Refer to Fig. 11-17, a medial view of the body of the mandible, and picture the lengths of the roots of the individual teeth. Now look at the mylohyoid line on the mandible and notice its location relative to the apices of the roots. You can see that, in general, the apices of the mandibular molar teeth are inferior to the mylohyoid line whereas the premolars and the anterior teeth have the apices of their roots above the mylohyoid line. Therefore a molar infection will tend to break out of the bone below the mylohyoid line and spread to the space beneath the chin, referred to as the

submental space. Infections of the premolars and the anterior teeth will tend to break out of bone above the mylohyoid line and spread to the spaces in the floor of the mouth, referred to as the sublingual space.

Infection spreading into the sublingual space causes a swelling into the floor of the mouth. If it spreads into the submental space, it will cause a swelling beneath the chin, sometimes referred to as **Ludwig's angina.** These infections continue to spread by gravity if not treated. Whether above or below the mylohyoid muscle, as they spread downward and backward, they reach the posterior end of the mylohyoid muscle. Both kinds of infection reach the same place, the side of the neck next to the pharynx, which is referred to as the **lateral pharyngeal,** or **parapharyngeal space.** This causes a swelling on the side of the neck if left untreated. From here the infection may spread around the pharynx to its posterior border, which is referred to as the **retropharyngeal space,** and from there to the **posterior mediastinum,** which is in the back of the chest, or thoracic, cavity. If it reaches this point, the person may die within a short period of time. With the advent of antibiotics, these infections are not so frequently seen as they were in the past, but occasionally they can still be found.

The importance of this section is not to be able to completely describe or define the boundaries of these spaces, or **potential spaces,** but to understand how the origin or location of the original infection determines the pathway it will follow and the potential outcome if left untreated.

OTHER MAXILLARY INFECTIONS

Maxillary infections react a little differently because of the anatomical features of the area. If the infection does not open into the maxillary buccal vestibule or onto the palate, it may spread toward three areas—the nasal cavity, the maxillary sinus, or the soft-tissue spaces of the cheek or the area below the eye. The area involved is, of course, related to the tooth involved. A swelling below the eye is usually related to infection from an anterior tooth, usually the maxillary canine, whereas swelling in the cheek area is usually related to infection in a posterior tooth. Although it is possible, as mentioned, for infection to spread to the nasal cavity or maxillary sinus, it is rather rare, especially in the nasal cavity. These maxillary infections around the eye or cheek can also spread to the lateral pharyngeal space and from there to other areas.

REVIEW QUESTIONS

1. What is the function of lymph nodes?
2. What are the major groups of lymph nodes in the head and neck?
3. Name the structures that drain primarily into each group of lymph nodes.
4. What are fascial spaces?
5. Submental space infections would come from which group of teeth? MAND. INCISORS
6. Swelling below the eye would come from infection in which teeth? MAX. ant tooth, usually a CANINE

1. function of lymph nodes - filters fluids, produces lymphocytes, combats infections

2. MAJOR groups of lymph nodes in head & NECK - submental, submandibular, upper deep cervical, lower deep cervical

3. Submental - Tip of tongue, lower lip, lower ant. teeth

   Submandibular - molars & premolars of mand, ant. & pre. & molars of max, floor of mouth, hard palate, ant. nasal cavity, cheek, most of tongue

   Upper deep cervicals - post. nasal cavity, soft palate, 3rd molars, base of tongue, retropharyngeal nodes in back of throat.

   Lower deep cervicals - drains upper deep cervicals & flow into junction of subclavian & internal jugular veins.

4. fascial spaces - spaces between muscle & tissue layers

DRAINS

TEST

1. Excluding the ear ossicles, there are ~~22~~ bones in the skull.
   a. 8
   b. 14
   c. 12
   d. 18
   e. none of the above
2. The nasal septum is formed by the _____ bone.
   a. sphenoid
   b. ethmoid ✓
   c. vomer ✓
   d. maxilla
   e. a and b
   f. b and c
3. Which of the following bones is *not* a part of the neurocranium?
   a. sphenoid
   b. ethmoid
   c. temporal
   d. frontal
   e. occipital
   f. all are a part of the neurocranium
4. The mental foramen is in the ~~Body of mAND.~~
   a. body of the maxilla
   b. ramus of the mandible
   c. alveolar process of the mandible
   d. alveolar process of the maxilla

e. none of the above
5. The posterior nasal spine is a part of the _____ bone.
   a. nasal
   b. maxilla
   c. mandible
   d. palatine
   e. none of the above
6. The hiatus semilunaris is found in the
   a. sphenoethmoidal recess
   b. superior meatus
   c. middle meatus
   d. inferior meatus
   e. none of the above
7. Which of the following opens into the inferior meatus?
   a. frontal sinus
   b. maxillary sinus
   c. anterior ethmoid sinus
   d. nasolacrimal duct
   e. all of the above
8. Which of the following teeth would *not* be found in proximity to the floor of the maxillary sinus?
   a. max. first molar
   b. max. lateral incisor
   c. max. first premolar
   d. max. third molar
   e. They would all be close to the floor of the sinus
9. The opening of the maxillary sinus into the nasal cavity is found
   a. in the floor of the sinus
   b. in the roof of the sinus
   c. two thirds of the way up the lateral wall
   d. two thirds of the way up the medial wall
   e. none of the above
10. The ethmoid bulla is found in the
    a. inferior meatus
    b. superior meatus
    c. sphenoethmoidal recess
    d. middle meatus
    e. none of the above
11. The temporalis muscle is a(n) _____ of the mandible.

a. depressor
b. elevator ✓
c. protrudor
d. retrudor ✓
e. a and c
f. b and d

12. Which of the following is *not* an origin of the medial pterygoid muscle?
    a. maxillary tuberosity
    b. pterygoid fossa
    c. medial wall of the lateral pterygoid plate
    d. lateral wall of the medial pterygoid plate

13. Which of the following muscles most directly affects TMJ movement?
    a. temporalis
    b. masseter
    c. medial pterygoid
    d. lateral pterygoid

14. The muscles of mastication are innervated by the _____ cranial nerve.
    a. V   *trigeminal*
    b. VII
    c. IX
    d. X
    e. none of the above

15. The muscle most directly affecting elevation of the larynx is the _____ muscle.
    a. sternohyoid
    b. sternothyroid
    c. thyrohyoid
    d. mylohyoid
    e. digastric

16. The disc of the TMJ is attached laterally and medially to the
    a. medial pterygoid muscle
    b. lateral pterygoid muscle
    c. poles of the condyle
    d. retrodiscal pad
    e. none of the above

17. The posterior collagenous lamina functions to
    a. pull the disc back
    b. pull the disc forward
    c. keep the disc from being pulled too far back

d. keep disc from being pulled too far forward
e. none of the above

18. The temporomandibular ligament is found in the
    a. posterior part of the capsule
    b. medial part of the capsule
    c. anterior part of the capsule
    d. lateral part of the capsule

19. Pain in the area of the TMJ coming from other areas is known as _____ pain.
    a. myofacial
    b. referred
    c. false
    d. none of the above

20. Dislocation of the TMJ is referred to as
    a. protraction
    b. retrusion
    c. subluxation
    d. depression
    e. none of the above

21. When the disc of the TMJ is deranged, it is usually _____.
    a. immobile
    b. displaced posteriorly
    c. displaced anteriorly
    d. none of the above

22. The muscles of facial expression are innervated by the _____ cranial nerve.
    a. V
    b. VII   *facial*
    c. IX
    d. X
    e. XI

23. The buccinator shares a common origin with the _____ muscle.
    a. orbicularis oris
    b. superior pharyngeal constrictor
    c. uvula
    d. levator veli palatini
    e. none of the above

24. Which of the following muscles plays a role in smiling?
    a. levator labii superioris
    b. depressor labii inferioris

c. zygomatic major

d. mentalis

e. orbicularis oris

25. Which of the following muscles plays a direct role in keeping the food on the occlusal surfaces during mastication? Buccinator

  a. orbicularis oris

  b. orbicularis oculi

  c. zygomaticus major

  d. mentalis

  e. none of the above

26. Which of the following palatal muscles is innervated by the fifth cranial nerve?

  a. uvula

  b. palatopharyngeus

  c. palatoglossus

  d. levator veli palatini

  e. tensor veli palatini

27. The stylopharyngeus muscle _____ the pharynx.

  a. elevates

  b. dilates

  c. depresses

  d. pulls forward

  e. a and b

28. Which of the following muscles pulls the soft palate into contact with the posterior pharyngeal wall?

  a. uvula

  b. palatopharyngeus

  c. palatoglossus

  d. levator veli palatini

  e. none of the above

29. Which of the following muscles would help move the bolus of food upward and backward to the oral pharynx?

  a. palatoglossus

  b. palatopharyngeus

  c. levator veli palatini

  d. tensor veli palatini

30. Which of the following arteries supplies blood to the oral cavity?

  a. lingual

  b. maxillary

  c. palatal

d. mental

e. they all do

31. Which of the following are branches of the internal carotid artery?

  a. lingual

  b. maxillary

  c. superficial temporal

  d. facial

  e. all of the above

  f. none of the above

32. The blood supply to the muscles of mastication is from the _____ artery.

  a. mental

  b. facial

  c. lingual

  d. maxillary

  e. superficial temporal

33. The vein that may be injured in anesthesia of the posterior superior alveolar nerve is the _____.

  a. retromandibular vein

  b. pterygoid plexus of veins

  c. facial vein

  d. temporal vein

  e. none of the above

34. The _____ gland's duct opens into the vestibule opposite the maxillary second molar.

  a. parotid

  b. submandibular

  c. sublingual

  d. buccal

  e. none of the above

35. Which of the following glands is mostly serous with some mucous acini?

  a. buccal

  b. sublingual

  c. parotid

  d. submandibular

  e. none of the above

36. The submandibular gland opens into the oral cavity

  a. opposite the maxillary second molar

  b. on the sublingual caruncle

  c. at the base of the labial frenum

  d. b and c

e. none of the above
37. The serous glands of von Ebner are found
    a. in the cheek
    b. in the palate
    c. in the floor of the mouth
    d. in the tongue
    e. none of the above
38. The nerve supply to all salivary glands comes from the
    a. autonomic nervous system
    b. parasympathetic nervous system
    c. sympathetic nervous system
    d. voluntary nervous system
    e. a and b
    f. a and c
39. There are _____ pairs of cranial nerves.
    a. 5
    b. 7
    c. 9
    d. 12
    e. none of the above
40. Which of the following cranial nerves is involved with taste?
    a. glossopharyngeal
    b. vagus
    c. facial
    d. all of the above
    e. none of the above
41. The second part of the trigeminal nerve is known as the _____ division.
    a. mandibular
    b. ophthalmic
    c. pharyngeal
    d. maxillary
    e. none of the above
42. The nerve supply to the maxillary central incisors is the _____ nerve.
    a. greater palatine
    b. inferior alveolar
    c. posterior superior alveolar
    d. nasopalatine
    e. none of the above
43. The nerve supply to the mucosa of the lower lip is the _____ nerve.
    a. lingual

b. anterior superior alveolar
    c. buccal
    d. mental
    e. none of the above
44. The nerve supply to the lingual gingiva of the maxillary central incisor is the
    a. anterior superior alveolar
    b. middle superior alveolar
    c. inferior alveolar
    d. lingual
    e. nasopalatine
45. Lymph nodes
    a. help return intercellular fluids to the bloodstream
    b. produce lymphocytes
    c. fight infection
    d. prevent spread of infection
    e. all of the above
    f. none of the above
46. A secondary node of involvement with infection of a maxillary premolar would be
    a. submental
    b. upper deep cervical
    c. submandibular
    d. lower deep cervical
    e. none of the above
47. The primary nodes of drainage for a maxillary central incisor are the
    a. submental nodes
    b. submandibular nodes
    c. retropharyngeal nodes
    d. upper deep cervical nodes
    e. none of the above
48. Fascial space infections in the region of the oral cavity could spread ultimately to the
    a. floor of the mouth
    b. side of the throat
    c. region behind the throat
    d. posterior chest region
    e. none of the above

SECTION THREE

REFERENCES

Friedman SM: Visual anatomy, vol 1, Head and neck, Hagerstown, Md, 1970, Harper & Row, Publishers.

McClintic JR: Human anatomy, St Louis, 1983, The CV Mosby Co.

Paff GH: Anatomy of the head and neck, Philadelphia, 1973, WB Saunders Co.

Reed GM and Sheppard VF: Basic structures of the head and neck, Philadelphia, 1976, WB Saunders Co.

Wischnitzer S: Outline of human anatomy, Springfield, Ill, 1972, Charles C Thomas, Publisher.

ILLUSTRATION SOURCES

Bhaskar SN: Synopsis of oral pathology, ed 5, St Louis, 1977, The CV Mosby Co.

Chusid JG and McDonald JJ: Correlative neuroanatomy and functional neurology, ed 17, Los Angeles, 1979, Lange Medical Publications.

DuBrul EL: Sicher's oral anatomy, ed 7, St Louis, 1980, The CV Mosby Co.

Goss CM: Gray's anatomy of the human body, ed 29, Philadelphia, 1973, Lea & Febiger.

Hollinshead WH: Anatomy for surgeons, vol 1, The head and neck, ed 2, New York, 1968, Harper & Row, Publishers.

Sections of Neurology and the Section of Physiology, Mayo Clinic and Mayo Foundation: Clinical examinations in neurology, ed 4, Philadelphia, 1976, WB Saunders Co.

Snell R: Gross anatomy dissector: a companion for atlas of clinical anatomy, Boston, 1976, Little, Brown & Co.

SUGGESTED READINGS

Anthony CP and Thibodeau GA: Textbook of anatomy and physiology, ed 11, St Louis, 1983, The CV Mosby Co.

Christensen JB and Telford IR: Synopsis of gross anatomy, ed 4, Hagerstown, Md, 1982, Harper & Row, Publishers.

DuBrul E: Sicher's oral anatomy, ed 7, St Louis, 1980, The CV Mosby Co.

Fried LA: Anatomy of the head, neck, face and jaws, ed 2, Philadelphia, 1980, Lea & Febiger.

DENTAL ANATOMY

21

The Tooth: Functions and Terms

OBJECTIVES

- To identify the different tissues that compose the teeth
- To differentiate between clinical and anatomical eruption
- To define single, bifurcated, and trifurcated roots
- To recognize how the functions of teeth determine their shape and size
- To understand the individual functions and therefore the individual differences that exist between incisors, canines, premolars, and molars
- To name and identify the location of the various tooth surfaces
- To name and identify the line angles of the teeth
- To name and identify the point angles of the teeth
- To define the terminology used in naming the landmarks of the teeth

The teeth are very important in many functions of the body. They are essential for protecting the oral cavity and in acquiring and chewing food, as well as in aiding the digestive system in breaking down food. They are necessary for proper speech, and their appearance can be a very positive sexual attraction. In dental anatomy the teeth are studied individually and collectively—their functions, anchorages, and relations to each other. Our study will therefore begin with a discussion of the individual tooth.

CROWN AND ROOT

Each tooth has a **crown** and **root** portion. The crown is covered with **enamel**, and the root portion is covered with **cementum.** The crown and root are joined at the **cementoenamel junction,** also called the **CEJ.** The line that demarcates it is called the **cervical line,** a line that is formed by the junction of the cementum of the root and the enamel of the crown (Fig. 21-1).

The crown portion of the tooth erupts through the **bone** and gum tissue. After eruption it will never again be covered with gum tissue. Only the cervical third of the crown in healthy young adults is partly covered by gingiva (gum tissue).

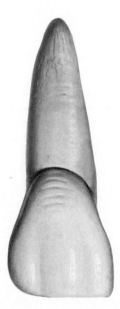

Fig. 21-1 Maxillary right central incisor. Crown and root are separated by cementoenamel junction. (Zeisz and Nuckolls.)

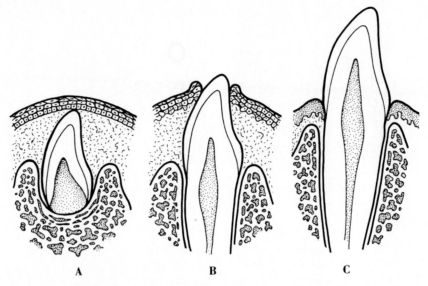

Fig. 21-2 **A,** Unerupted tooth. **B,** Beginning eruption. **C,** Young adult; eruption almost completed.

The tooth continues to erupt from the bone and **gingival tissue** until all the crown is exposed (Fig. 21-2).

There is a clinical difference between the amount of crown that could be erupted and the actual amount that is visible in the mouth. The **anatomical crown** is the whole crown of the tooth that is covered by enamel, whether erupted or not. The **clinical crown** is only that part seen above the gingiva. Any nonerupted area is not a part of the clinical crown of the tooth. Therefore, if all the anatomical crown does not erupt, the part that is visible is considered the clinical crown, and the unerupted portion is part of the **clinical root** (Fig. 21-3). **Eruption** of a tooth is thus the moving of that tooth through its surrounding tissues so that the clinical crown gradually appears longer. The root portion of the tooth may be **single** (see Fig. 21-1) or **multiple** with **bifurcation** or **trifurcation,** that is, division of the root portion into two or three roots (Figs. 21-4 and 21-5). Each root has one **apex,** or terminal end. The root portion is held in its position

relative to the other teeth in the **dental arch** by being firmly anchored in the bony process of the jaw. The portion of the jaw that supports the teeth is called the **alveolar process.** The bony socket in which the tooth fits is called the **alveolus** (Fig. 21-6). Teeth in the upper part of the jaw are called **maxillary** teeth because they are anchored in the maxillary bone. In the lower jaw they are called **mandibular** teeth because they are anchored in the bone called the mandible.

TOOTH TISSUES

The four tooth tissues are enamel, **dentin,** cementum, and **pulp** (Fig. 21-7). The first three are **hard tissues;** the pulp is **soft tissue.**

Enamel

The enamel forms the outer surface of the anatomical crown. It is thickest over the tip of the crown and becomes thinner until it ends at the cervical line. The color of enamel varies with its thickness and mineralization. The thicker the

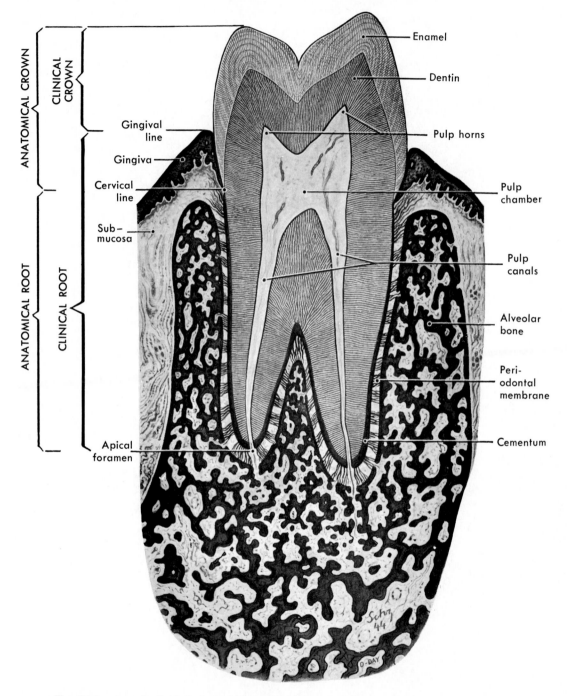

Fig. 21-3   Longitudinal section of tooth. Clinical crown and root can change, but anatomical crown−root ratio must always remain same. (Zeisz and Nuckolls.)

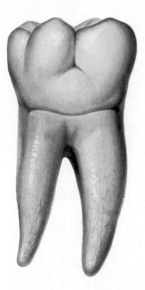

Fig. 21-4 Bifurcated root. (Zeisz and Nuckolls.)

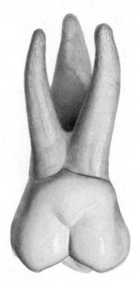

Fig. 21-5 Trifurcated root. (Zeisz and Nuckolls.)

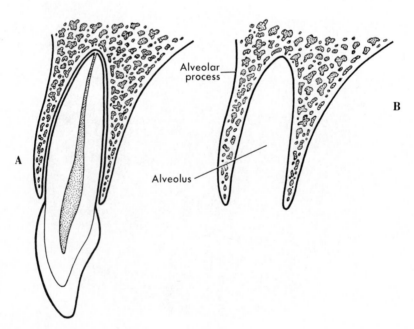

Fig. 21-6 **A,** Tooth surrounded by bony alveolus. **B,** Alveolus is tooth socket in alveolar process.

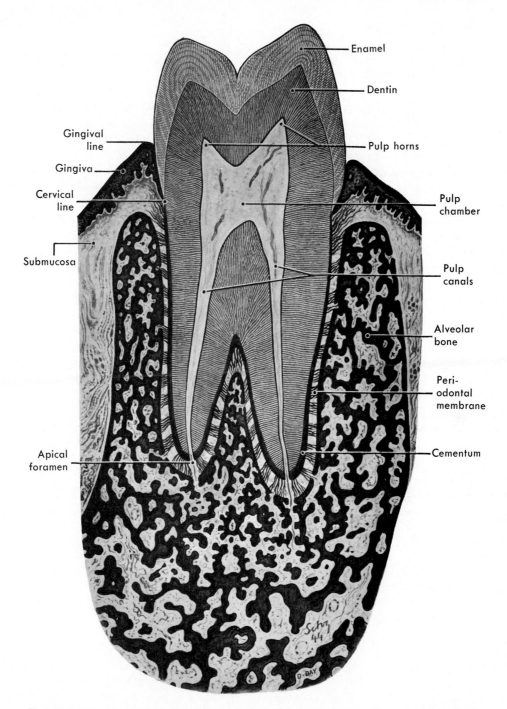

Enamel

Dentin

Gingival line

Pulp horns

Gingiva

Cervical line

Pulp chamber

Submucosa

Pulp canals

Alveolar bone

Peri- odontal membrane

Apical foramen

Cementum

Fig. 21-7   Pulp cavity is composed of pulp chambers, pulp horns, and root canals. (Zeisz and Nuckolls.)

enamel, the whiter it appears. The thinner the enamel, the more it varies, from grayish white at the crown cusps' edges, to white in the middle of the tooth, and to yellow-white at the cervical line, where the thin enamel covering is translucent enough to show the yellow tint of the dentin. The more mineralized the enamel, the more it lends itself to translucency. These two factors— the mineralization and thickness of enamel— coupled with the skin pigmentation, tend heavily to determine the color of the enamel.

Enamel is the most densely mineralized and hardest tissue in the human body. The chemical composition of enamel is 96% inorganic and 4% organic matter and water. This dense mineralization gives enamel the ability to resist the wear that the crown of a tooth is subjected to. The hard enamel does not wear very readily; rather it wears down, grinds up, and crushes almost anything that a person subjects it to—nuts, seeds, ice cubes, even particles of bone, grit, and leather. In addition to being durable, the densely packed enamel is smooth. This smoothness gives the crown of the tooth a certain self-cleaning ability, making it difficult for food particles, bacteria, sticky carbohydrate material, and other debris to adhere to the surface of the tooth crown. This self-cleaning ability of enamel and its extreme hardness and resistance to wear make it a nearly perfect outer covering for the crown.

Dentin

Dentin forms the main portion, or body, of the tooth. It is wrapped in an envelope of enamel, which covers the crown, and an envelope of cementum, which covers the root. The greatest bulk of the tooth is composed of dentin because it forms the largest portion of the crown and root.

Dentin is a hard, dense, calcified tissue. It is softer than enamel but harder than cementum or bone. It is yellow in color and elastic in nature. Its chemical composition is 70% inorganic and 30% organic matter and water. Unlike enamel, dentin is capable of adding to itself. When it does

this, the new dentin is called **secondary dentin.**

Secondary dentin is formed throughout the pulp chamber after the tooth erupts. In time, secondary dentin could completely fill the pulp chamber. **Reparative dentin** is the dentin laid down in response to caries or trauma. Dentin, then, is one tooth tissue that continues to be formed after the tooth has erupted.

Cementum

The cementum is a bonelike substance that covers the root. Its main function is to provide a medium for the attachment of the tooth to the alveolar bone. It is not as dense or as hard as enamel or dentin but is denser than bone, to which it bears a physiological resemblance. The chemical composition is 45% to 50% inorganic and 50% to 55% organic components. The cementum is quite thin at the cervical line but increases slightly in thickness at the apex of the root. The union of cementum and dentin is called the **dentinocemental junction.**

There are two types of cementum: **cellular** and **acellular.** The acellular cementum covers the entire anatomical root. The cellular cementum is confined to the apical third of the root and can reproduce itself, thereby compensating for the attrition (wear) that occurs on the crown of the tooth. The nutrition for cementum is derived from the outside of the tooth through blood vessels that come directly from the bone.

Cellular cementum derives its name from the fact that the very cells that lay down and form the cementum become trapped within this cementum. The cells that produce cementum are called **cementoblasts.**

Cellular cementum has cementocytes trapped within it. Acellular cementum has no cells trapped within it.

Cementum is another tooth tissue that continues to be formed after the tooth has erupted.

Cementum gives the tooth a mechanism of anchorage that protects and supports the teeth, yet it is self-adjusting and independent of the tooth's main nourishment system.

Pulp

The pulp is the nourishing, sensory, and dentin-reparative system of the tooth. It is composed of blood vessels, lymph vessels, connective tissues, nerve tissue, and special dentin formation cells called **odontoblasts.**

The pulp is housed in the center of the tooth, with the dentin surrounding the pulp tissue. The walls of the **pulp cavity** are lined with odontoblasts, the chief function of which is to lay down primary and secondary dentin. The odontoblasts form secondary dentin when the tooth is subjected to trauma from chemical, mechanical, or bacterial causes. Blood vessels bring in the nourishment necessary to activate and support the formation of secondary dentin. In addition, the blood vessels also supply the white blood cells necessary to fight bacterial invasion within the pulp. The lymph tissue filters the fluids within the tooth; the nerve tissue is sensory in function and responds only to pain.

Anatomically the pulp is divided into two areas: the **pulp chamber** and the **pulp canal,** or **root canal.** The pulp chamber is housed within the coronal portion of the tooth. The pulp canals are located within the roots of the tooth. Together the pulp chamber and pulp canals are referred to as the pulp cavity; thus the pulp cavity runs the entire length of the interior of the tooth from the tip of the pulp chamber, the **pulp horns,** to the apex of the root canal (Fig. 21-7).

TYPES OF TEETH

The functions of the teeth vary, depending on their individual shape and size and their location in the jaws. The three basic functions of the teeth are cutting, holding or grasping, and grinding.

Incisors

The **incisors** are designed to cut (incisor means that which makes an incision, or cut), and

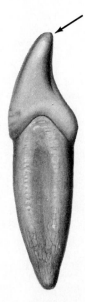

Fig. 21-8   Mandibular central incisor. Notice incisal edge *(arrow),* which incises, or cuts, food. (Zeisz and Nuckolls.)

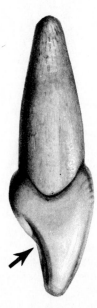

Fig. 21-9   Arrow points to shoveled-out lingual aspect of maxillary right central incisor. (Zeisz and Nuckolls.)

the biting edge is called an incisal edge (Fig. 21-8). The tongue side, or lingual surface, is shaped like a shovel, to aid in guiding the food into the mouth (Fig. 21-9).

Canines

The **canines** are designed to function as holding or grasping teeth. The importance of these teeth can be seen in dogs, for example, whose animal family is named for these teeth. The dog uses the canines as a weapon, or fighting tool. With them it pierces and then holds its victim.

The canines are also used as a tearing tool.

The canines are the longest teeth in human dentition. They are also some of the best anchored and most stable teeth, since *they have the longest roots* (Fig. 21-10). Canine roots are shaped triangularly in **cross section.** This triangular root shape makes it possible for a canine to hold its place in the corner of the mouth. The shape resists both anterior and posterior forces of displacement, as well as forces that would rotate or turn the tooth within its bony socket (Fig. 21-11).

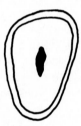

Fig. 21-11 Triangular cross-sectional shape of maxillary canine resists forces that would dislodge it.

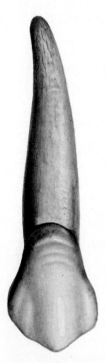

Fig. 21-10 Maxillary canine. Bulk of canine root affords resistance to displacement. (Zeisz and Nuckolls.)

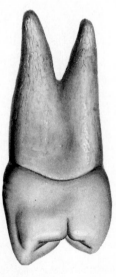

Fig. 21-12 Maxillary first premolar with two cusps. (Zeisz and Nuckolls.)

Premolars

There are four maxillary and four mandibular **premolars.** Premolars are a cross between canines and molars. They are not as long as canines, and they usually have at least two **cusps** rather than one large ridge. Like canines they aid in holding food, and they also help grind rather than incise it. Their pointed buccal cusps hold the food while the lingual cusps grind it, making their function similar to that of the molars.

Premolars are sometimes referred to as **bicuspids.** The term "bicuspid" is not accurate, however, since it implies only two cusps, and some premolars have three. Therefore the term "premolar" is preferred (Fig. 21-12).

Molars

Molars are much larger than premolars, usually having four or more cusps. Also, molars are located more posteriorly than the premolars.

The function of the 12 molars is to chew or grind up food. They do not incise food, and, like

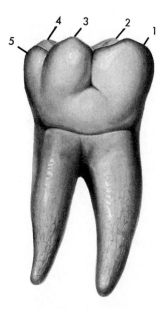

Fig. 21-13 Mandibular first molar. This lower molar has five cusps. (Zeisz and Nuckolls.)

premolars, they do not have incisal edges. Instead they have cusps, which are designed to interlock the upper and lower molars. There are four or five cusps on the occlusal surface of each molar, depending on its location and the occurrence of normal variations (Fig. 21-13). Maxillary (upper) and mandibular (lower) molars differ greatly from each other in shape, size, number of cusps, and roots.

The incisors and canines are called **anterior** teeth because they occupy the anterior, or front, of the dental arch. Premolars and molars occupy the back portion of the arch and are called **posterior** teeth.

SURFACES OF TEETH

The crowns of the teeth are divided into **surfaces,** which are named according to the direction in which they face. Anterior teeth (incisors and canines) have four surfaces and a ridge, whereas posterior teeth (premolars and molars) have five surfaces.

If the surface of a tooth faces the tongue, it is called the **lingual surface.** If facing the cheek or lip, it is called the **facial surface,** also known as the **labial** (lip) **surface** if it is an anterior tooth or the **buccal** (cheek) **surface** if it is a posterior tooth (Fig. 21-14).

The surface of a tooth that faces the neighboring tooth's surface in the same arch (next to each other) is called a **proximal surface.** Each tooth has two proximal surfaces: mesial and distal. The **mesial proximal surface** of a tooth is closest to the **midline** of the face. The **distal proximal surface** faces away from the midline.

The fifth surface of the posterior teeth is called the **occlusal surface**—the biting surface of the tooth. It is also the **occluding,** or chewing, surface. The occlusal surfaces of the lower posterior teeth hit against the occlusal surfaces of the upper teeth when the jaw closes (Figs. 21-14 and 21-15).

There is a question as to whether the anterior teeth have a fifth surface. They have a biting edge

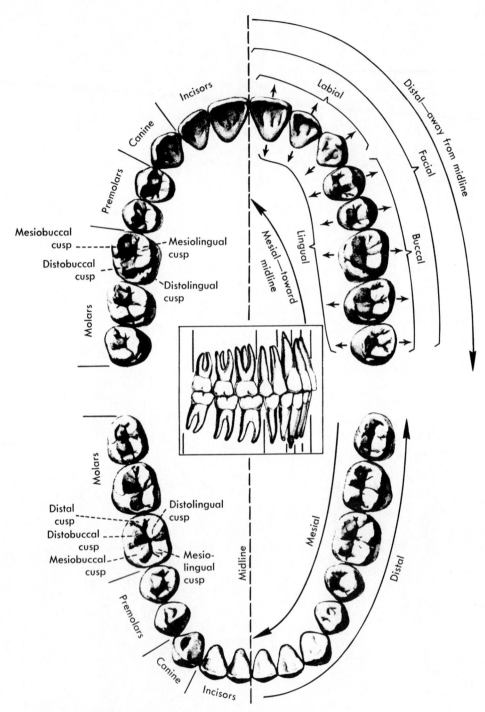

Fig. 21-14 Permanent arch (terms of orientation). (Kraus et al.; after Massler and Schour, 1958.)

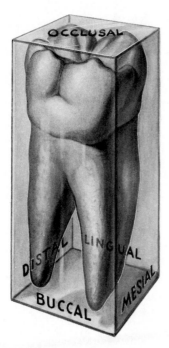

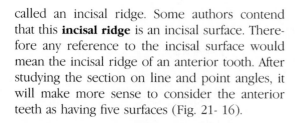

Fig. 21-15 Surfaces of a mandibular right first molar. (Zeisz and Nuckolls.)

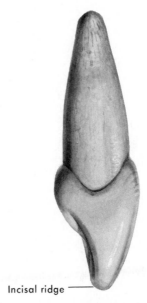

Incisal ridge ——

Fig. 21-16 Incisal ridge of central incisor. Even though incisal ridge is small, it is treated independently. (Zeisz and Nuckolls.)

called an incisal ridge. Some authors contend that this **incisal ridge** is an incisal surface. Therefore any reference to the incisal surface would mean the incisal ridge of an anterior tooth. After studying the section on line and point angles, it will make more sense to consider the anterior teeth as having five surfaces (Fig. 21- 16).

DIVISION OF SURFACES

For the purpose of facilitating the location of various areas within a specific surface of a tooth, the surface is divided into thirds. The lingual surface of a tooth is divided into a **mesial,** a **middle,** and a **distal third.** The facial (labial and buccal) surfaces are divided in the same manner (Fig. 21-17). The proximal (mesial and distal) surfaces of

a tooth are divided into a **facial,** a middle, and a **lingual third.**

The teeth can be divided into divisions perpendicular to these, so that any of the proximal, facial, or lingual surfaces can be further divided into an **incisal,** a middle, and a **cervical third.** On posterior teeth the incisal third is called the **occlusal third.**

LINE ANGLES

A **line angle** separates two surfaces of a tooth by forming the junction of the two surfaces. For instance, the junction of the buccal surface and the occlusal surface of a tooth is a line angle. Since the line angles are named according to the surfaces they join, the line angle that separates

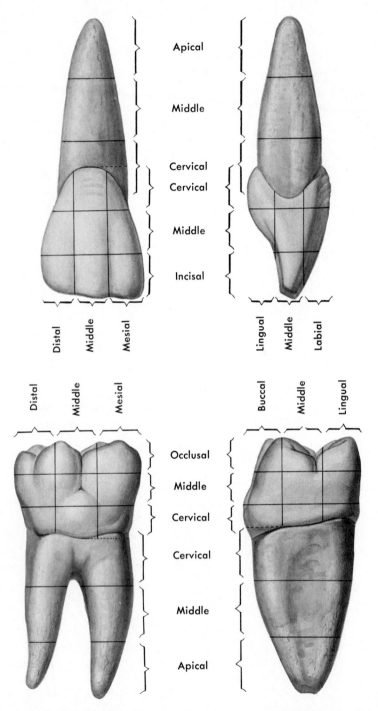

Fig. 21-17 Maxillary right permanent central incisor and mandibular right permanent first molar. (Zeisz and Nuckolls.)

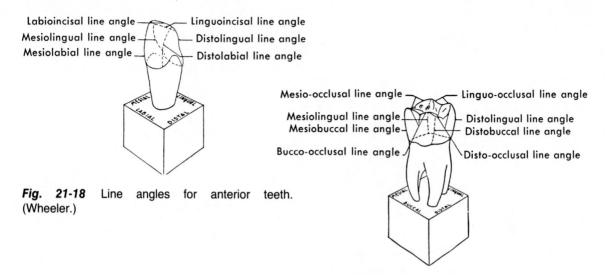

Fig. 21-18 Line angles for anterior teeth. (Wheeler.)

Fig. 21-19 Line angles for posterior teeth. (Wheeler.)

the buccal and the occlusal surfaces is called the bucco-occlusal line angle (Figs. 21-18 and 21-19). Following are the various combinations.

Line angles for anterior teeth

Distolabial	Mesiolingual
Mesiolabial	Linguoincisal
Distolingual	Labioincisal

Line angles for posterior teeth

Distobuccal	Distoocclusal
Mesiobuccal	Mesioocclusal
Distolingual	Buccoocclusal
Mesiolingual	Linguoocclusal

POINT ANGLES

A **point angle** is the point at which three surfaces meet. For instance, the point at which the mesial, labial, and incisal surfaces join is called the mesiolabioincisal point angle (Figs. 21-20 and 21- 21).

Point angles for anterior teeth

Mesiolabioincisal
Distolabioincisal
Mesiolinguoincisal
Distolinguoincisal

Point angles for posterior teeth

Mesiobuccoocclusal
Distobuccoocclusal
Mesiolinguoocclusal
Distolinguoocclusal

LANDMARKS

The student must know basic landmarks to be able to study individual teeth.

When the crowns are formed, they develop from four or more growth centers, or **lobes.** These lobes grow and eventually fuse, but a line remains on the erupted tooth where fusion of the primary parts, or lobes, took place. These shallow grooves or lines that separate primary parts of the crown or root are called **developmental grooves** (Fig. 21-22).

Incisors, canines, and most premolars are developed from three facial lobes and one lingual lobe. Second molars are developed from four lobes, two facial and two lingual. First molars are developed from five lobes. The upper has two facial and three lingual lobes. The lower has two lingual and three facial lobes. In Fig. 21-22 the

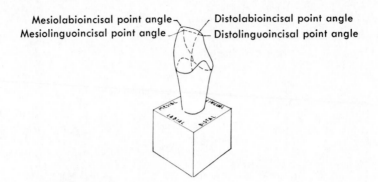

Mesiolabioincisal point angle
Mesiolinguoincisal point angle
Distolabioincisal point angle
Distolinguoincisal point angle

Fig. 21-20 Point angles for anterior teeth. (Wheeler.)

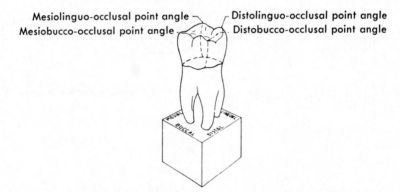

Mesiolinguo-occlusal point angle
Mesiobucco-occlusal point angle
Distolinguo-occlusal point angle
Distobucco-occlusal point angle

Fig. 21-21 Point angles for posterior teeth. (Wheeler.)

lines separating the lobes represent developmental grooves and the lobes are numbered.

A **tubercle** is a small elevation of enamel on some portion of the crown of the tooth. It does not always occur on the lingual surface of a tooth but can occur on an area such as the labial or occlusal surface (Fig. 21-23).

A **fossa** of a tooth is a depression or concavity, an area on the tooth that is indented, or concave. Fossae is the plural. The fossae are named for their location. For instance, a lingual fossa is on the lingual surface of a tooth.

On the anterior teeth there is a lingual fossa between the marginal ridges and incisal to the **cingulum.** These terms are discussed under the subject of anterior teeth. When there is a pinpoint hole within the fossa, this depression is called a **pit.** A small pinpoint depression located anywhere on the tooth is called a pit. Pits usually occur along the developmental grooves or in the fossae. On canines there are two lingual fossae; on premolars there are triangular fossae on the occlusal surfaces, mesial or distal to the marginal ridges (which shall be discussed shortly), and between cusps along the central developmental groove. Pits are named for their location on a

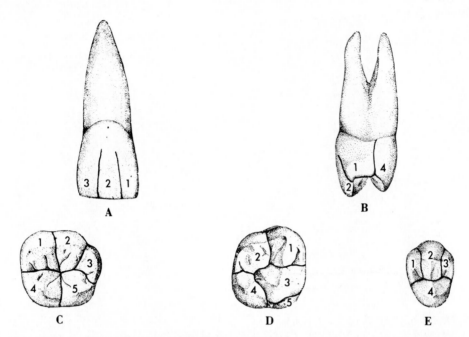

Fig. 21-22 Lobes of teeth. **A,** Maxillary central incisor. **B,** Maxillary first premolar. **C,** Mandibular first molar. **D,** Maxillary first molar. **E,** Maxillary premolar. Lines separating lobes are developmental grooves. (Wheeler.)

tooth; thus a lingual pit occurs on the lingual surface of a tooth, and a buccal pit occurs on the buccal surface of a tooth.

A **cusp** is a mound on the crown portion of the tooth that makes up a major division of its occlusal or incisal surface. Cusps are found on premolars and molars and on canines. They are not, however, found on incisors. The difference between a tubercle, which is a smaller elevation on a tooth, and a cusp is that a cusp makes up a major, or divisional, part of the occlusal or incisal surface, and a tubercle does not.

A **ridge** is an elevated portion of a tooth that runs in a line. Ridges are named for their location, such as the linguocervical ridge or the distal and mesial marginal ridges. All cusps have four ridges—buccal (or labial), lingual, mesial, and distal.

Marginal ridges are the rounded borders of enamel that form the mesial and distal shoulders of the occlusal surfaces of the posterior teeth and the mesial and distal shoulders of the lingual surface of the anterior teeth. (See Fig. 21-24).

A **concavity** is a carved-out section or area, like a cave. The opposite of concavity is **convexity,** a bulging out. The ridges of a tooth and a cusp tip are convex (Fig. 21-25).

Anterior Teeth

Anterior teeth show two developmental grooves on their labial surfaces. These two grooves separate the three lobes that formed the labial surface (Fig. 21-22, *A*).

The fourth developmental lobe of anterior teeth occurs on the lingual surface of the crown (Fig. 21-26). This fourth lobe is called the **cingulum,** and it makes up the bulk of the cervical third of the lingual surface of an anterior tooth.

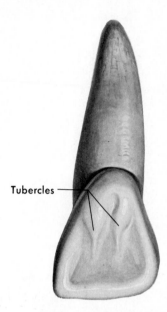

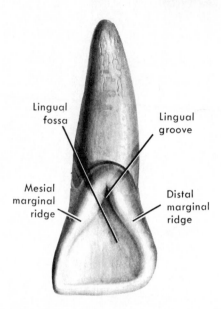

Fig. 21-23 Maxillary central incisor, lingual view. Tubercles of an anterior tooth extend from cingulum onto lingual fossa. (Zeisz and Nuckolls.)

Fig. 21-24 Lingual view of central incisor. (Zeisz and Nuckolls.)

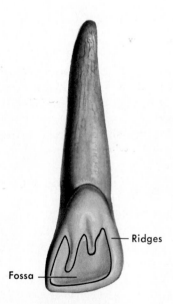

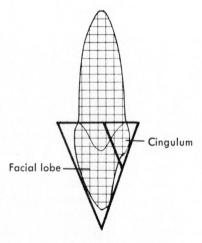

Fig. 21-25 Fossa and ridges of tooth. Fossa is concavity, or depression, and ridge is convexity, or bulge. (Zeisz and Nuckolls.)

Fig. 21-26 Fourth developmental lobe, or cingulum, of anterior tooth. Lingual fossa separates cingulum from three facial lobes. (Wheeler.)

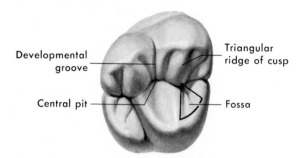

Fig. 21-27   Maxillary second molar. (Zeisz and Nuckolls.)

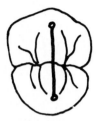

Fig. 21-28   Maxillary right first premolar. The transverse ridge is formed by lingual ridge of buccal cusp and buccal ridge of lingual cusp.

The developmental line that separates this fourth lobe, the lingual lobe, or cingulum, from the labial lobes is called the **lingual groove** or grooves (there may be more than one). The lingual fossa separates the lingual lobe from the other three lobes. A lingual developmental·groove may not always be a single groove; rather, it may be several grooves interrupted by a tubercle, or finger-like projection of enamel (Fig. 21-23).

Posterior Teeth

The most obvious landmarks on the posterior teeth are the cusps. The number will vary according to the tooth, and these are discussed under the individual teeth.

Aside from the marginal ridges on a posterior tooth, there are several other types of ridges (Fig. 21-27).

Triangular ridges are the main ridges on each cusp that run from the tip of the cusp to the central part of the occlusal surface. Thus the triangular ridge of the mesiobuccal cusp is the lingual ridge of the cusp that runs to the center of the occlusal surface, whereas the triangular ridge of the mesiolingual cusp is the buccal ridge that runs from the tip of the cusp to the center of the occlusal surface (Fig. 21-27).

A **transverse ridge** is the union of two triangular ridges, a buccal and a lingual, that cross the occlusal surface of a posterior tooth (Fig. 21-28).

REVIEW QUESTIONS

1. What line separates the enamel from the cementum of the tooth? *Cervical line*
2. How could a portion of the anatomical crown be a part of the clinical root? *Not fully erupted*
3. Which has more roots, a _trifurcated_ or a bifurcated tooth?
4. Are maxillary teeth _upper_ or lower jaw teeth?
5. Which tooth tissue composes the bulk of the tooth? *Dentin*
6. Which tooth tissue is the hardest? *enamel*
7. Which tooth tissue is the softest? *pulp*
8. Which tooth tissues have their own nourishment system? *cementum*
9. Which tooth tissue is most like bone? *cementum*
10. What is the main nourishing system of the tooth? *pulp*
11. Name the different parts of the pulp cavity.
12. Is the pulp horn a part of the _pulp chamber_ or the pulp canal?
13. What is the pulp tissue comprised of?
14. A bifurcated tooth has how many roots? *2*
15. Which is larger, the alveolus or the _alveolar process?_ *alveolus = socket only*
16. Which is seen in the mouth first, the _clinical_ or the anatomical crown?
17. What is the percentage of inorganic material in enamel? in dentin? in cementum?
18. Enamel is harder than dentin; dentin is

13. pulp is made of blood vessels, lymph vessels, connective & nerve tissue, & odontoblasts

17. Enamel is 96% inorganic & 4% organic
    Dentin is 70%   "   + 30%   "
    Cementum 45-50% "   50-55% "

harder than cementum. How does this correlate to the percentages of inorganic versus organic materials present in these tissues?

19. What are the basic functions of the teeth? What determines which teeth have which functions?

20. What are the longest teeth in human dentition? Why are they considered the longest?

21. Why is the term "bicuspid" inaccurate? *implies only 2 cusps*

22. What is the function of the molars, and how do the cusps perform this function?

23. How many premolars and how many molars are there in the permanent dentition?

24. How many surfaces are on a posterior tooth? Name them.

25. Which proximal surface is farther away from the midline, and which is closest to the midline? *Distal* *mesial*

26. If the anterior teeth do not have a fifth surface, what do they have that replaces the fifth surface? *incisal edge*

27. What is a line angle? List the six line angles for the anterior teeth and the eight for the posterior teeth.

28. What is a point angle? *where 3 surfaces meet*

20, *canines are longest & have the longest roots*

27, *line angle - where 2 surfaces meet*

35, *grooves separate development parts of crown or roots.*
pits are pinpoint holes w/in a fossa.

29. The developmental grooves separate the lobes of a tooth. How many lobes does an anterior tooth have?

30. What separates the cingulum on an anterior tooth from the labial lobes? *lingual fossa*

31. A small elevation of enamel on some portion of the crown of a tooth is called a *Tubercle*

32. A small pinpoint depression that occurs along a developmental groove is a *pit* .

33. Explain the difference between a tubercle and a cusp.

34. Which of the following are convex, and which are concave?
    a. empty swimming pool
    b. empty soup bowl
    c. cave
    d. ridge of a mountain
    e. cusp tip
    f. valley between two hills
    g. empty bathtub
    h. lingual fossa of an anterior tooth

35. Explain the difference between a developmental groove and a pit.

36. Identify the distal, lingual, and occlusal surfaces of the mandibular lower right first molar in Fig. 21- 29.

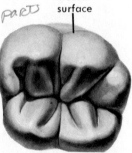

Buccal surface

Mesial surface

Fig. 21-29   (Zeisz and Nuckolls.)

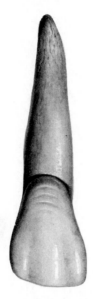

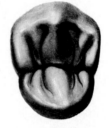

Fig. 21-30   (Zeisz and Nuckolls.)

Fig. 21-31   (Zeisz and Nuckolls.)

37. Label the mesiolabioincisal point angle and the distolabial line angle of the upper right maxillary lateral incisor in Fig. 21-30.
38. Label the distal marginal ridge, the mesial pit, and the transverse ridge of the maxillary right first premolar in Fig. 21-31.

We suggest that you turn to the sections in Chapter 5 concerning enamel composition, dentin composition, formation of regular dentin, and formation of secondary dentin and the section in Chapter 6 concerning cementum formation. These discussions contain much more detailed information about the material covered.

22

Fundamental and Preventive Curvatures

PROXIMAL ALIGNMENT OF THE TEETH AND PROTECTION OF THE PERIODONTIUM

OBJECTIVES

- To understand the importance of the shape of teeth in regard to preservation of the dentition
- To identify the proximal contact areas
- To identify contact points

EVOLUTION OF FUNDAMENTAL AND PREVENTIVE CURVATURES AND PROXIMAL ALIGNMENT OF THE TEETH

Over millions of years of evolution the teeth have gradually developed a specific shape, with fundamental curvatures at certain areas on each tooth—representing successful adaptation toward the maintenance of the teeth within the dental arch. In other words, the curvatures aid the teeth in preventing disease, damage, bacterial invasion, and calculus buildup; dispersing excessive occlusal trauma and biting forces; and protecting the gingiva and periodontium—therefore increasing the life expectancy of the tooth within the dental arch.

These curvatures, by preserving the teeth, also increased the life and productivity of the possessor. As the life expectancy of the animal or person increased, so did the number of potential offspring. Thus through the process of evolution, through successful traits outnumbering, outlasting, and outproducing the less successful traits, the teeth of modern man possess certain success-

ful characteristics of shape and **alignment** (their position in the jaw). Some of these successful adaptations and characteristics follow:

1. Specific location and size of proximal (mesial or distal) contact areas of various teeth
2. Size and location of interproximal spaces formed by the proximal contact surfaces
3. Location and effectiveness of the embrasures, or spillways
4. Facial and lingual **contours** on the labial, buccal, and lingual surfaces of crowns
5. Amount of curvature of the cementoenamel junction on the mesial and distal surfaces of the various teeth
6. Self-cleaning qualities of the tooth; smoothness of the enamel; overall shape of the tooth to meet its function
7. Occlusal and incisal curvatures and contours

Proximal Contact Areas

The **proximal** (mesial or distal) **contact areas** of the teeth are situated in a way that food debris is prevented from packing between them. The actual contact areas themselves touch each other so that the surfaces are not large enough to create a buildup of excessive amounts of bacteria or food debris but are large enough to be an effective barrier and prevent food from packing between the teeth. Finally, because the teeth do slightly touch each other, they offer support and

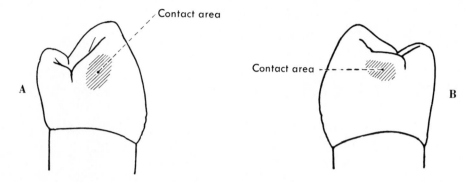

Fig. 22-1 Contact areas. *Shaded area,* Where distal contact area of mandibular first premolar, **A,** touches mesial contact area of second premolar, **B.** (Zeisz and Nuckolls.)

anchorage to each other as well as resistance to displacement from traumatic forces.

The proximal contact areas are located on the mesial and distal surfaces of each tooth, at the widest portion and at the greatest curvature. The **distal contact area** of one tooth touches the **mesial contact area** of the tooth posterior to it. For example, the distal contact area of the lower first premolar touches its neighbor, the lower second premolar.

In Fig. 22-1, observe how the two premolars touch each other. Where they touch is called a contact area—the contact area on the distal surface of the first premolar is called the distal contact area. What would the contact area on the mesial surface of the second premolar be called? The contact area is not just a point, but rather a flattened portion of the tooth. **Contact point** refers to the occlusal cusp of a tooth that touches the occlusal portion of another tooth in the opposing arch. Thus a contact area and a contact point are *not* the same (Fig. 22-2).

Looking at a buccal view of the tooth in Fig. 22-3, notice that the contact area occurs at the portion of the tooth that has the greatest curvature. In other words, the distal contact area occurs at the part of the distal portion of the tooth that bulges or curves out the most.

Even from the occlusal view it is apparent that although the proximal contacts do not touch the entire surface, at least a considerable portion of the proximal surface does touch the adjacent tooth.

Interproximal Spaces

Interproximal spaces are V-shaped spaces between the teeth formed by the proximal surfaces and their contact areas. These spaces are normally filled with gingival tissue called **papillary gingiva** or **interdental papilla.** By its presence the interdental papilla keeps food from collecting cervically to the contact areas between the teeth. In addition to this preventive function, the interdental space provides a place for a bulk of bone, thus affording better anchorage and support. The space is wider cervically than occlusally. This allows vascular support to nourish the interdental bone and papillary tissue. When gingival recession occurs between the teeth, the interdental papilla and bone no longer fill the entire interproximal space; then a void exists cervically to the contact area. This void is called a **cervical embrasure.** It occurs frequently as a pathological consequence of periodontal or orthodontic causes and offers a place in which bacteria and food debris can accumulate (Fig. 22-4).

Embrasures

Embrasures (spillways) are the spaces between the teeth that are occlusal to the contact

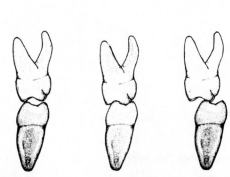

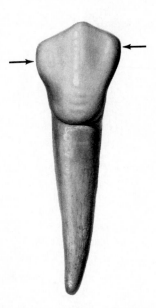

Fig. 22-2 Contact points. Contact points of a maxillary molar occluding with a mandibular molar in three different positions. NOTE: A *contact area* is where two teeth in the same arch touch; a *contact point* is where a tooth in one arch touches a tooth in the opposite arch. (Wheeler.)

Fig. 22-3 Buccal view of a lower first premolar. Contact areas, *arrows.* (Zeisz and Nuckolls.)

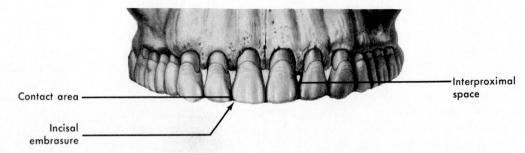

Contact area

Incisal embrasure

Interproximal space

Fig. 22-4 *Arrow,* Incisal embrasure. Area cervical to contact area is gingival embrasure, also called interproximal space. *Triangle,* Interproximal space. (Zeisz and Nuckolls.)

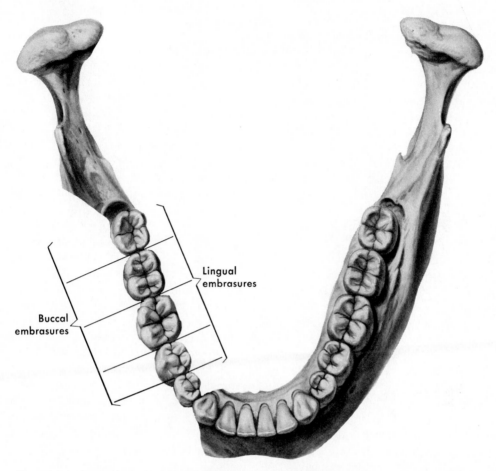

Fig. 22-5 Occlusal view of proximal contact areas and embrasures. Width of contact areas is not just a small point but an area of contact. Notice position of contact area with respect to buccolingual dimensions of tooth. (Zeisz and Nuckolls.)

areas (Fig. 22-5). They allow for the passage of food around the teeth so that food is not forced into the contact area between the teeth. These embrasures, or spillways, are named for their location in relation to the contact area. For instance, the space buccal to the contact area is the **buccal embrasure;** the **lingual embrasure** is lingual to the contact area. The names of the embrasures are **facial** (buccal or labial), **lingual, incisal,** or **occlusal.** There is also a **gingival embrasure,** but only if the interproximal space is not occu-

pied by any gingiva or bone. The gingival embrasure is gingival to the contact area and not usually present. The gingival embrasure and the cervical embrasure are the same. The embrasures have the following purposes:

1. They allow food to be shunted away from contact areas and thus keep food from being packed between the teeth.
2. By doing this, the embrasures reduce the forces of occlusal trauma brought to bear on the teeth—they dissipate and reduce occlusal forces.

3. They are self-cleaning because of the rounded smooth surfaces of the teeth that form the embrasures, allowing food to be swished away by saliva, ingested liquids, the cleaning action of other foods, and the friction of the tongue, cheeks, and lips.

4. They permit a slight amount of stimulation to the gingiva by frictional massage of food while at the same time protecting the gingiva from undue trauma. A poorly contoured embrasure leads to gingival irritation and breakdown.

Location of the Contact Areas, Embrasures, and Interproximal Spaces

Facial view. The contact areas of the anterior teeth are located closer to the incisal surfaces of the teeth. The posterior teeth have their contact areas nearer to the middle third of the teeth. The more posterior the tooth, the more cervical is the location of its contact area. *The one exception* is the distal contact area of the maxillary canine, the location of which is in the center of the middle third of the tooth. This is more cervical than that of the first and second premolars, where the contact areas are just cervical to the junction of the occlusal and middle thirds of the tooth.

The more posterior the location of the tooth, the wider the embrasures, at least in comparison to the occlusocervical dimensions of the tooth. The interproximal spaces become shorter occlusocervically. Although the contact areas are at the same location, the teeth are shorter.

Occlusal view. The location of the contact areas and embrasures, as seen from the occlusal surface, shows that the contact areas of the anterior teeth are located in the center between the labial and lingual surfaces of the tooth. The posterior teeth have contact areas slightly buccal to the center of the teeth. Buccolingually the lingual embrasures are wider than the facial embrasures; the reason is that from their contact point outward the teeth are narrower on the lingual than on the facial side.

Facial and Lingual Contours

Facial and **lingual contours** of the teeth also afford the correct amount of frictional massage to the gingiva by directing food off the tooth and against the gingiva at a proper angle (Fig. 22-6). Too much deflection of the food would leave some gingiva without the right amount of stimulation, whereas too little deflection would allow some food to be forced into the gingival crevice, the space that separates the tooth from the gingiva. Food packed into this crevice could cause gingival inflammation, periodontal disease, or tissue recession.

The correct degree of facial or lingual curvature allows for the proper deflection of food, so that the right amount of tissue stimulation occurs and the gingival crevices are protected. In addition to this, the contour on the lingual surface should allow the tongue to rest against the tooth to promote the most efficient cleaning. Likewise, the facial height of contour allows for maximum cleaning of the lips and cheeks.

It should be apparent that this contour must vary in degree from tooth to tooth, but in general the location of the **buccal height of contour** of anterior and posterior teeth will always be the same—at the cervical third of the tooth. The lingual height of contour of anterior teeth will also

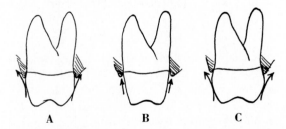

Fig. 22-6 Angle at which food is deflected from tooth surface is determined by buccal and lingual contours. Height of curvature is on buccal and lingual surfaces. **A,** Normal contour. **B,** Undercontoured. **C,** Overcontoured. (Wheeler.)

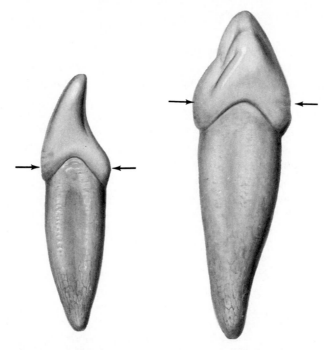

Fig. 22-7 Labial and lingual heights of curvature of mandibular and maxillary incisors and canines are located within cervical thirds of teeth. *Arrows,* Facial and lingual crests of curvature. Also notice curvature of cervical lines (CEJ). (Zeisz and Nuckolls.)

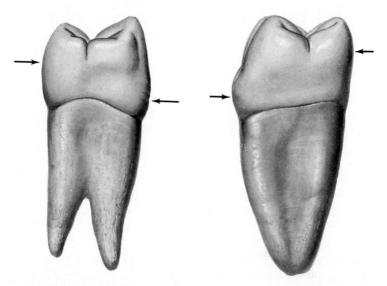

Fig. 22-8 Buccal height of curvature is at cervical third, and lingual height of curvature is at middle third on maxillary and mandibular premolars and molars. *Arrows,* Buccal and lingual crests of curvature. Notice curvatures of cervical lines (CEJ). (Zeisz and Nuckolls.)

be at the cervical third of the tooth, but the **lingual crest of curvature** of posterior teeth will be at or near the middle third (Figs. 22-7 and 22-8). The crest of curvature refers to the widest part of the crown of the tooth. It is the most convex bulge of the tooth. It is the same thing as height of contour of the tooth.

In young people most curvatures, buccal and lingual, lie beneath the gingiva. As the teeth erupt, the curvature becomes more clinically apparent. In the normal adult whose tooth eruption has been completed, the **gingival crest** is cervical to the buccal and labial contours of all maxillary teeth and the lingual contour of anterior teeth. The **free gingiva** of the **cervical crest** covers the cervical enamel of the tooth. The normal amount of curvature found on most facial contours is approximately 0.5 millimeter (mm) and somewhat less lingually on the anterior teeth.

On the lingual side of posterior teeth the crest of the gingiva is considerably more cervical than the lingual contour of the tooth. This is true because the height of contour on the lingual side of posterior teeth is located on the middle third of the crown. The amount of curvature on the lingual side of maxillary posterior teeth averages approximately 0.5 mm, and on the mandibular posterior teeth, approximately 1 mm (Figs. 22-7 and 22-8). The height of contour is the same as the crest of curvature and refers to the buccal or lingual width of a tooth. The contact areas refer to the mesial or distal crest of curvatures of the tooth.

Curvature of the Cementoenamel Junction

As defined earlier, the cementoenamel junction (CEJ) is the line that marks the junction of the enamel and the cementum. It is also called the cervical line.

The curvature of the cervical lines (cementoenamel junction) on the mesial and distal surfaces of the teeth depends on the height of the contact area above the crown **cervix** and on the diameter of the crown labiolingually or buccolingually. The crowns of anterior teeth show greater curvature to the cervical line than the posterior teeth

do. The anterior teeth are narrower labiolingually, and, to afford more anchorage and bony support, nature may have allowed interdental bone between the teeth to protrude more incisally. The posterior teeth, which are wider buccolingually, have more bone support and therefore need not have this raised portion of bone between the teeth. Because of their cervicoincisal length, the anterior teeth need this added portion of bone for anchorage. The tooth crown is shaped on the mesial and distal surfaces to accommodate this needed bone. The enamel does not go so far gingivally on the mesial and distal surfaces as it could; instead, the cementum rises in an incisal direction in the middle of the tooth. This affords more cementum on which the bone can attach itself. The periodontal attachment follows the cervical line and connects the gingiva and the cementum. The periodontal ligament attaches the cementum to the bone.

The maxillary anterior teeth show the greatest amount of curvature of the cervical line. The more anterior the tooth, the greater the curvature. On the other hand, *the mesial curvature of a tooth is greater than the distal curvature of the same tooth.* The mandibular anterior teeth show less curvature than their maxillary counterparts do, generally less than 1 mm variation in cervical curvatures.

The posterior teeth in both arches show little variation. The mesial curvature of all posterior teeth usually averages about 1 mm, and the distal curvature is generally nonexistent or at least very slight, less than 0.5 mm. As a general rule, *the curvature of the cementoenamel junction is usually about 1 mm less on the distal surface of the tooth than on the mesial.* If a maxillary incisor has a 3.5 mm mesial curvature of the cementoenamel junction, the distal curvature may be 2.5 mm (Fig. 22-9).

Self-Cleaning Qualities of the Teeth

To a large extent the teeth are self-cleaning in that the crowns of the teeth are covered by a very smooth enamel. As mentioned previously, the smoothness of this enamel helps food and sticky

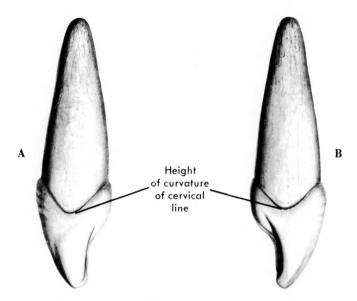

A   B

Height
of curvature
of cervical
line

Fig. 22-9   Mesial curvature of cementoenamel junction is greater than distal curvature. **A,** Mesial view. **B,** Distal view. (Zeisz and Nuckolls.)

substances slip off the crown of the tooth and allows the tooth to remain relatively free of bacteria, thus lessening decay and periodontal disease.

The shape of the crown also aids greatly in the prevention of periodontal disease by stimulating and cleaning the gingival tissue. It does this by deflecting the food onto the gingival tissue at a specific and proper angle. For instance, the shape of the incisors is like a shovel, and accordingly the incisor cuts its way through food and forces it toward the lingual surface onto the gingiva. In the case of the upper teeth, the food is directed toward the gingiva and onto the palate. Thus the food is directed by the shape of the incisor, off the incisor and onto the gingiva.

It is evident that the shapes of the teeth reflect their functions and their self-cleaning ability as well. As you know, the canine is a piercing tool. Like a spear it pierces through food. Because it is wedge shaped, it forces the food off the pointed canine cusp onto the cingulum and the gingiva. The premolars are shaped in such a way that food is deflected onto the occlusal surface of the

premolar, where it is ground up by the cusps of the teeth in the opposing arch.

When food is introduced into the mouth, it is aided by the tongue and cheek in pushing the previously pulverized food back onto the surface of the molars. This process continues from molar to molar until the food reaches the back of the mouth and is swallowed. If there are deep pits and **fissures** on the occlusal surface of the tooth, some of the food debris will remain after eating. It would seem that deep pits, fissures, or holes in the enamel of the teeth would make cleaning difficult. Yet these pits and fissures do provide a method of dissipating the extreme occlusal forces that result from the interdigitation of the cusps in the process of grinding up food. These little pits and fissures act as spillways on the occlusal surfaces of the teeth. Should these pits and fissures be too deep, nature has devised a way to eliminate them.

Primitive people, by eating natural raw foods, wore down some of the enamel of their teeth in the process of chewing. This resulted in the gradual obliteration of the pits and fissures. The wearing down of these pits and fissures could only be accomplished by the diet chosen. For over a million years humans chose to eat foods that were semiraw or uncooked. In this form the food presented a certain amount of roughage in that it was hard and course and helped wear down the enamel. But the modern approach has found a way to avoid all this. Our diet of soft, overcooked, tacky, and sticky foods has resulted in an inability to wear down enamel; additionally, the stickiness of the food allows it to adhere to the tooth surface even when pits and fissures are not present. If our diet leaves a lot to be desired, it must also be said that our ingenuity does not—modern dentistry has found many more painless ways to obliterate the pits and fissures of teeth than through the abrasive action of eating.

PERIODONTIUM

The **periodontium** is the supporting tissue adjacent to the teeth. It consists of the free gingiva, **attached gingiva,** and **alveolar mucosa,** as well as the cementum, periodontal ligament, and bone. These tissues are essential for the support and anchorage of the teeth. The curvatures and contact areas of the teeth must be shaped in such a way that they not only protect these tissues from

excessive trauma but also keep them free of bacteria and offer frictional massage and stimulation.

The buccal and lingual **contours** of the tooth are shaped so that food is deflected off the tooth and onto the gingival tissue. The angle at which the food is deflected is specific (Fig. 22-10). The mechanical friction of the food must not place extreme pressure on the free gingiva, since this part of the gingival apparatus cannot tolerate extreme trauma.

If the curvature is too extreme, the food will be deflected in such a way that the gingival tissue will not be stimulated and cleaned by the frictional action of the food that deflects off it. In this situation, bacteria will not be removed from the free gingival collar around the tooth, and the bacteria could then begin to destroy the gingival tissue. The tissue would become edematous, puffy, and inflamed and would bleed easily, eventually leading to the periodontal breakdown of these supporting structures.

The contact areas are equally essential to the health and maintenance of the periodontal tissue in the interproximal spaces. If **open contacts** are present, the teeth do not touch each other at their contact areas, and food is allowed to pack between the teeth and remain there. The bacteria captured on and in the **gingival crevice** could then cause a periodontal breakdown of these tis-

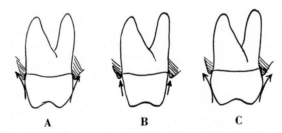

Fig. 22-10 **A,** Normal curvatures as found on maxillary molar. *Arrows,* Path of food as it is deflected over these curvatures onto gingiva. **B,** Molar with little curvature and underdeveloped contours. Gingiva is likely to be stripped or pushed apically through lack of protection and consequent overstimulation. **C,** Molar with excess curvature. Gingiva will be protected too much and will suffer from lack of proper stimulation. Food and bacteria may lodge under these curvatures, promoting pathological disturbances. (Wheeler.)

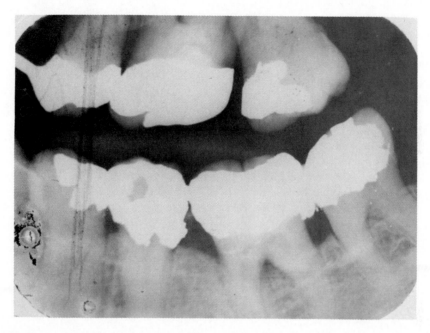

Fig. 22-11   Large open contact between two upper molars and large overhanging restorations on bottom teeth.

sues. If the contact area is so wide open that food can be forced into the interproximal space but not remain in this area because of the extremely large size of the space, the bacteria would be flushed out by the frictional massage of the food. Here again, if the deflection of the food is at an extreme angle, a **recession** of the tissues away from the crown of the teeth could result. When gingival tissue recedes from the tooth, the root of the tooth becomes exposed.

When the missing part of a tooth is restored by some type of dental material, it is very important that the margins of the restoration be smooth and approximate as much as possible the normal shape of the tooth. If the margins are rough, they will allow bacteria to be retained around the restoration and thus cause gingival inflammation and decay. If the margin of the filling or restoration is such that it extends far beyond the tooth, it will cause a condition known as **overhanging restoration.** This condition allows for the buildup of plaque, bacteria, and food. Such a response would damage the gingival tissue (Fig. 22-11). Chapter 27 would be helpful in understanding the clinical implications of Chapter 22.

REVIEW QUESTIONS

1. What is the relationship between the size of embrasures and the location of the contact areas of two adjacent teeth?
2. Name the embrasures and explain their function. Which embrasure is not always present and why?
3. Which teeth have the greater curvature of the cementoenamel junction, anterior or posterior? Why is there a difference?
4. What terms are synonymous with "cementoenamel junction"?
5. Does the diet a person chooses have any effect on the gums and teeth?
6. What happens if a tooth is restored so that it has an overhanging restoration?
7. What happens if two adjacent teeth have open contact areas?

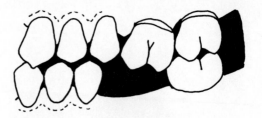

Fig. 22-12

8. What is the difference between a contact area and a contact point?
9. Identify the following in Fig. 22-12:
    a. occlusal embrasure
    b. contact area
    c. interproximal space

23

Dentition

OBJECTIVES

- To understand the difference between primary dentition, secondary dentition, and mixed dentition
- To understand the arrangement of the teeth into dentitions, arches, and quadrants
- To name and code any individual tooth
- To code teeth using the Universal system, the Palmer notation system, and the FDI system
- To identify a tooth when given a code from one of the three systems

ARRANGEMENT OF TEETH

The general arrangement of teeth is referred to as the **dentition. Primary dentition** refers to the twenty **deciduous** teeth, often called baby teeth. **Secondary dentition** refers to the thirty-two permanent teeth (Figs. 23-1 and 23-2).

The dentition is divided into two **arches:** upper and lower. The teeth anchored within the upper jaw belong to the **maxillary arch.** The mandible is the bone that supports the lower arch of teeth, hence the name **mandibular arch.**

The mandibular and maxillary arches each compose one half the dentition. In the permanent dentition of 32 teeth, each arch is composed of 16 teeth. How many teeth are in an arch of the primary dentition? How many teeth compose the total primary dentition?

Each arch is further divided into a right and a left half. Thus there are four **quadrants,** two in each arch. The quadrants are determined by the intersection of a vertical and a horizontal line, which bracket the entire quadrant in the Palmer notation system. The maxillary quadrants are represented by numbers or letters above the horizontal line; the mandibular, below the line.

The technical term for the dividing line between the right and left sides of the body is the **midsagittal plane.** In dentistry this is called the **midline,** or **median line,** of the face. The right and left quadrants are separated by this vertical line, which represents the midline of the skull when facing the patient.

Thus each quadrant consists of one fourth of the dentition and has a mirror image on the other side of the arch, as well as an opposing quadrant in the opposite arch.

Note that a permanent dentition quadrant has eight teeth—a central and lateral incisor, a canine, a first and second premolar, and a first, second, and third molar. A deciduous quadrant has five teeth—two incisors, a canine, and a first and second molar. There are no deciduous premolars.

The permanent teeth that replace or succeed the deciduous teeth are called **succedaneous** teeth. The permanent molars are called **nonsuccedaneous** teeth. They do not have predecessors, and they do not succeed or replace deciduous (primary) teeth. The permanent premolars replace the deciduous molars. How many teeth in the secondary dentition are nonsuccedaneous? How many are in each arch? How many are in each quadrant?

A **mixed dentition** refers to one that is composed of some permanent teeth and some deciduous teeth. After a child's permanent teeth begin to erupt, there are several years of mixed denti-

MAXILLARY

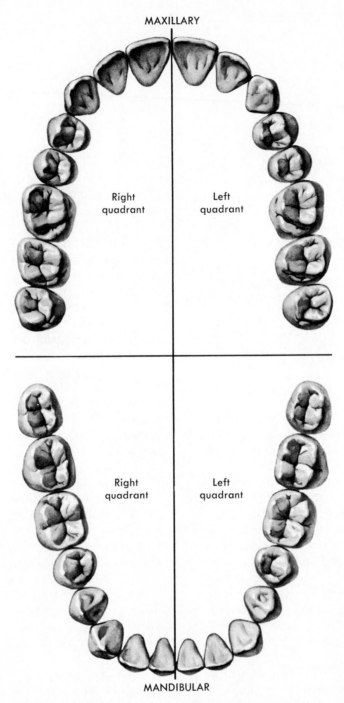

Right
quadrant

Left
quadrant

Right
quadrant

Left
quadrant

MANDIBULAR

Fig. 23-1 Permanent teeth, or secondary dentition. Horizontal and vertical lines divide arches into quadrants. (Massler and Schour.)

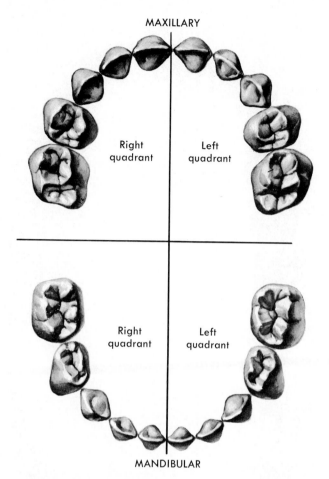

MAXILLARY

Right
quadrant

Left
quadrant

Right
quadrant

Left
quadrant

MANDIBULAR

Fig. 23-2   Deciduous teeth, or primary dentition.
(Massler and Schour.)

tion. Not all the deciduous teeth are replaced at one time. Some adults may also have a mixed dentition; this occurs when a deciduous tooth is retained although the remainder of the teeth are permanent.

NAMING AND CODING TEETH

When identifying a specific tooth, list the dentition, arch, quadrant, and tooth name in that order. For example:

permanent	mandibular	right	central incisor
(dentition)	(arch)	(quadrant)	(tooth)
primary	maxillary	left	lateral incisor

Therefore, for example, we would refer to a "permanent mandibular right central incisor," *not* a "right mandibular permanent central incisor."

It is essential that each dental team be familiar with the various systems of naming and coding teeth. Although each office may use only one system, it is necessary that the personnel be familiar

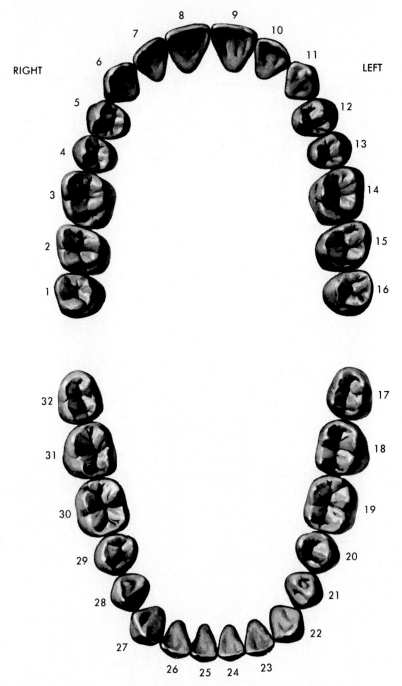

RIGHT

LEFT

Fig. 23-3 Universal system of permanent teeth. (Massler and Schour.)

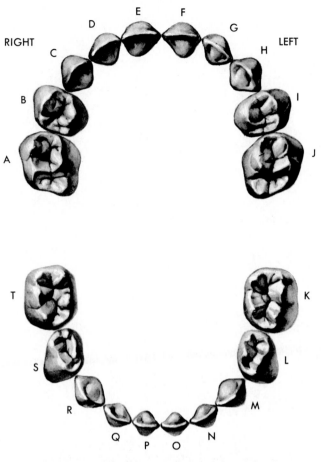

Fig. 23-4 Universal system of deciduous teeth. (Massler and Schour.)

with all systems so that communication between dental offices is possible. Therefore the most popular systems will be considered here.

Universal System

The **Universal system** uses the arabic numerals 1 through 32 for permanent teeth; the letters A through T are used for the primary teeth. The number 1 is assigned to the most posterior molar on the upper right, the permanent maxillary right third molar. The highest number is given to the permanent mandibular right third molars (Fig. 23-3). Likewise, the letter A is given to the

primary maxillary right second molar and the letter T to the primary mandibular right second molar (Fig. 23-4).

What symbol would represent each of the following?

1. Secondary mandibular left first molar
2. Secondary maxillary right first premolar
3. Primary maxillary right first molar
4. Primary mandibular left central incisor

What tooth is represented by each of the following symbols of the Universal system?

19   5   B   O

Palmer Notation System

In the **Palmer notation system** each of the four quadrants is given its own prefix symbol. For instance, if the tooth is a maxillary tooth, the number or letter should be placed above the line of the prefix symbol, thus indicating an upper tooth. Oppositely, a mandibular tooth symbol should be placed below the line, indicating a lower tooth. Teeth from the right quadrant should be placed in a bracket with a line to their immediate right. This line indicates the midline or the midsagittal plane (refer to the diagram below).

The number or letter assigned to the tooth depends on its position relative to the midline; for example, the central incisors, the teeth closest to the midline, have the lowest number—the number 1 for permanent teeth and the letter A for deciduous teeth.

After studying the diagram, notice that there are thirty-two individual numbers, four of each with numbers ranging from 1 to 8. In the Palmer notation system, the lowest number is closest to the midline. For instance, all central incisors, maxillary and mandibular, right or left, are given the same number—1. All lateral incisors are given the number 2, all canines the number 3, and the number 8 is assigned to the third molars. The farther from the midline, the higher the number assigned to the tooth. The number 6 is assigned to the first molars, since it is the sixth tooth from the midline.

The tooth is further identified as being maxillary or mandibular by its position above or below the horizontal maxillary–mandibular dividing line. In the diagram notice that the number 1 appears at the four locations closest to what is called the midline. Number 1 in all instances refers to a central incisor. By studying the midline bracket, we can identify whether the tooth belongs to a right or left quadrant. If the bracket is to the left of the letter or number, the tooth belongs to the left quadrant. The teeth are placed in relation to the midline as if one were *looking* at the patient, not looking from within the patient's mouth.

Study the following symbols:

$$\frac{}{3}\Big|\,1\ 2\ 4$$

What can be determined from this diagram?
1. We know that three of the symbols (1, 2, and 4) are maxillary teeth because they are above the horizontal line.
2. One of the teeth (3) is a mandibular tooth. Why?
3. Number 1, 2, and 4 belong to the patient's maxillary left quadrant because the vertical line is to the immediate left of these numbers. This would also be the relationship of the vertical line to the teeth in the patient's

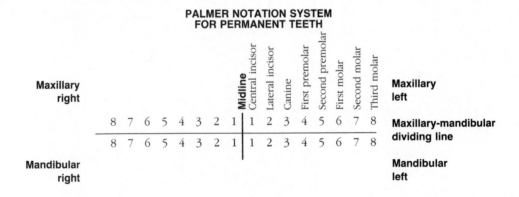

**PALMER NOTATION SYSTEM
FOR PERMANENT TEETH**

	Central incisor	Lateral incisor	Canine	First premolar	Second premolar	First molar	Second molar	Third molar	
Maxillary right									**Maxillary left**
8 7 6 5 4 3 2 1	1	2	3	4	5	6	7	8	**Maxillary-mandibular dividing line**
8 7 6 5 4 3 2 1	1	2	3	4	5	6	7	8	
Mandibular right									**Mandibular left**

mouth if one were *looking at* the patient.

4. Number 3 refers to a tooth in the mandibular right quadrant. Why?

5. Since number 1 refers to a central incisor, number 2 to a lateral incisor, and number 4 to the first premolar, these numbers refer to the maxillary left central and lateral incisors and the first premolar.

6. Since number 3 refers to a canine, number 3 in this diagram refers to the mandibular right canine.

If we wanted to represent only one tooth, such as the secondary maxillary left lateral incisor, the following symbol would be used:

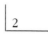

All that we have done is eliminate some of the horizontal and vertical lines. The original symbol would have looked like this:

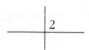

So far we have been using secondary (permanent) teeth in our examples of the Palmer system. Remember that the numbers 1 to 8 are used for permanent teeth and capital letters A to E for primary (deciduous) teeth. Refer to the diagram below for deciduous teeth.

Which tooth is represented by each of the following?

What is the symbol for the primary mandibular right first molar?

FDI System

In the **FDI system** (from the Fédération Dentaire Internationale) each tooth, deciduous or permanent, is given a two-digit number. No letters or duplicate numbers are used. It is similar to the Palmer system in that the second digit indicates the position of the tooth relative to the midline. The first digit indicates the quadrant and whether the tooth is permanent or deciduous.

Looking at Fig. 23-5, notice that each tooth has its own specific two-digit number. The permanent maxillary right quadrant teeth are assigned numbers from 11 to 18; the permanent maxillary left quadrant teeth, numbers in the twenties (21 through 28). The permanent mandibular teeth are numbered 31 to 38 in the left quadrant and 41 to 48 in the right.

Each quadrant is symbolized by a specific first digit, and all teeth in that quadrant have the same first digit. The second digit depends on the position the tooth occupies relative to the midline. The lowest number is given to the tooth closest to the midline.

Likewise, the deciduous teeth have their own first-digit number identifying each specific quadrant. Similar to the above, the second digit denotes the position the tooth occupies relative to the midline. See Fig. 23-6 for quadrant numbers.

PALMER NOTATION SYSTEM
FOR PRIMARY TEETH

					Central incisor	Lateral incisor	Canine	First molar	Second molar		
Maxillary right										**Maxillary left**
	E	D	C	B	A	A	B	C	D	E	
Mandibular right	E	D	C	B	A	A	B	C	D	E	**Mandibular left**

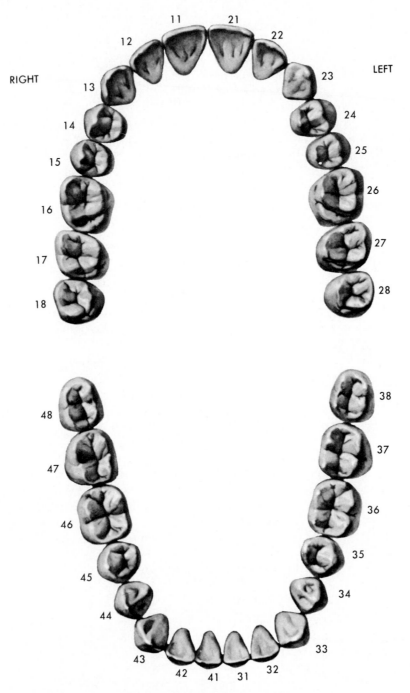

RIGHT

LEFT

Fig. 23-5 FDI system of permanent teeth. (Massler and Schour.)

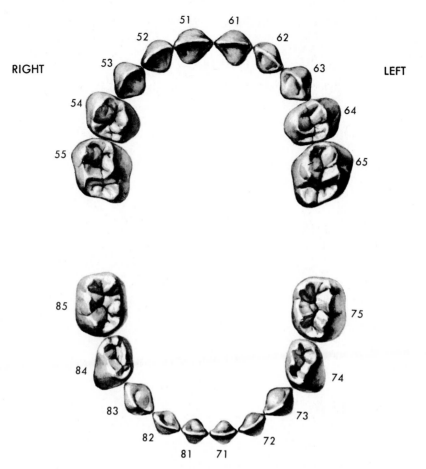

Fig. 23-6   FDI system of deciduous teeth. (Massler and Schour.)

REVIEW QUESTIONS

1. Name two types of dentition and the number of teeth in each.
2. Name the different arches. How many teeth are present in a primary arch and how many in a secondary mandibular arch?
3. How many different quadrants are there?
4. Are any primary teeth succedaneous? If not, why not?
5. Name all the succedaneous teeth.
6. Are secondary molars nonsuccedaneous?
7. A dentition composed of both primary and secondary teeth is called a _____ dentition.
8. How many dentitions are there?
9. Identify the following in the Universal system:
   a. numbers 1, 5, 17, 20, 28, 32
   b. letters A, G, L, M, T
10. Give the correct Universal system symbol for the following:
    a. primary maxillary left central
    b. primary mandibular right first molar
    c. primary maxillary right canine

d. permanent maxillary right second premolar

e. permanent mandibular right central incisor

11. Identify the following by dentition, arch, and quadrant:
    a. $\underline{8}$
    b. $\underline{E}|$
    c. $\underline{1}$
    d. $\underline{6}|$

12. Translate the above four symbols of the Palmer system into the symbols of the Universal system.

13. Give the Palmer, Universal, and FDI symbols for the permanent mandibular right first molar.

14. Give the Palmer, Universal, and FDI symbols for the deciduous mandibular right first molar.

15. Give the Palmer, Universal, and FDI symbols for the permanent mandibular right first premolar.

16. Identify the following symbols. Which systems are they derived from and which teeth do they represent?
    a. 8
    b. $8|$
    c. $\underline{E}|$
    d. $\underline{1}|$
    e. 11
    f. 18

24

Development, Form, and Eruption

OBJECTIVES

- To understand how the tooth germs develop within the crypts
- To understand how the growth centers, or lobes, fuse and form a tooth
- To understand that this fusion can take a variety of forms, which result in different types of teeth—incisors, premolars, and molars
- To know how many lobes form each type of tooth and where the lobes are located
- To understand the eruption schedule of the deciduous and permanent teeth
- To understand some general rules about the eruption of teeth
- To understand the phenomena of mesial drift, root resorption, and exfoliation
- To understand the implications of the following terms: impacted teeth, congenitally missing teeth, attrition, occlusal plane, and curve of Spee
- To understand the periods of primary, mixed, and permanent dentition

DEVELOPMENT AND FORM

During the sixth week of fetal life (7 or 8 months before birth), tiny tooth buds, sometimes called **tooth germs,** begin to grow within the alveolar process of the fetus. Tooth germs are small clumps of cells that have the ability to form tooth tissues (dentin, enamel, cementum, and pulp). Both the primary and secondary teeth develop from these tooth germs, which later are located within cavities of the alveolar process called **crypts.** (See Chapter 4 text and Figs. 4-1 to 4-4.)

At this time the dentin and enamel begin to form, followed later in development by the cementum. The type of dentin formed at this early stage is called primary dentin, and it occurs before root completion. Secondary dentin is continually formed within the tooth by the same odontoblasts that form regular dentin. This process continues throughout one's entire lifetime. It differs from reparative dentin in that reparative dentin is laid down locally as protection for the pulp from irritation, caries, or trauma (see Chapter 5, p. 66).

The permanent teeth show no evidence of development until about the fourth month of fetal life. At this time their formation begins.

The primary teeth begin to calcify about the fourth or fifth month of fetal life. The process of **calcification** is the hardening of the tooth tissues by the deposition of mineral salts within these tissues (Fig. 24-1). This process continues until about the third or fourth year after birth, when the deciduous roots become fully formed.

Soon after birth the permanent teeth begin to calcify and continue until about the twenty-fifth year, when the roots of the third molars become calcified. The last tissue to become calcified is the apex of the root. (See Chapters 14 and 15.)

Developmental Lobes

Each tooth begins to develop from four or more growth centers. These centers grow out from the tooth germ and are known as **developmental lobes.** The anterior teeth and the maxillary premolars develop from four of these lobes, three labial and one lingual. The lobes grow and

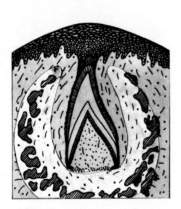

Fig. 24-1 Beginning of tooth calcification. Small hole in bone in which tooth bud germ forms is called a crypt. It later will become tooth socket, which will house root of tooth. (Massler and Schour.)

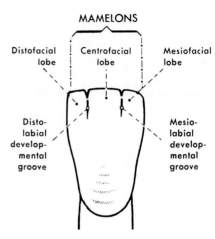

Fig. 24-2 Incisal ridge of three labial lobes is formed from mamelons. (Zeisz and Nuckolls.)

develop within their bony crypt until they fuse, or unite. This fusion of the lobes is called **coalescence.** The junction that forms the union of these lobes is marked by lines on the tooth called developmental grooves, which can be seen on the tooth after it has erupted.

The number of developmental lobes necessary for the formation of a tooth depends on the particular tooth and how many cusps it may have. For instance, all the anterior teeth develop from four lobes, three labial and one lingual. The three labial lobes form the labial surface of the tooth. The **mamelons,** which are evident after the eruption of incisor teeth, are the incisal ridges of these three labial developmental lobes. The lines separating these mamelons are the **developmental grooves.**

In Fig. 24-2 notice how the three labial lobes fuse to form the entire labial surface. The only evidence that there ever were three separate lobes is at the incisal ridge, where the mamelons are distinct and separate, and on the labial surface of a tooth, where there are developmental lines or grooves. The three labial developmental

lobes are called the mesiofacial, centrofacial, and distofacial. The sole lingual lobe is called, appropriately, the lingual lobe and makes up the entire cingulum on the lingual surface of the tooth.

Lobes and Cusps

The maxillary premolars are like the anterior teeth in that they have three facial lobes and one lingual lobe. Unlike the anterior teeth, the three facial lobes form one high buccal cusp instead of an incisal ridge, and the single lingual cusp forms a large lingual cusp rather than a cingulum. The names of the lobes are the same as those for the anterior teeth (Fig. 24-3).

The mandibular first premolar has the same number and arrangement of lobes as the maxillary premolars have. The lingual cusp of the mandibular first premolar is smaller than its maxillary counterpart. These teeth are termed bicuspids, since they have only two cusps, a buccal and a lingual. The mandibular second premolar varies—it may be a two-cusped or three-cusped form. Because not all these premolars have only two cusps, the term "premolar" is preferred.

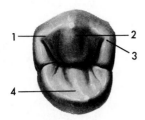

Fig. 24-3 Four lobes of maxillary second premolar. (See also Fig. 21-22, *B* and *E*.) (Zeisz and Nuckolls.)

The two-cusp variety of the mandibular second premolar is exactly the same in number and arrangement of lobes as the mandibular first premolar. The lingual cusp of this bicuspid type is longer than that of the mandibular first premolar. The facial lobes and cusps of the three-cusp variety are exactly the same as on the first premolar, but the lingual lobes are quite different. First, there are two lobes instead of a single lobe: a mesiolingual and distolingual lobe. Second, this results in two separate lingual cusps, with the mesiolingual usually being larger than the distolingual. Third, there is a considerable difference in the number and location of the developmental grooves, with an additional groove located between the two lingual cusps. Further differences

in anatomy are discussed in Chapter 31 (Figs. 31-44 to 31-49).

All molars have two facial and two lingual lobes, except the first molars, which usually have a fifth or minor lobe. For example, the maxillary first molar generally has five developing lobes: two major facial lobes (mesiobuccal and distobuccal) and a mesiolingual lobe; one minor lobe, the distolingual; and one **rudimentary lobe,** called the **lobe of Carabelli,** or commonly called the **cusp of Carabelli.** Each of the four major and minor lobes develops into a cusp, which is named according to its lobe; for example, the mesiobuccal lobe forms the mesiobuccal cusp. The fifth lobe, the lobe of Carabelli, is more appropriately termed a tubercle than a cusp. It is located on the lingual surface of the mesiolingual cusp. The lobe of Carabelli is not a cusp located on a cusp; rather, it is a tubercle (a small cusp-like elevation) located on a cusp formed from its own individual lobe.

The maxillary second molar often does not have a cusp of Carabelli; if it is present, it is much smaller in proportion to the other lobes. This molar will be much smaller in all cusp proportions as a rule, and the distolingual cusp (which is a minor cusp) is often even smaller in proportion.

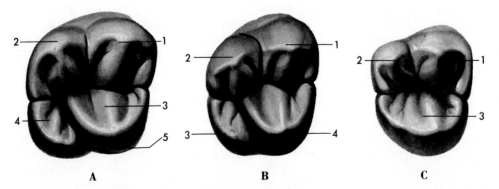

Fig. 24-4 **A,** Maxillary first molar with five lobes. **B,** Maxillary second molar with four lobes. **C,** Maxillary third molar with three lobes. (Zeisz and Nuckolls.)

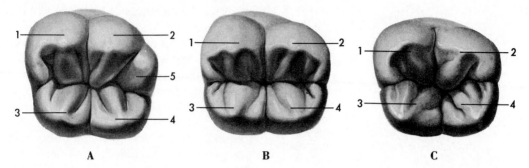

Fig. 24-5 **A,** Mandibular first molar with five cusps. **B,** Mandibular second molar with four cusps. **C,** Mandibular third molar. Each cusp is formed from one lobe. (Zeisz and Nuckolls.)

As a rule, maxillary and mandibular second molars are smaller than the first molars. The minor cusp becomes smaller as the location becomes more posterior. Therefore it is not unusual that the third molars may have only major cusps and no minor cusps. In such instances a maxillary third molar might have only three cusps, with little or no distolingual cusp. The crown is usually smaller and its roots shorter than those of the second or first molar (Fig. 24-4).

The mandibular first molar has four major cusps, mesiobuccal, distobuccal, mesiolingual, and distolingual, as well as one minor cusp, the distal.

The third molars are usually smaller than the second molars. As a general rule, the more posterior the molar, the smaller it is. The distal cusp is generally missing on both (Fig. 24-5).

Special mention should be made about third molars in general. They are the most unpredictable of all the teeth. For instance, it is quite possible to have extremely well-developed mandibular third molars that are better proportioned and larger than the first molars in the same mouth, but they are more likely to be poorly formed and vary from three to eight cusps. They are also most likely to be not only deviated in form but also missing entirely. With this in mind, any general rule that applies to the regression of minor cusps or the size of teeth must be limited by the extreme variability of third molars.

ERUPTION

The first teeth to emerge into the oral cavity are the deciduous or baby teeth. Calcification of these teeth begins around the fourth month of fetal life. By the end of the sixth month, all the deciduous teeth have begun to develop. Normally no teeth are visible in the mouth at birth. Occasionally infants are born with erupted incisor teeth, but these premature teeth are usually lost soon after birth.

The calcification process first forms the crown of the tooth, and root formation follows later. No two persons are exactly alike in calcification, crown and root formation, or eruption schedules. The human dentition varies somewhat in all persons, but certain approximations or averages are recognizable.

During the development of the enamel and dentin of the teeth, minerals are deposited in the forming tooth germs. Any fever, metabolic dysfunction, childhood or nutritional disease, or physical illness or trauma can alter the formation of the teeth and even stop their formation or mineralization completely.

There are twenty deciduous teeth, ten in each jaw. Following is a list of deciduous teeth and approximate eruption times. It represents more recent data on eruption times than Fig. 24-6.

Central incisors	8 to 12 months
Lateral incisors	9 to 13 months
First molars	13 to 19 months
Canines	16 to 22 months
Second molars	25 to 33 months

The first general rule concerning eruption is that individual mandibular teeth usually precede the maxillary teeth in this process. The second rule is that the teeth in both jaws erupt in pairs, one on the right and one on the left. The third rule is that teeth usually erupt slightly earlier in girls than in boys. Remember that these rules are not firm, and exceptions are numerous.

The first teeth to appear in the mouth are usually the deciduous mandibular central incisors. They generally erupt at the age of approximately 8 months. A month or so later the maxillary central incisors can be seen.

The deciduous mandibular lateral incisors emerge about the ninth month, followed by the maxillary laterals about a month later.

To illustrate the variety that can exist, I have seen many instances in which the first two teeth to erupt were the maxillary central incisors. I have also seen an equal number of instances in which three or more of the mandibular incisors erupted before any of the maxillary incisors.

Next to erupt are the mandibular first deciduous molars, at approximately 13 to 19 months of age, closely followed by the maxillary first deciduous molars. The deciduous canines erupt between 16 and 22 months of age, followed by the second molars between the twenty-fifth and thirty-third months. They are often called the 2-year-old molars. Much of the cantankerous attitude of 2-year-olds is credited to the fact that the eruption of these large molars is painful.

All the deciduous teeth are expected to have been erupted by the time the child is 2¾ years old. For the next 36 months, as the child continues to grow, so too do the jaws, which support the teeth. The teeth that have erupted, however, do not become any larger. Consequently, by 5 years of age it is normal to have spaces and separations between the teeth, caused by the increased growth of the jaws.

Unfortunately, many people do not realize the importance of the deciduous teeth. They believe that since these teeth will be lost in the process of making way for the permanent teeth, they are unimportant and are left to suffer dental neglect. Terms such as "baby teeth" or "milk teeth" lend credence to this fallacy and should be discouraged.

With premature loss of deciduous teeth, the normal jaw growth and development may not take place. The deciduous teeth must remain intact to retain the proper spacing for the permanent teeth that will replace them. So too must the deciduous dental arch help guide the first permanent molars into their normal position. These molars act as the foundation for the rest of the permanent dentition. To a large extent the proper position and location of the other permanent teeth are dependent on the first permanent molars being in their proper position (Fig. 24-6).

Normal growth and development of the jaws also depend on daily exercise. Premature loss of a deciduous tooth results in one side of the jaw developing differently from the other because a normal amount of exercise is not divided equally when one tooth is missing.

PERMANENT DENTITION

The first teeth of the permanent dentition to emerge into the oral cavity are the first molars. They emerge immediately distal to the deciduous second molars. Often they are called the 6-year molars because they erupt at approximately 6 years of age. Much larger than the deciduous molars, they cannot emerge into the oral cavity until sufficient jaw growth has occurred to allow space for them.

Along with the eruption of the permanent molars comes the phenomenon of **mesial drift.** Me-

DECIDUOUS DENTITION

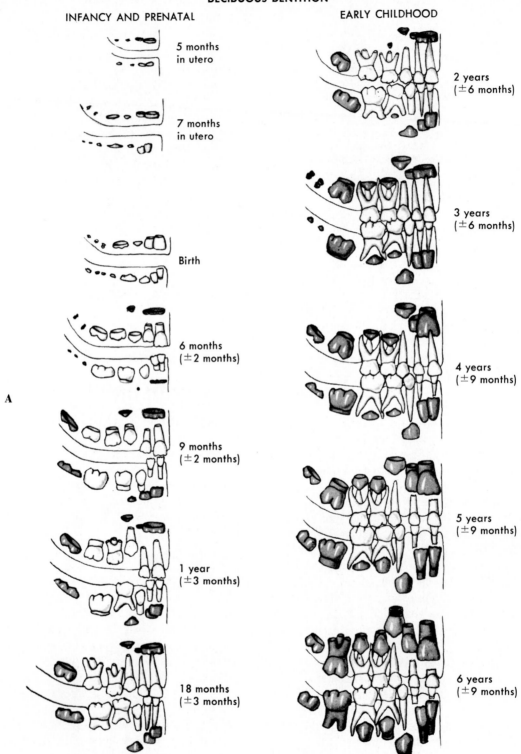

INFANCY AND PRENATAL

5 months
in utero

7 months
in utero

Birth

6 months
(±2 months)

9 months
(±2 months)

1 year
(±3 months)

18 months
(±3 months)

EARLY CHILDHOOD

2 years
(±6 months)

3 years
(±6 months)

4 years
(±9 months)

5 years
(±9 months)

6 years
(±9 months)

A

Fig. 24-6 Development of human dentition. **A,** Deciduous dentition. (Massler and Schour.)

Continued.

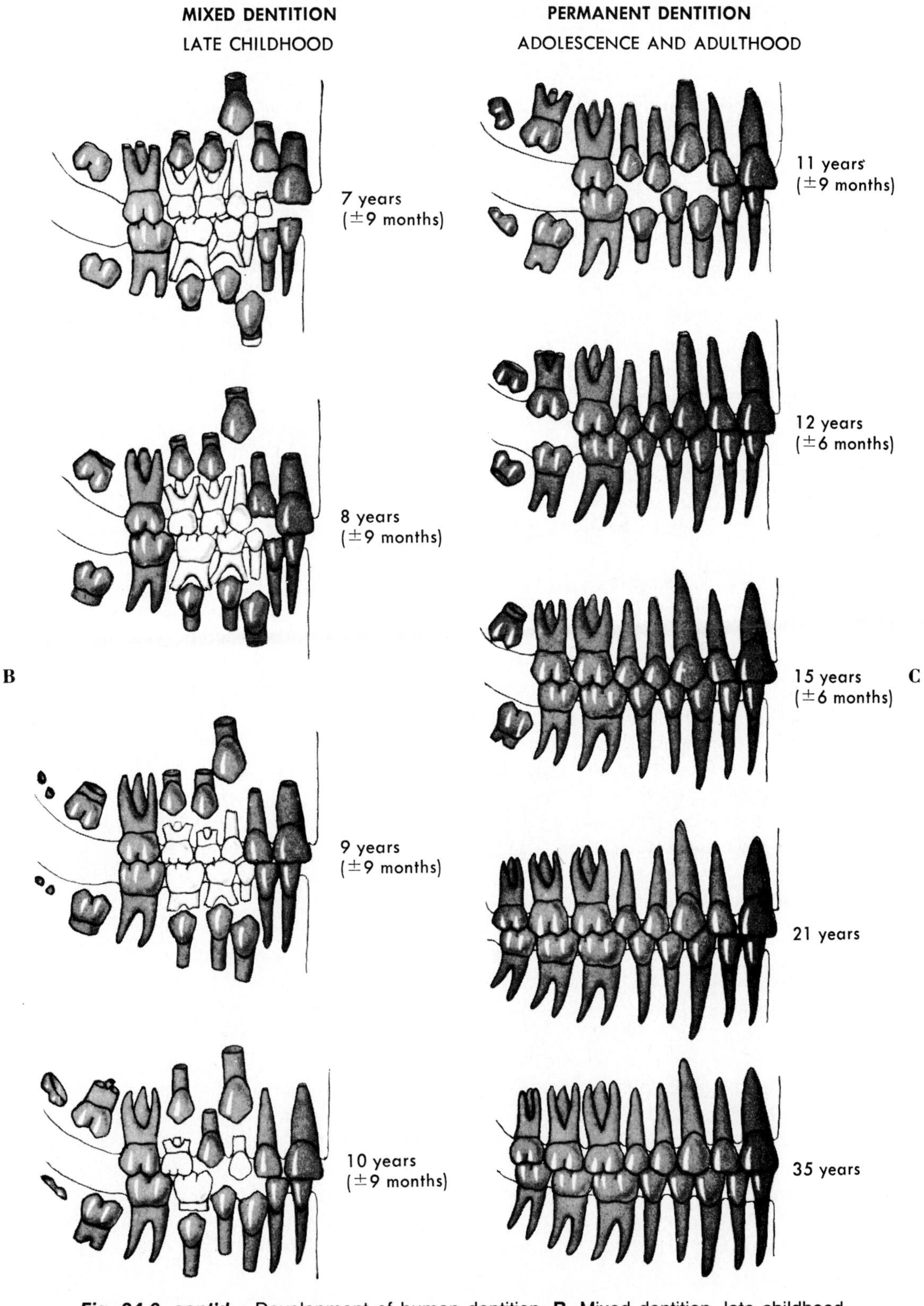

MIXED DENTITION
LATE CHILDHOOD

PERMANENT DENTITION
ADOLESCENCE AND ADULTHOOD

7 years (±9 months)

8 years (±9 months)

9 years (±9 months)

10 years (±9 months)

11 years (±9 months)

12 years (±6 months)

15 years (±6 months)

21 years

35 years

B

C

Fig. 24-6, cont'd Development of human dentition. **B,** Mixed dentition, late childhood. **C,** Permanent dentition, adolescence and adulthood. (Massler and Schour.)

sial drift is the tendency of the permanent molars to have an eruptive force toward the midline. This means that the permanent molars not only erupt occlusally to meet their antagonists in the opposite arch, but they also have an eruptive force that causes them to move mesially. This force is strong enough to move the permanent molars into any available space mesial to them. The phenomenon has two direct effects on the deciduous dentition: (1) the spaces between the deciduous teeth are closed as the first molar pushes the deciduous molars together; (2) if a deciduous tooth is prematurely lost or if interproximal decay on the deciduous molar is not restored, the permanent first molar moves mesially into the available space. Since there is very little extra space left to allow room for the eruption of premolars and canines, the infringement of the permanent molar into this space may keep a premolar or canine from erupting.

The next permanent teeth to erupt are the central incisors, the mandibular at about 6 or 7 years of age and the maxillary at about 7 or 8 years.

The permanent incisors take over the position that the deciduous incisors held. This is made possible because the deciduous incisors are exfoliated. **Exfoliation** is the process by which the roots of a baby tooth are resorbed and dissolved until so little root remains that the baby tooth falls out. As the permanent tooth erupts, osteoclastic cells destroy the root of the deciduous tooth. This phenomenon is called **resorption.** The pressure brought to bear on the deciduous root by the eruption of the permanent tooth triggers the body to activate certain bone-destroying cells called **osteoclasts.** These cells destroy the roots of the deciduous teeth. As each deciduous root is destroyed, the tooth loses its anchorage, becomes loose, and finally exfoliates. During this process, the permanent tooth moves into the space that was occupied by the deciduous tooth.

It is not uncommon for the permanent incisors to erupt lingually to the deciduous incisors. Sometimes both central incisors are still in place, with the permanent central incisor located immediately lingual to the deciduous tooth. When the deciduous tooth is finally lost, pressure from the tongue forces the permanent tooth facially until it occupies its correct position, in a balance between the forces of the tongue lingually and the lips facially.

The next teeth to erupt are the lateral incisors at 7 to 9 years of age, followed by the mandibular canines at 9 or 10 years. The maxillary canines *do not erupt* at this time. The developing incisors and canines are in a position lingual to the deciduous roots. Like the central incisors they can erupt lingual to their predecessors.

The mandibular canines are followed by the mandibular first premolars, at 10 to 12 years of age. Maxillary first premolars erupt soon after, at 10 or 11 years of age. The mandibular canines and the first premolars often erupt simultaneously.

The second premolars erupt at 10 to 12 years of age, with the maxillary teeth often preceding the eruption of the mandibular teeth. This is the most common exception to the rule of mandibular teeth preceding the maxillary.

The maxillary canine then erupts at 11 or 12 years of age. It is very important that the deciduous teeth have maintained the proper amount of space for the canine to erupt. If the space is insufficient, the canine is forced to erupt facially toward the cheek or possibly is unable to erupt at all. In the latter situation the tooth is blocked out by the already erupted teeth, and there is little available room.

At about the same time, 11 to 13 years of age, the mandibular second molars emerge, followed within the year by their maxillary counterparts. The permanent second molars are often called 12-year molars.

The third molars do not appear in the oral cavity until 17 years of age or later. There is much variation in the eruption of third molars, especially when one considers that third molars are the most likely teeth to be **impacted.** Impacted teeth are those that do not completely erupt but remain embedded in bone or soft tissue. Man-

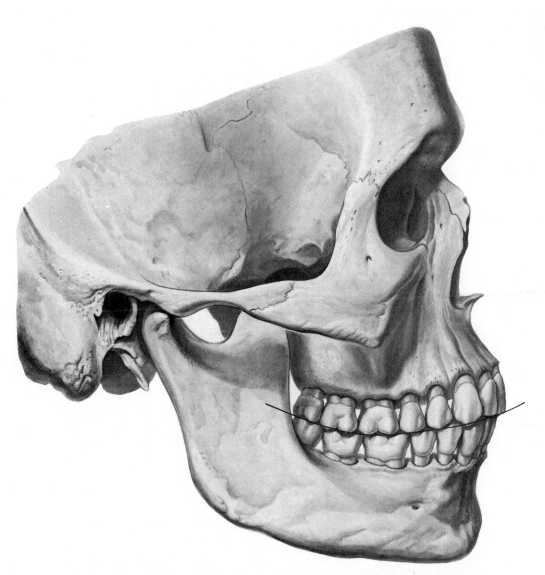

Fig. 24-7 Occlusal plane (curve of Spee) rises to meet incisors and third molars. It dips down in area of first molars and second premolars. (Zeisz and Nuckolls.)

dibular third molars are most often affected because the mandible has to grow enough to accommodate them. The maxillary third molars are the next most likely teeth to be impacted.

The third molars, maxillary and mandibular, are also the most common teeth to be **congenitally missing.** A congenitally missing tooth is one that never forms because a tooth bud was never produced from which to form it. This can be a hereditary trait.

After the eruption of the third molars, the eruptive forces do not cease. Eruption continues because of **attrition,** the wearing away of the tooth through contact of its functioning surfaces.

As the teeth erupt and meet their antagonist in the opposite arch, they form what is known as the **occlusal plane.** Von Spee noted that the cusps and incisal ridges of the teeth tended to follow a curved line when the arches were observed from a point opposite the first molars. This line of the occlusal surfaces is known as the occlusal plane. The curved alignment of the occlusal plane is named after von Spee and is called the **curve of Spee** (Fig. 24-7).

Following is an approximate breakdown of permanent tooth eruption:

Maxillary

Central incisor	7 to 8 years
Lateral incisor	8 to 9 years
Canine	11 to 12 years
First premolar	10 to 11 years
Second premolar	10 to 12 years
First molar	6 to 7 years
Second molar	12 to 13 years
Third molar	17 to 22 years

Mandibular

Central incisor	6 to 7 years
Lateral incisor	7 to 8 years
Canine	9 to 10 years
First premolar	10 to 12 years
Second premolar	11 to 12 years
First molar	6 to 7 years
Second molar	11 to 13 years
Third molar	17 to 22 years

PERIODS OF DENTITION

The period of primary dentition begins with the eruption of the first deciduous tooth. This first deciduous tooth, a central incisor, usually erupts 8 months after birth, but some erupt as early as 6 months or as late as 12 months after birth. The period of primary dentition lasts as long as only deciduous teeth are present. When the first permanent molar erupts, the period of primary dentition ends.

At about 6 years of age the period of **mixed dentition** begins. This period exists while both primary and secondary (permanent) teeth are simultaneously present. This period ends when the last deciduous tooth is exfoliated and only permanent teeth remain.

The period of permanent dentition begins when the last primary tooth is lost and ends when the last permanent tooth is lost. This period usually begins at about 12 years of age and hopefully does not end.

If all of the permanent teeth are lost, no other period of dentition exists because no dentition is in existence. Such a condition is termed **edentulous,** meaning 'no teeth.' Refer to Chapters 4 and 5 for discussion of the formation of enamel, dentin, and pulp and to Chapter 33 for information concerning deciduous teeth.

REVIEW QUESTIONS

1. Only primary teeth begin to develop in utero (during fetal life). True or false?
2. Name the first hard tissue of the tooth that is formed.
3. What does the term "coalescence" mean?
4. How do developmental lines occur?
5. From what lobe does the cingulum of an anterior tooth form?
6. What is a rudimentary lobe of the maxillary first molar called?
7. Which teeth erupt first, the deciduous first molars or the canines?
8. Which of the following statements are usually true about eruption?

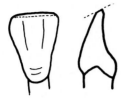

Fig. 24-8

Fig. 24-9

a. Girls' teeth erupt earlier than boys' teeth.
b. Maxillary teeth erupt before their mandibular counterparts.
c. Teeth in both jaws do not erupt in pairs.
d. The eruption sequence varies little from person to person.

9. Name the first permanent tooth to erupt in the oral cavity.

10. If a child has spaces between the deciduous teeth at 5 years of age, these spaces will always remain, even after the permanent teeth have erupted. True or false?

11. Of the following, which is the only acceptable dental term?
   a. bicuspid   c. milk teeth
   b. premolar   d. baby teeth

12. Explain all the various problems connected with premature loss of a deciduous molar.

13. With which teeth does the phenomenon of mesial drift occur, and what does it do?

14. Explain the following terms.
   a. exfoliation
   b. resorption
   c. congenitally missing
   d. attrition

15. The mamelons of the mandibular right central incisor in Fig. 24-8 have worn off, forming an incisal edge from what was once the incisal ridge. Redraw the mamelons.

16. Label and name the developmental lobes of the mandibular premolar in Fig. 24-9. (*Hint:* It has three cusps that take their names from the developmental lobes from which they were formed.)

17. What periods of dentition might a 12-year-old boy be in? Give two possible reasons for each period of dentition.

18. When does the period of primary dentition end?

19. What deciduous teeth might an 11-year-old still have?

20. An orthodontist asks you to refer a patient back to him when the patient is out of mixed dentition. When would you send the patient back to him? What marks the end of the period of mixed dentition?

25

Occlusion

OBJECTIVES

- To understand how the eruption schedule, growth, and ultimate alignment of the teeth are related
- To understand how muscle forces affect the alignment of the teeth
- To understand what the curve of Spee, the curve of Wilson, and the sphere of Monson are
- To understand in what way the teeth are aligned vertically—maxillary to mandibular
- To understand what centric occlusion is
- To understand the meaning of overjet, overbite, cross-bite, and open bite, as well as some idea of how they occur
- To know and identify the three occlusal classifications
- To understand the relationship that exists between the teeth during lateral excursive movements

POSITION AND SEQUENCE OF ERUPTION

In the preceding chapter we studied the eruption patterns of the teeth. It is easy to see how the eruption schedule helps the permanent teeth emerge in their proper position. The loss of certain deciduous teeth at the proper time allows the permanent teeth to move into key positions.

What about the deciduous teeth? What allows them to take their position for alignment? When we look at the deciduous teeth, they not only appear in a certain position that is normal for each tooth but also are arranged in a row or line. This is referred to as being in alignment.

Normally, the eruption schedule helps the de-

ciduous teeth to take their proper position. For example, the central incisors come into position anterior to the lateral incisors because the centrals erupt before the lateral incisors. The facial development and growth of the person help the teeth to erupt properly. The anterior teeth are not covered by as much bone, and the tooth buds begin their formation earlier than those of the posterior teeth; the result is that most of the anterior teeth erupt before the posterior teeth. Some of the posterior teeth must actually wait until growth has occurred in the mandible; otherwise the **ramus of the mandible** would cover them. Thus the eruption pattern, growth and facial development, and sequence in which the tooth buds begin their formation all play an important part in the eventual relationship of the teeth and jaws.

The development of the **occlusion** begins with the eruption of the primary teeth (see Fig. 24-6, development of human dentition, 6 months [± 2 months]). Usually the first teeth to erupt are the central incisors, with the mandibular teeth erupting slightly before the maxillary. The eruption of the lateral incisors, which occurs next, follows the same sequence.

The primary molars erupt next around the sixteenth month of age. This is an important event in that these primary molars establish the vertical height of the primary occlusion. These primary molars also establish the **intercuspation,** the mesial-distal and buccal-lingual relationships determining how the upper teeth will touch, hit, and interlock with the lower teeth. These upper primary molars then establish the anteroposterior

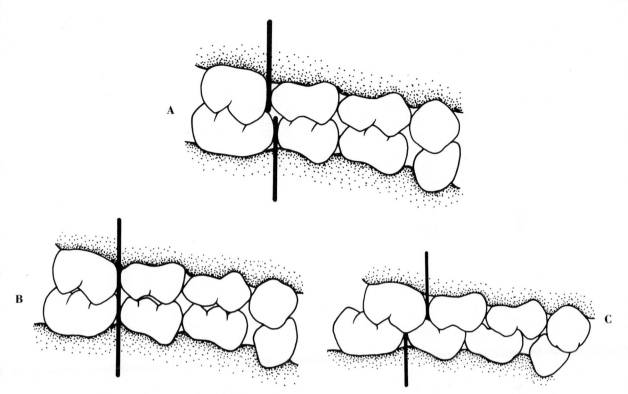

Fig. 25-1 **A-C,** Relationship of first permanent molars to each other is what determines step or plane.

(mesial-distal) relationship of the remaining deciduous teeth because their presence causes the canines and second deciduous molars to erupt around them.

The primary teeth erupt in a more upright position than their secondary teeth replacements. The average overjet is 3.0 mm, and the average overbite is 2.5 mm.

The primary dentition is usually complete around 2½ years of age. This primary occlusion has one of three possible anteroposterior molar relationships called steps or planes.

The majority of children have a **mesial step** between the distal surfaces of the second primary molars (Fig. 25-1, *A*). The mandibular molars are situated more mesially than their maxillary counterparts. Thus they form a mesial step.

A smaller but still large group of children exhibit a **flush terminal plane,** i.e., the distal surfaces of the deciduous second molars are even with each other (Fig. 25-1, *B*).

A still smaller minority have a **distal step** (Fig. 25-1, *C*). How would you describe this distal step in comparison with the mesial step or flush terminal plane? Note the large diastema, or space, in the mandibular arch between the canine and first molar.

As the child grows in height and weight, so too does the size of the jaws. This growth of the mandible and maxillary results in horizontal and vertical growth of the dental arches. The teeth, however, remain the same size. Thus as the arches grow, spaces are formed between the teeth called **diastemas.**

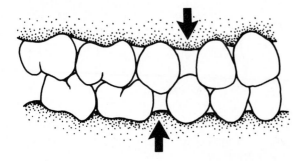

Fig. 25-2 Primate spaces. These spaces occur in primary dentition. In maxillary arch they are anterior to canine. In mandibular arch they are distal to canine.

The largest spaces are often found mesial to the maxillary primary canines and distal to the mandibular canines. These spaces are called **primate spaces** and although not always present are characteristic of all primates such as man, apes, and monkeys (Fig. 25-2). As growth continues, diastemas also develop between the incisors.

DEVELOPMENT OF THE MESIAL STEP

The permanent molars erupt, follow, and eventually touch up against the distal surfaces of the deciduous molars. As the permanent molars push up against the deciduous molars, they cause a chain reaction that pushes all of the spaces between the teeth closed.

A mesial step occurs in the majority of individuals because closing the primary space allows room for the lower molars to move mesially.

This trend toward a mesial step is further enhanced as the deciduous molars exfoliate and are replaced by permanent premolars. Extra space, **leeway space,** is gained from the exchange of the narrower premolars. The earlier eruption cycle of the mandibular teeth allows them to capitalize on this exchange before the maxillary teeth. This further helps establish the mesial step (Fig. 25-3).

Finally the head of the condyles of the mandi-

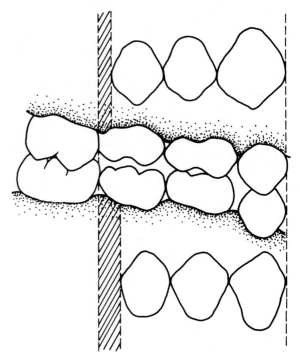

Fig. 25-3 Leeway space is extra space that deciduous canines and molars occupy to help save room for their permanent successors. These permanent teeth take up less space. Difference between space deciduous teeth take up and that of their permanent replacements is called leeway space.

ble continue to grow later than the maxilla allowing even further mesial mandibular advancement and ensuring in most instances a mesial step heading the patient toward a class I relationship (see Fig. 25-17.)

Further growth of the condyle head could push the patient into an extreme mesial step resulting in a class III relationship (see Fig. 25-21).

A class II relationship (see Fig. 25-18) could result if the mandible does not continue to grow or if the maxilla outgrows the mandible. A class II relationship could result on just one side whereas the other side could be a class I relationship.

A deep bite (see Fig. 25-15, *C*) could result if

the condyle head is displaced distally in the glenoid fossa, if the posterior teeth do not erupt enough, if the muscles are so hyperactive that they prevent the eruption of the posterior teeth, or if the condyle grows at an angle that allows the jaw to develop in a less mesial direction.

The development of the occlusion is further influenced by hereditary factors such as congenitally missing teeth, empacted teeth, or the size and shape of muscle and bone. Finally, there are factors we can control that affect occlusal devel-opment such as premature loss of deciduous teeth, decayed teeth that were not restored, and harmful habits.

HORIZONTAL ALIGNMENT

After the teeth erupt in the oral cavity, the tongue acts as a huge internal force, pushing the teeth toward the lips and cheeks. What prevents the teeth from being pushed out of the mouth? Resistance from the muscles that form the cheeks

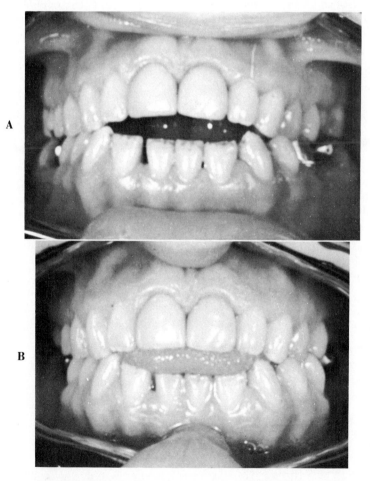

Fig. 25-4 Open bite resulting from tongue thrusting. **A,** Posterior teeth touch when jaws are closed, but space exists between anterior teeth. **B,** During swallowing, tongue closes space. (Ross.)

and lips is the controlling factor that prevents the teeth from moving too far facially. At this point the teeth have reached the point of equilibrium between the muscles of the tongue and the muscles of the cheeks and lips. The balance, or relative equilibrium, between these two forces allows the teeth not only to be brought into proper alignment but also to maintain this alignment once they have erupted.

If this balance of forces is disturbed, a **malocclusion** (that is, an abnormal alignment of the teeth within the dental arches) can result. Abnormal forward thrusting of the tongue against the anterior teeth can cause such an imbalanced state (Fig. 25-4). Tongue thrusting pushes the maxillary anterior teeth labially out of the mouth—they **protrude.** This is especially true if there is an underdeveloped upper lip along with the tongue thrust.

An opposite situation can also occur if the lower lip is overdeveloped; the **retrusion** of the lower anterior teeth occurs. The patient is constantly tightening the lower lip against the lower anterior teeth. These lip muscles are so strong that the lower teeth will be pushed back into the mouth by this overdeveloped lower lip.

The lip, tongue, and cheek muscles and their relationship to each other are not the only factors that determine the alignment of the teeth. The intercuspation of the teeth helps prevent tooth deviations in a buccal or lingual direction. The maxillary posterior teeth have a buccal and a lingual cusp, and when the jaws are closed, the buccal cusps of the mandibular posterior teeth are interlocked between the buccal and lingual cusps of the maxillary teeth. This interlocking is similar to the interlocking of two gears.

The alignment of previously erupted teeth also affects the alignment of successive teeth. Adequate space between teeth allows the complete and unhindered eruption of more teeth. If a tooth does not have room enough to erupt, it will deflect off the obstructing tooth and erupt out of alignment. It could also be blocked out entirely by the obstruction and never erupt.

Other factors also influence the alignment of the teeth. Mesial drift could account for the closure or loss of space necessary for tooth eruption. The size and shape of the jaws, the shape of the teeth, and the amount of lingual convergence of each tooth not only affects the alignment of the teeth but also the curvature of the dental arch and the spacing or lack of space necessary for incoming teeth.

CURVE OF SPEE, CURVE OF WILSON, AND SPHERE OF MONSON

Usually the buccal cusp tips of posterior teeth, seen in alignment from a lateral view (see Fig. 24-10), conform to a fairly even curve in an anterior to posterior direction. This curve is known as the **curve of Spee.**

An occlusal curve exists for posterior teeth in a direction from right to left as seen from a posterior view (Fig. 25-5). This transverse occlusal

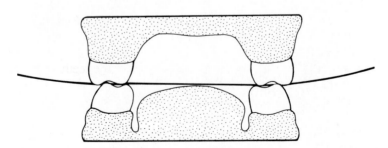

Fig. 25-5 Curve of Wilson.

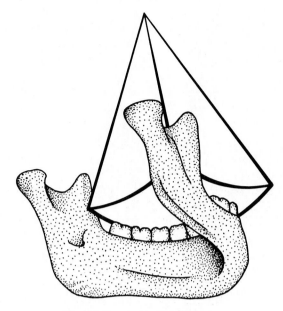

Fig. 25-6   Sphere of Monson.

curve is called the **curve of Wilson.**

It has long been the belief that the occlusal surfaces of the natural dentition are aligned in such a way that a spherical curve 8 inches in diameter could rest on the buccal cusp tips of the mandibular posterior teeth. The two curves of Wilson and Spee, when studied simultaneously in three-dimensional alignment, demonstrate an illusion of the cusp tips of the mandibular posterior teeth resting on a sphere known as the **sphere of Monson** (Fig. 25-6). This theory has yet to be proved.

VERTICAL ALIGNMENT

We tend to think of the teeth as being vertically straight, but this is not true. The teeth are not positioned straight up and down in the mouth. As we have seen, the mandibular posterior teeth have a tendency to tip their crowns lingually and their roots laterally (Fig. 25-7). The maxillary posterior teeth tend to keep the crown straighter, with a slight buccal inclination, as well

as a lingual inclination of the root (Fig. 25-8). From a lateral view, we can see that all the teeth, maxillary and mandibular, anterior and posterior, show a slight mesial inclination, with the possible exception of the maxillary third molar. Notice that the anterior teeth (Figs. 25-9 and 25-10) have a slight labial protrusion (a condition of being tipped forward), and from a frontal view their crowns incline laterally. In other words, the anterior teeth tip out to the side and toward the front.

OCCLUSION

Occlusion is the term used to describe the relationship of the mandibular and maxillary teeth when the teeth are closed together or during excursive movements when the teeth are touching.

When the jaws are completely closed together, there are two possible relationships. Either there is a relationship of the upper jaw to the lower jaw, centric relation, or there is a relationship of the upper teeth to the lower teeth, centric occlusion.

Centric Relation

Centric relation refers to the position of the mandible relative to the maxilla that is determined by the maximum contraction of the muscles of the jaw. This relationship of the mandible to the maxilla occurs during strong muscle contractions such as swallowing. It is the most stable and most braced position that affords the strongest muscle contractions. It is a relationship of bone to bone brought about by allowing the muscles to contract in their most natural posture to their most comfortable and effective position.

It does not have anything to do with the interdigitation of the teeth. Indeed, it may not be the position that allows the greatest intercuspation of the teeth.

Centric relation is defined as the most retruded relationship of the mandible to the maxillae when the condyles of the temporal mandibular joint are in their most upward, back-

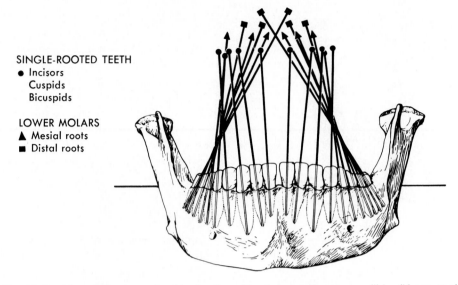

SINGLE-ROOTED TEETH
● Incisors
  Cuspids
  Bicuspids

LOWER MOLARS
▲ Mesial roots
■ Distal roots

Fig. 25-7   Lines indicate angle of inclination of teeth in relation to mandible. (Kraus et al.)

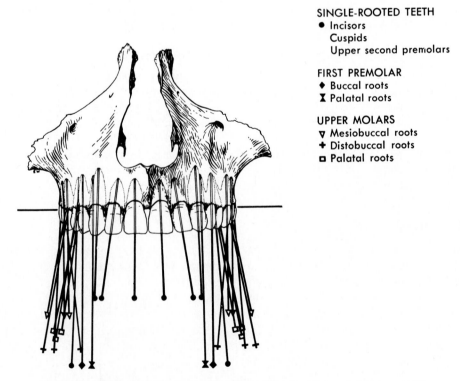

SINGLE-ROOTED TEETH
● Incisors
  Cuspids
  Upper second premolars

FIRST PREMOLAR
♦ Buccal roots
✗ Palatal roots

UPPER MOLARS
▽ Mesiobuccal roots
✛ Distobuccal roots
▫ Palatal roots

Fig. 25-8   Lines indicate inclination of maxillary teeth in relation to maxilla.

SINGLE-ROOTED TEETH
- Incisors
  Cuspids
  Upper second premolars

FIRST PREMOLAR
- Buccal roots
- Palatal roots

UPPER MOLARS
- Mesiobuccal roots
- Distobuccal roots
- Palatal roots

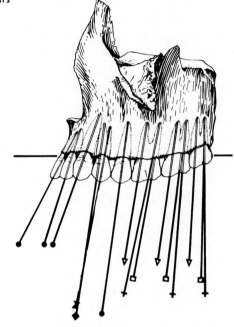

Fig. 25-9   Inclination of maxillary teeth, lateral view. (Kraus et al.)

SINGLE-ROOTED TEETH
- Incisors
  Cuspids
  Bicuspids

LOWER MOLARS
- Mesial roots
- Distal roots

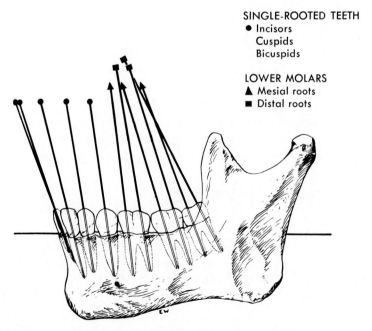

Fig. 25-10   Inclination of mandibular teeth, lateral view. (Kraus et al.)

ward, and unstrained position in the glenoid fossae. It is a relationship also of the structural features of the temporal mandibular joint.

If you wish to experience centric relation, let your head tip as far back as possible and gently close your teeth together. Let your mandible go back as far as possible. You will notice this is different than your **habitual occlusion.** If you tip your head forward and close your teeth together as you usually do, this is your centric occlusion. Is your mandible further forward in your habitual centric occlusion or in your centric relation?

Centric Occlusion

Centric occlusion also refers to a position when the jaws are closed, but this position is determined by the way the teeth fit together. It is the jaw position that affords the greatest interdigitation of the teeth. It depends on the position that allows the most intercuspation. It is related to tooth occlusion and not determined by muscle or bone. It is the habitual way that the teeth come together. Centric occlusion is sometimes called **acquired occlusion,** habitual occlusion, **convenience occlusion,** or **intercuspal position** (ICP). This is the way your teeth fit together out of habit without planning or forethought. The teeth usually occlude better in this position because this position is determined by how your teeth interlock or occlude. With the jaws closed, the occlusal surfaces of the maxillary teeth touch

the occlusal surfaces of the mandibular teeth. The lingual cusps of the maxillary premolars and molars rest in the deepest parts of the occlusal sulci of the mandibular premolars and molars, and the buccal cusps of the mandibular premolars and molars rest in the deepest parts of the sulci of the maxillary premolars and molars (Figs. 25-11 and 25-12).

When the jaws are closed in centric occlusion, the cusps of the maxillary teeth overlap the cusps of the mandibular teeth so that the maxillary teeth are facial to the mandibular teeth. Although

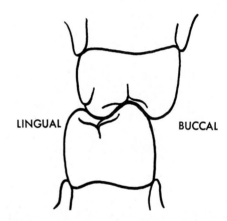

Fig. 25-12 Left first molars, mesial view. In centric relation, teeth interconnect to their greatest potential. (Ross.)

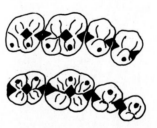

Fig. 25-11 Centric relation. Contacting marginal ridge areas are indicated by triangles, central fossae by diamonds, and occluding cusp tips by circles. Buccal cusp tips of mandibular teeth contact maxillary marginal ridges and central fossae of maxillary molars. Lingual cusp tips of maxillary teeth contact marginal ridges and central fossae of mandibular molars.

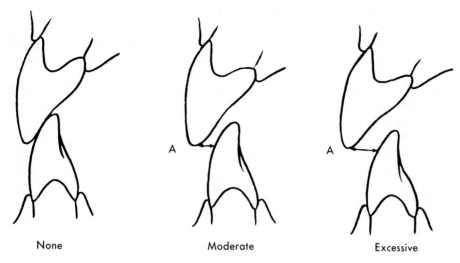

Fig. 25-13 Overjet.

the cusps of the maxillary teeth do not directly touch the cusps of the mandibular teeth on closure of the jaw, it is possible for the cusps to come into contact when the mandible slides from side to side. Notice that the maxillary cusps are located facial to the mandibular cusps. Does that mean that the maxillary cusps are on the outside of the mandibular cusps?

The amount of facial horizontal overlap of the maxillary teeth is called an **overjet** (Fig. 25-13). Notice that the maxillary incisors are facial to the mandibular incisors. Line *A* is the amount of horizontal overlap, or overjet.

In Fig. 25-14 notice that the maxillary incisors also vertically overlap the mandibular incisors. Line *A* indicates the amount of vertical overlap, or **overbite.** Overbite is the extension of the incisal edges of the maxillary anterior teeth below the incisal edges of the mandibular anterior teeth in a vertical direction (Fig. 25-15).

If one or more teeth in the mandibular arch are located facial to their maxillary counterparts, a condition known as **cross-bite** occurs. Fig. 25-16 illustrates a mandibular right first molar in cross-bite. Notice that the buccal cusp of the mandibular molar is located facial to the buccal

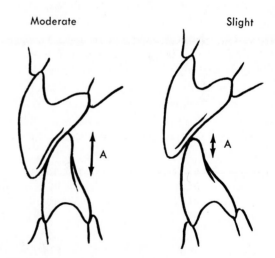

Fig. 25-14 Moderate and slight overbite. Line A indicates difference in overbite; amount of overjet is same. (Ross.)

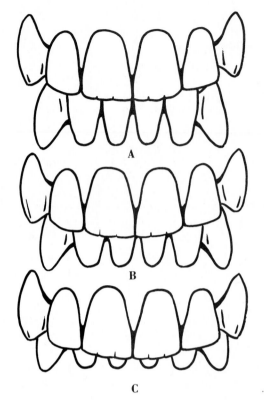

Fig. 25-15 **A,** Slight overbite, **B,** Moderate overbite. **C,** Excessive overbite. (Ross.)

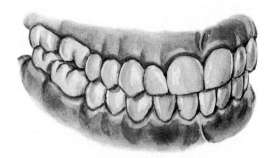

Fig. 25-16 Posterior cross-bite of right first molars. (Massler and Schour.)

cusp of the maxillary molar. A cross-bite condition can exist between any number of teeth. It can be caused by a loss of space in the deciduous arch so that the maxillary second premolar, which is one of the last teeth to replace a deciduous tooth, might be blocked out to the lingual side of the other maxillary teeth. Then, if the lower premolar erupted normally, a maxillary cross-bite of the second premolar could occur. A cross-bite of all the mandibular teeth can occur if there is a disease that causes the patient's mandible, but not the maxilla, to continue growing. Such a condition is **acromegaly.** In this disease, growth hormone causes the mandible to grow faster than the maxilla. As a result, the mandibular teeth are eventually positioned in cross-bite with the maxillary teeth.

OPEN BITE

When the teeth are in centric occlusion, the maxillary and mandibular teeth should touch each other. The occlusal surfaces of the posterior teeth should touch. The anterior teeth should touch in such a way that the incisal edges of the mandibular anterior teeth touch against the lingual surfaces of the maxillary anterior teeth. If the anterior teeth do not touch but are widely separated when in centric occlusion, the condition known as **open bite** exists. An open bite exists when the anterior teeth of the maxillary arch do not overlap the mandibular teeth in a vertical direction. Such a condition can be caused by either a thumb-sucking or a tongue-thrusting habit. In either situation a powerful force is exerted against the anterior teeth when the jaws close. In thumb-sucking the patient's thumb or fingers rest between the anterior teeth, maxillary and mandibular. As the patient sucks on the thumb, the jaws are closed but the anterior teeth are prevented from touching each other. Thus a force is exerted that pushes the anterior teeth back into the bone and prevents them from erupting. The outcome is a wide separation of the anterior teeth when the jaws close (Fig. 25-4).

The tongue-thrusting habit places the tongue between the anterior teeth every time the patient swallows. The act of swallowing requires the jaws to come together and the lips to close. This seals off air spaces, and a negative pressure can result. If the patient has poor tongue placement or open spaces exist between the front teeth, the following sequence occurs. First the patient places the tongue against these open spaces or against the anterior teeth. When the patient swallows, closing the jaws, the tongue pushes against the anterior teeth. The result is a protrusion of the maxillary anterior teeth, with the pressure preventing the teeth from erupting normally. In the normally developed swallowing pattern this situation is prevented because the tongue is placed against the roof of the mouth, not against the teeth. When the tongue thrusts during jaw closure, it exerts pressure on the palate rather than on the teeth.

OCCLUSAL CLASSIFICATION

There are two basic ways to consider occlusion. The first is based on the relationship of the bone of the maxilla relative to the bone of the mandible. This system, since it is related to the bones, is referred to as the **skeletal classification.**

The second system is based on the relationship of the teeth of the mandible to the teeth of the maxilla. It is called the "dental classification," since it is concerned with the teeth.

The skeletal classification is divided into three classes of relationship.

Class I—The maxilla and mandible are in the normal relationship to each other.

Class II—The mandible is retruded, thus retrognathic. The mandible has a distal relationship with the maxilla.

Class III—The mandible is protruded, thus prognathic. The mandible has a mesial relationship with the maxilla.

The dental classification is based on the relationship of the teeth. Usually the canines or the first permanent molars are used in dental classifications.

Angle's classification system is the most popular dental classification system in use today. His system is based primarily on the relationship of the permanent first molars to each other and to a lesser degree on the relationship of the permanent canines to each other.

In centric occlusion there are three relationships that can exist between the first molars. In the normal relationship the maxillary first molar is slightly posterior to the mandibular first molar. The mesiobuccal cusp of the maxillary first molar is directly in line with the buccal groove of the mandibular first molar. Such a relationship is called a **class I occlusal relationship, neutroclusion** (Fig. 25-17).

A **class II occlusal relationship, distoclusion,** exists when the maxillary first molar is even with or anterior to the mandibular first molar. In this relationship the buccal groove of the mandibular

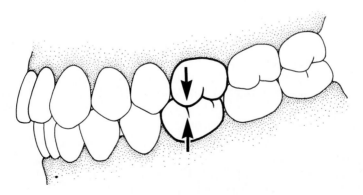

Fig. 25-17 Class I occlusal relationship.

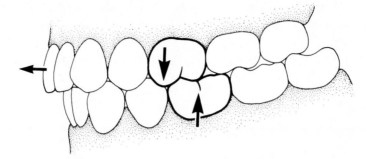

Fig. 25-18 Class II, Division I occlusal relationship.

first molar is posterior to the mesiobuccal cusp of the maxillary first molar (Fig. 25-18). Could such a relationship be present if the maxillary teeth protruded or the mandibular teeth were retruded?

There are two separate class II divisions. Class II, division I, occurs when the permanent first molars are in class II and the permanent maxillary central incisors are in their normal slightly protruded position (Figs. 25-17 and 25-18). Class II, division II, occurs when the permanent first molars are in class II relationship and the permanent maxillary central incisors are retruded and inclined lingually (Figs. 25-17 and 25-18).

A class II, division II, relationship frequently occurs when the following scenario is present:

1. Deep overbite
2. Crowded maxillary anteriors
3. Normal overjet
4. Excessive masseter muscle development

A **class III occlusal relationship, mesioclusion,** exists when the buccal groove of the mandibular first molar is more anterior than normal to the mesiobuccal cusp of the maxillary first molar (Fig. 25-19). This relationship would be present if the maxillary teeth were retruded or if the mandibular teeth protruded.

It is possible for one side of the mandible to be in class I, II, or III and the other side to be in a different class.

The canines can be used in a dental classification system as follows:

Class I—The distal surface of the mandibular canine is within one premolar's width of the mesial surface of the maxillary canine.

Class II—The distal surface of the mandibular canine is distal to the mesial surface of the maxillary canine by a width of at least one premolar.

Class III—The distal surface of the mandibular canine is mesial to the mesial surface of a maxillary canine by at least a width of one premolar.

LATERAL MANDIBULAR GLIDE (LATERAL EXCURSION)

In **lateral excursion** the mandible moves toward the right or left side. The side to which the mandible moves is referred to as the **working side.** The side away from which the mandible is moving is referred to as the **nonworking side.** On artificial teeth this nonworking side is referred to as the **balancing side.** (See Fig. 25-20.)

A working-side contact exists when the mandible is moved to one side, with buccal cusps of the maxillary and mandibular teeth touching each other and the lingual cusps directly over each other.

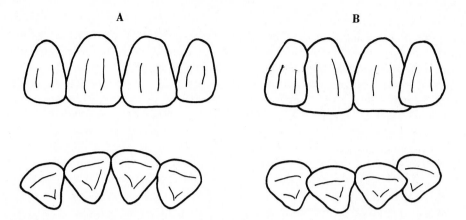

Fig. 25-19   A, Class II, Division I—maxillary incisors are in good alignment. **B,** Class II, Division II—maxillary central incisors are retruded lingually behind laterals.

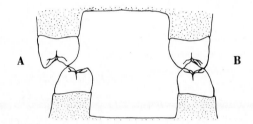

Fig. 25-20   Lateral excursion. A, Balancing side. **B,** Working side.

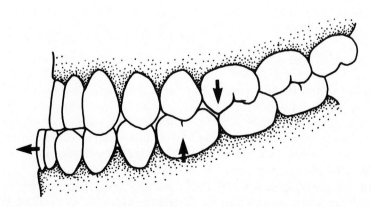

Fig. 25-21   In natural dentition in protrusion, only incisors should touch.

In lateral mandibular glide only a few pairs of interlocking cusps make occlusal contact. The canines carry the bulk of the contact. This is referred to as a canine rise because the mandibular canine opens the bite by gliding down the lingual surface of the maxillary canine. In lateral excursion the last two teeth to touch, in an almost cusp tip-to-cusp tip arrangement, should be the canines. If the lateral glide is to the right, the last two teeth to touch should be the right canines. Try it.

In natural dentition the cusps on the nonworking side rarely touch at all. In artificial teeth they do touch, but that is to prevent the denture from dislodging. Dividing the forces equally in artificial teeth keeps the dentures from tipping or displacing during lateral movement of the jaw.

PROTRUSION

When the mandible moves forward from centric occlusion **(protrusion),** the only teeth that should touch are the anterior teeth. The mandibular anterior four incisors should glide across the maxillary four incisors. The canines may touch slightly, but no posterior teeth should touch in a mandibular protrusive movement (Fig. 25-21).

PREMATURE CONTACT

When the jaw closes, all of the teeth should come into contact at the same time. If one tooth hits ever so slightly more than the others, this tooth will bear more force. It is called a **premature contact.**

A premature contact will cause the jaw to deflect before allowing the rest of the teeth to occlude. If the path of the lower jaw movement deflects from its true course, the temporal mandibular jaw joint must be put into a stretched or abnormal position. This has the following results.

1. The temporal mandibular joint is under abnormal stress causing damage to the ligament or the muscles of the joint. Often the jaw joint affected is the one from the opposite side of the premature contact.
2. The muscles that act as **antagonists** to the muscles of mastication become tired, sore, and tender. If one set of muscles is forced to be overexerted because of a premature contact, eventually that set of muscles will become tender and sore.
3. The tooth that is hitting prematurely becomes sensitive to percussion and tender when chewing. It may become mobile, and x-ray examination may reveal a widening of the periodontal ligament.
4. The responsible tooth may become cracked or broken. Even under the normal stress of occlusion, when all of the teeth are hitting at the same time, the occluding cusps undergo a contact pressure of 300 pounds per square inch. In premature contact the force extended to the offending cusp could be thousands of pounds per square inch.

FUNDAMENTALS OF IDEAL OCCLUSION IN PERMANENT DENTITION

The ideal occlusion is the result of the maxillary bones and the mandibular bone in proper harmony with each other. The condyles of the mandible are in their most favorable location within the glenoid fossae. At the same time the muscles of the face and jaws must be in balance with each other and the above mentioned bones. Finally the occlusion of the teeth and how they interlock or interdigitate would be the most stable when all of the above mentioned bones, muscles, and joints are synchronized to be in balance and harmony with each other.

Is ideal occlusion a matter of luck, wishful thinking, or a dream? No, it actually happens. The function of these structures helps guide and balance the other structures, and finally a harmony of forces results in a balanced occlusion not by accident but rather by the design and function and symmetry of these structures as they interrelate. When these all occur in a well-balanced, harmonious environment, a well-balanced, harmonious occlusion results.

E. H. Angle found that the most ideal occlusion was a class I occlusion. The class I molar relationship exists when the mesiobuccal cusps of the first permanent molar falls within the groove between the mesiobuccal and middle buccal cusps of the lower first molar.

A class I canine relationship exists when the distal surface of the mandibular canine is within one premolar's width of the mesial surface of the maxillary canine. The lower canine should then be positioned in the embrasure located between the upper canine and the upper lateral incisor.

In centric occlusion all of the posterior teeth should hit at the same time with no teeth prematurely hitting. The anterior incisors may also hit but not harder than the posteriors. If the anteriors hit in centric occlusion, it is called **anterior coupling.** The upper canines touch the lower canines in lateral excursive movements to one side or the other. This is called **canine rise.** If the premolars also touch in excursive movements, it is called **group function.** Only the anterior teeth hit when the teeth go in protrusion. The laterals may also hit in lateral excursions but only after the canines have performed most of the guidance.

In the ideal occlusion the occlusal plane is almost flat with a slight curve of Spee, which deepens with age. The teeth have good tight proximal contacts with no spaces between teeth. There are no rotated teeth, and the upper and lower arches are symmetrical and well formed. If the crown angulation of the gingival portion of the long axis of all crowns is more distal than the incisal portion, it is called mesial tip. The crown inclination labiolingually and buccolingually is such that the incisors flair labially and the rest of the teeth flair lingually. Finally the maxillary first molar touches the mandibular second molar. This is called a **stolarized** molar, and in the ideal occlusion the distal marginal ridge of the permanent maxillary first molar touches the mesial marginal ridge of the permanent mandibular second molar. Thus

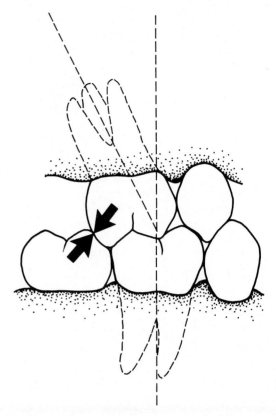

Fig. 25-22 Stolarized molars. Upper first molar is tipped forward so that the distal marginal ridge of the upper touches mesial marginal ridge of the lower second molar.

the maxillary first permanent molar is slightly tipped mesially so that it touches the mesial surface of the mandibular second molar (Fig. 25-22).

Since all humans are as different as snowflakes, only a few experience ideal occlusion. However, it is easier to discover malocclusions when familiar with the ideal.

REVIEW QUESTIONS

1. What affects the alignment of the teeth?
2. Which muscle forces affect the alignment of the teeth?

3. What is the difference between the curve of Spee and the curve of Wilson?
4. Define the following terms:
   a. open bite
   b. overbite
   c. overjet
   d. centric occlusion
   e. working side
   f. balancing side
5. Pattern a drawing after Fig. 25-13 depicting the condition you would expect to find in a patient with a severe thumb-sucking habit. Label the overjet, overbite, and open bite.
6. Mark in Fig. 25-23 the anatomical features that determine the class of occlusal relationship. Is this a class I, II, or III relationship?
7. Test out the theory that people as a rule do not have a bilaterally balanced occlusion.
   a. If this theory were true, the fact that a right-handed person would use a fork to place food on the left side of his mouth could have a bearing on his occlusion.
   b. Do your own survey: ask people which side of their occlusion interlocks best.
8. What is meant by mesial step?
9. If an occlusion with a mesial step proceeds without problems, which of the following will most likely result?
   a. class I
   b. class II

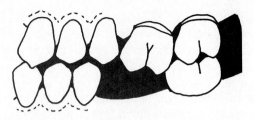

Fig. 25-23   Premature occlusal contact of maxillary first molar. To avoid premature occlusal contact, mandible moves backward when closing.

   c. class III
   d. a distal step
10. Which factors influence occlusion?
    a. heredity
    b. unrestored deciduous decayed molars
    c. impacted deciduous teeth
    d. congenitally missing teeth
    e. growth of the condyles
    f. eruption sequence of teeth
    g. leeway space
    h. primate space
11. Outline the elements of the ideal occlusion.

26

Dental Anomalies

An **anomaly** is defined as something that is noticeably different or deviates from that which is ordinary or normal. A dental anomaly is a deviation of dental tissue origin. A dental anomaly therefore would be derived from dental tissues such as enamel, dentin, or cementum.

Anomalies can be extreme variations or just slight deviations. They could be caused by a multitude of things or just by one small variation in the environment. When concerning ourselves with anomalies, it is important to differentiate the origins of such diversification. In general anomalies are caused by a combination of several things.

Some abnormalities result from **intrinsic** factors (heredity, metabolic dysfunction, mutations); other causes are more **extrinsic** (such as physical or chemical trauma, biological agents, nutritional deficiencies, stress, habits, or environmental conditions). In many instances anomalies result from a combination of intrinsic and extrinsic factors.

If a condition occurs because of characteristics resulting from the individual's genetic make-up, we term the condition **hereditary.** If the condition occurs at or before birth, it is termed **congenital.** A congenital condition is sometimes the result of heredity, and sometimes a hereditary condition does not become evident until years after birth. If a condition exhibits some evidence of an inherited tendency but such evidence is inconclusive, we sometimes refer to it is as a **familial tendency.**

If a condition results during the formation and development of the structure, it is referred to as a developmental anomaly. A developmental anomaly occurs during the developmental stage of the structure.

CLASSIFICATION OF DENTAL ANOMALIES

Anomalies resulting in a variation in the size of teeth are called **macrodontia** (teeth are too large) (Fig. 26-1) and **microdontia** (teeth are too small) (Fig. 26-2).

Anomalies resulting in a variation in the number of teeth are **hyperdontia** (multiple or extra teeth) (Fig. 26-3) and **anodontia** (too few teeth) (Fig. 26-4).

Total anodontia exists if no teeth are present at all. Partial anodontia exists if less than the normal number of teeth are present. True anodontia is the congenital absence of teeth. It may involve the permanent dentition, primary dentition, or both. If the primary teeth are congenitally missing, their permanent replacements will also be absent.

Hyperdontia is not an uncommon anomaly. It has been reported that from 0.1% to 3.6% of individuals from various populations have too

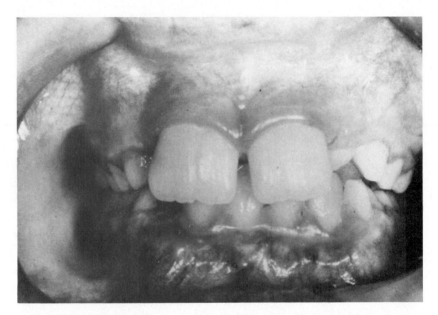

Fig. 26-1 Macrodontia. Incisor teeth are too large for size of oral cavity.

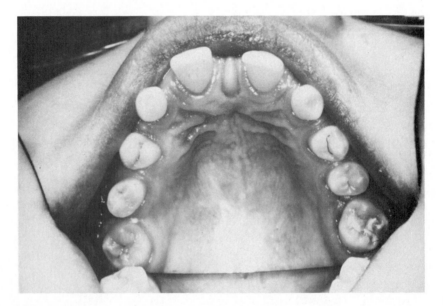

Fig. 26-2 Microdontia. Although some lateral incisors are missing, teeth are too small for size of oral cavity.

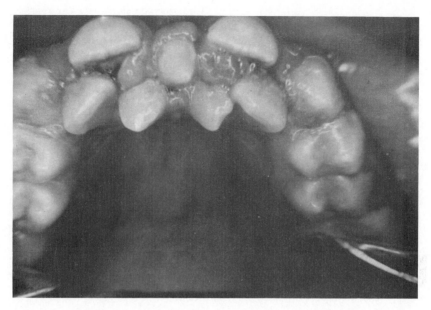

Fig. 26-3   Hyperdontia, or supernumerary teeth. Notice extra teeth to lingual of regular dentition.

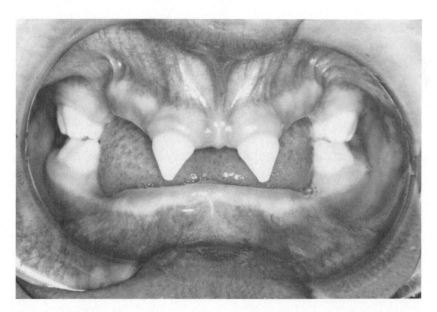

Fig. 26-4   Anodontia. In this case it is partial anodontia. Notice large number of missing teeth.

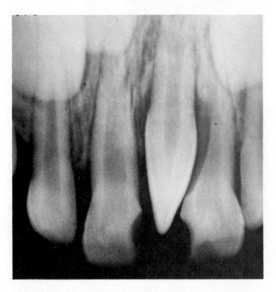

Fig. 26-5 Mesiodens. Peg-shaped supernumerary tooth between maxillary incisors; this is mesiodens.

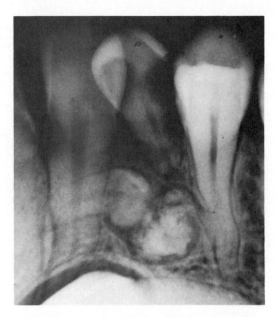

Fig. 26-6 Odontoma. Two odd-shaped, calcified structures in middle of field; these are odontomas.

many teeth. These extra teeth are referred to as **supernumeraries.** Supernumary teeth are most commonly found in the midline and molar regions of the maxilla, followed by the premolar region of the mandible, whereas other sites are only rarely involved. Maxillary supernumerary teeth outnumber mandibular nine to one.

Supernumerary teeth arising in the midline of the maxilla are termed **mesiodens** (Fig. 26-5). Mesiodens are the most common supernumeraries. The maxillary distomolars are the next most common supernumerary teeth. These distomolars are also called fourth molars and are located distal to the maxillary third molars. Mandibular distomolars do occur but not nearly as often. A supernumerary tooth situated buccally or lingually to a molar is called a **paramolar.** They are usually small and rudimentary. The next most likely location for supernumaries is the premolar area of the mandible. Only 10% of all supernumeraries occur in the mandible.

If a supernumerary resembles a regular tooth, it is termed **supplemental.** If it is cone shaped, it is called **conical.** If it is very small, it is called **tubercle.**

Supernumerary teeth are much more common in the permanent than in the primary dentition.

ANOMALIES IN SHAPE

An **odontoma** (Fig. 26-6) is a tumorous anomaly of calcified dental tissues (enamel, dentin, cementum, and pulp). There are two types of odontoma: complex, which consists of a single mass of dentin, cementum, and enamel in a large blob or unspecified shape (not recognizable as tooth shaped); and compound, consisting of several small masses that more or less resemble rudimentary teeth. Although compound odontomas may sometimes resemble multiple mesoderms because they resemble small supplemental teeth, they are smaller and multiple.

Dens in Dente

Dens in dente (Fig. 26-7) is a developmental variation that is thought to occur when the outer surface of the tooth crown invaginates, turns itself inward, prior to mineralization, rather than a tooth splitting into two or two teeth fusing into one. This allows communication between the oral cavity and the inner enamel-lined cavity. This inner enamel-lined cavity could be considered an extremely deep pit. Permanent maxillary lateral incisors are the teeth most frequently involved as dens in dente.

The name, *dens in dente,* means tooth within a tooth. An X-ray of a dens in dente appears to be a tooth actually within a tooth (Fig. 26-7, A).

Dilaceration

A **dilacerated** tooth (Fig. 26-8) is a tooth that has a sharp bend or curve in the root or crown. It appears as if a tooth suddenly was bent or de-

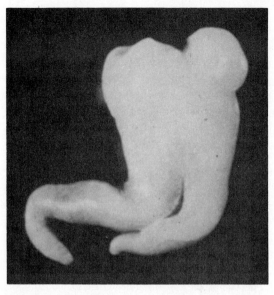

Fig. 26-8 Dilacerated tooth with numerous bends in root. This anomaly makes tooth extraction very difficult.

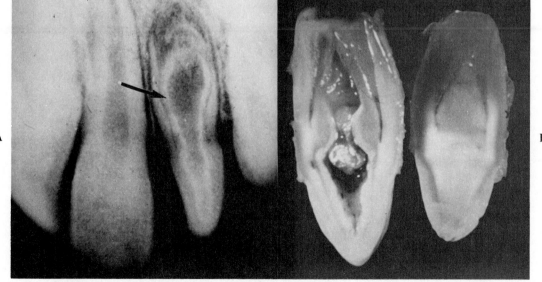

A   B

Fig. 26-7 **A,** Radiograph of dens in dente. Enamel growing within tooth *(arrow),* or "tooth in tooth". **B,** Dens in dente has been extracted and sectioned in half showing enamel growing within tooth.

formed under pressure. The term dilaceration should only be used to describe teeth with very sharp bends.

Dwarfed Roots

Dwarfed roots (Fig. 26-9) are a condition in which the roots of the teeth are extremely short in comparison with their crowns.

Gemination

Gemination (Fig. 26-10) is an anomaly that arises when a tooth attempts to divide itself, or partially twin itself, by splitting its tooth germ. It therefore is a developmental anomaly. Gemination could occur if a tooth completely divided into two separate entities or twin teeth. In most cases, however, geminated teeth are only partially split. Usually the geminated teeth have a single root and a common pulp canal. A tooth split into two crowns with one root would be termed a "bifid" tooth, or bifurcated crown.

Fusion

Fusion (Fig. 26-11) occurs when two adjacent tooth germs unite. The two teeth may be united along a part of or the entire length. They may be joined by their crowns or their roots. The fusion of the teeth must be made at the dentin. If the teeth are only connected by their cementum then it is not fusion but concrescence that has occurred. For fusion to exist, two teeth must be joined; therefore there is one less tooth than the normal complement.

Concrescence

Concrescence (Fig. 26-12) is a form of fusion that occurs after the roots have formed. It is thought to occur sometimes as a result of trauma.

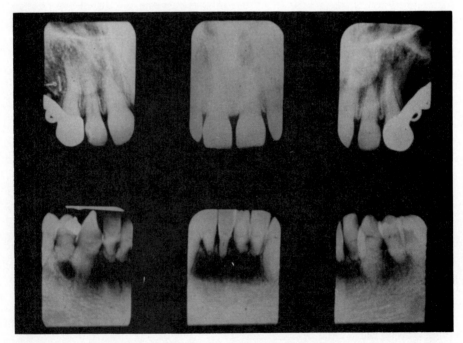

Fig. 26-9 Dwarfed roots. Most roots in this patient have never fully developed.

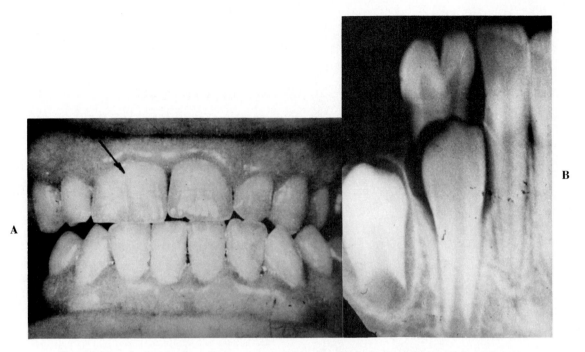

Fig. 26-10   **A,** Gemination. Groove in central incisor *(arrow)* where two teeth have begun development. **B,** Gemination. This radiograph shows how two teeth have grown from one tooth. Much more obvious anomaly than in **A.**

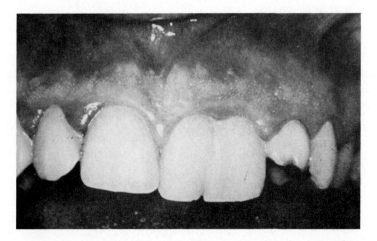

Fig. 26-11   Fusion. Central and lateral incisors have fused in their development. They are fused at both enamel and dentin.

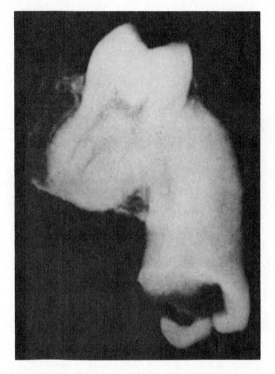

Fig. 26-12 Concrescence. Teeth grew separately but then fused at their cemental surfaces and were joined together.

It occurs when two approximating roots contact and fuse by a deposition of cementum. It can occur before or after eruption.

Hypercementosis

Hypercementosis (Fig. 26-13) is the deposition of excessive amounts of secondary cementum. This usually occurs at the apex of the tooth and often along the entire length of the root.

Cementoma

Cementoma (Fig. 26-14) is a form of hypercementosis that is also associated with localized destruction of the bone.

Enamel Pearls

Enamel pearls (Fig. 26-15) are small masses of excess enamel on the surface of the teeth located apically to the cementoenamel junction. They are frequently found at the bifurcation or trifurcation area and are formed by a small misplaced group of ameloblasts.

Hutchinson's Incisors

Hutchinson's incisors (Fig. 26-16) are notched incisors, sometimes called screwdriver shaped, that are formed as a result of prenatal syphilis. The notched incisors are characteristic of congenital syphilis, as are **mulberry molars**—irregular-shaped molars with poorly formed cusps.

Enamel Dysplasia

Enamel dysplasia includes two types of abnormal enamel development: **enamel hypoplasia** and **enamel hypocalcification.** Enamel hypoplasia is caused by any condition that inhibits enamel formation (Fig. 26-17). Enamel hypocalcification is caused by a condition that inhibits the calcification of enamel.

Enamel hypoplasia may leave small pits or grooves at different levels in the crown. They are formed by a local disturbance in the enamel formation. Such situations can be caused by inflammation, fever, systemic disease, and even heredity.

Enamel Fluorosis

One of the most common forms of enamel hypocalcification is enamel fluorosis (Fig. 26-18). Enamel fluorosis is a discolored enamel caused by an excessive amount of fluoride in the tooth structure. This could occur naturally from well water with excess amounts of fluoride. It could occur accidentally by a child taking vitamins with fluoride, fluoride mouthwashes, or fluoride supplements either in excess or in combination with fluoridated water. The enamel discoloration can range from small white flecks to large opaque areas to brownish spots sometimes with pits. In the more severe cases, the large areas of the crown are a brownish color. These more discolored areas are called mottled enamel.

Look at the chart on pages 258-259 and see at

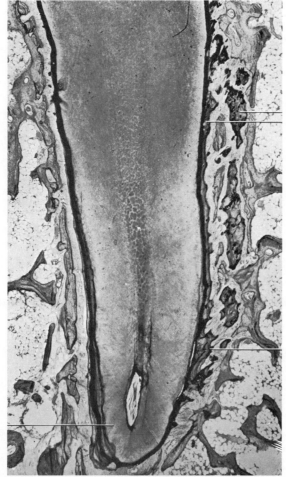

Remnants of
fractured cementum
Hyperplastic cementum

Hyperplastic cementum

Apex

Fig. 26-13 Hypercementosis. Note localized area of hypercementosis, which may be referred to as hyperplastic cementum (From Bhaskar SN: Orban's oral histology and embryology, ed 10, St Louis, 1986, The CV Mosby Co.)

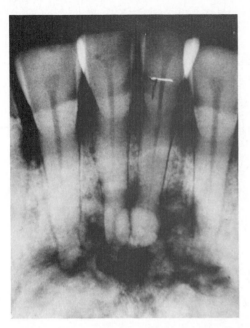

Fig. 26-14 Cementoma. Thickened radiopaque area of cementum at apex of central incisors with localized bone destruction around them.

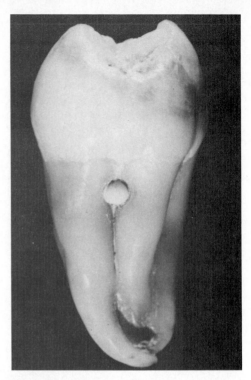

Fig. 26-15 Enamel pearl. Notice small ball of enamel in bifurcation of this molar. It virtually always is found in bifurcations or trifurcations of teeth.

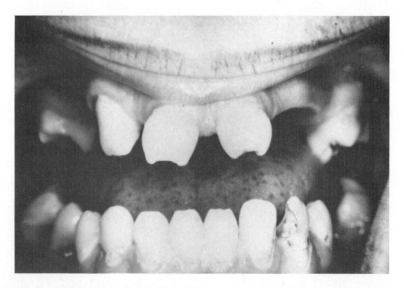

Fig. 26-16 Hutchinson's incisors. Note typical notching of incisal edge of incisors as a result of congenital syphilis.

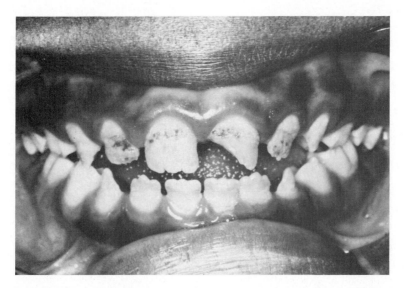

Fig. 26-17   Enamel hypoplasia. Note pitting on surfaces of maxillary central and lateral incisors. Enamel is thin in these areas.

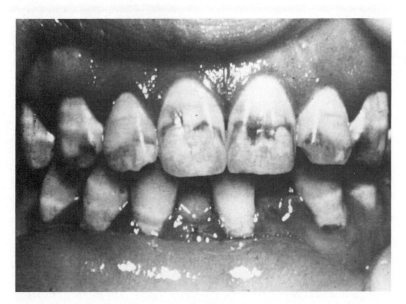

Fig. 26-18   Enamel fluorosis. Discoloration to teeth from too much fluoride. This usually results from drinking natural well water with high fluoride content.

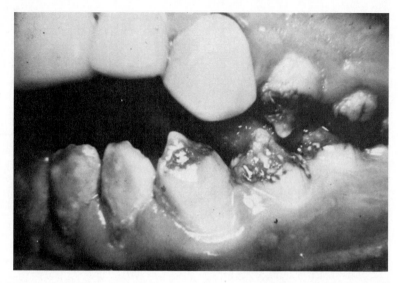

Fig. 26-19   Amelogenesis imperfecta. Enamel is soft and chips off easily. Note chipped and misshapen areas.

what age a developmental anomaly could occur to a maxillary permanent central incisor.

Amelogenesis Imperfecta

Amelogenesis imperfecta (Fig. 26-19) is another developmental anomaly, but one that is hereditary. It affects the calcification of the enamel, so it is a form of enamel hypocalcification. It differs from other forms because it is a hereditary condition passed on to other family members. In its typical form the enamel of the permanent and deciduous teeth are affected. Sometimes only the permanent teeth are affected. The enamel when present is very thin. It is stained various shades of yellow and brown and easily fractures away.

Turner's Teeth

Turner's teeth (Fig. 26-20) is a hypocalcification of a single tooth, usually a maxillary incisor. The condition occurs if a developing permanent tooth is affected by a local infection or trauma.

Something, bacteria or trauma, disturbs the ameloblastic layer. This results in a hypoplasia of the enamel.

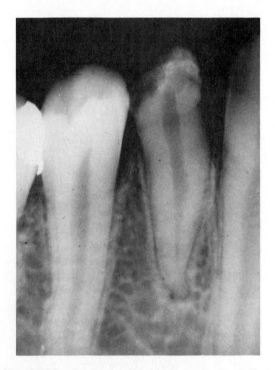

Fig. 26-20   Turner's tooth. Note lack of calcification of crown of this tooth. Tooth was affected while crown was forming but was not affected later when root was forming.

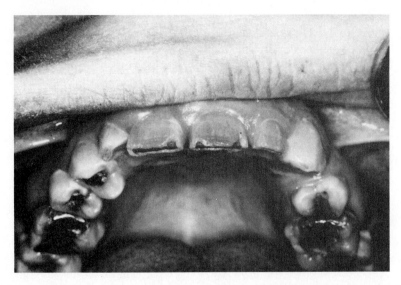

Fig. 26-21   Dentinogenesis imperfecta. Discoloration of maxillary anterior teeth. Enamel frequently chips away because poorly developed dentin beneath it does not support it.

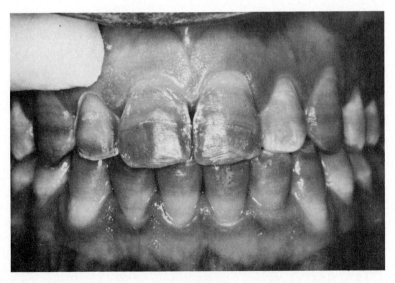

Fig. 26-22   Tetracycline staining. Note discolored banding of all teeth. This individual was taking tetracycline for extended period of time, and most teeth were affected.

Dentinogenesis Imperfecta

Dentinogenesis imperfecta (Fig. 26-21) is a hereditary dentinal developmental abnormality. The dentin is colored grey, brown, or yellow but the tooth exhibits an unusual translucent hue. The most striking feature of this condition is the fact that the pulp chambers and root canals are completely filled in with dentin. This total obliteration of the pulp tissue occurs because the dentinal tissue continues to form dentin until all of the root canal and pulp chambers are completely filled.

Tetracycline Staining

Another dentinal developmental condition is **tetracycline staining** (Fig. 26-22). This condition occurs when an expectant mother, or a young child whose tooth crowns are still developing, takes the antibiotic tetracycline. The teeth of the developing fetus or the young child discolors, ranging from yellow to brown or greyish blue.

REVIEW QUESTIONS

1. What is an anomaly?
2. Name some extrinsic and intrinsic factors that may cause anomalies.
3. What is the difference between hereditary and congenital factors?
4. What is the difference between hyperdontia and anodontia?
5. What is an odontoma?
6. What is the difference between gemination and fusion?
7. What is the cause of Hutchinson's incisors and mulberry molars?
8. What is the difference between amelogenesis imperfecta and dentinogenesis imperfecta?
9. What is tetracycline staining and when does it occur?

27

Supporting Structures

THE PERIODONTIUM

OBJECTIVES

- To understand the relationships within the gingival unit, a supporting structure of the teeth
- To understand the terminology of the gingival unit and to identify its various parts
- To understand how the gingival unit functions
- To understand how the attachment apparatus is related to the gingival unit
- To understand the relationship of cementum, periodontal ligament, and alveolar bone
- To understand how the fibers of the periodontal ligament function in tooth movement and shock absorption

The periodontium consists of those tissues that support the teeth. It is divided into a **gingival unit** and an **attachment unit** or **attachment apparatus:**

I. Gingival unit
   A. Gingiva
      1. Free gingiva
      2. Attached gingiva
   B. Alveolar mucosa
II. Attachment unit
   A. Cementum
   B. Alveolar bone
   C. Periodontal ligament

GINGIVAL UNIT

The gingiva is made up of free and attached gingiva (Fig. 27-1). Composed of very dense mucosa, called **masticatory mucosa,** it has a thick **epithelial** covering and is **keratinized.** The underlying **mucosa** is composed of dense collagen fibers. (See the tabular listing on p. 296.)

This type of masticatory mucosa is also found on the hard palate. Masticatory mucosa is well designed to withstand the trauma it is subjected to in grinding food. The rest of the mouth is lined with a different type of mucosa, called **lining mucosa.** This type makes up the alveolar mucosa. It is thin, freely movable, and tears or injures easily. The epithelium covering this lining mucosa is thin and nonkeratinized. Its mucosa is composed of loose connective tissue and muscle fibers.

Free Gingiva

Free gingiva is the gum tissue that extends from the gingival margin to the base of the **gingival sulcus.** The attached gingiva extends from the base of this sulcus to the **mucogingival junction.** Alveolar mucosa is found apical to the mucogingival junction, contiguous with the rest of the mucous membrane of the cheeks and lips, as well as the floor of the mouth. Free gingiva is usually light pink in color and averages between 0.5 and 2 mm in depth.

The free gingival margin around a fully erupted tooth is located next to the enamel about 0.5 to 2 mm coronal to the cementoenamel junction. It forms a little collar, which is separated from the tooth by the gingival sulcus. This gingival sulcus is the space between the free

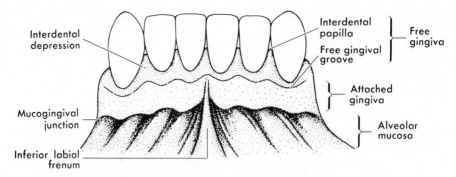

Fig. 27-1   Anatomy of normal gingival unit.

gingiva and the tooth. The bottom of the sulcus is influenced by the curvature of the cervical line of the tooth. A healthy gingival sulcus will rarely exceed 2.5 mm in depth.

The **gingival papilla** is the free gingiva located in the triangular interdental spaces. The apex in the anterior teeth is rather sharp, whereas in the posterior teeth the apex is more blunt. The shape of gingival papilla is greatly affected by the location of the contact area of the adjacent teeth, by the shape of the interproximal surfaces of the adjacent teeth, and by the cementoenamel junction of the adjacent teeth.

Inflammation is easily recognized, since the area takes on a redder color and exhibits a more puffy appearance, with some blunting of its apex.

A gingival groove often corresponds to the base of the gingival sulcus. This groove is not always present but is to be considered a normal part of the anatomy when present.

The inner portion of the gingival sulcus is lined with nonkeratinized epithelium. The outer portion of this gingival sulcus is the free gingiva, covered with keratinized epithelium. The attached gingiva begins at the base of the gingival sulcus. A gingival groove often occurs on the outside of the free gingiva and, as mentioned before, corresponds to the base of the sulcus. The attached gingiva extends apically from the base of the sulcus and is attached to the bone and the cementum by a dense network of collagenous fibers. It often has a stippled texture, resembling the dimpled surface of an orange. Stippling becomes evident before the teeth erupt and be-

Characteristics of gingiva and alveolar mucosa

Tissue characteristics	Free and attached gingiva	Alveolar mucosa
Type of mucosa	Masticatory	Lining
Tone	Tightly bound	Movable and elastic
Epithelium	Thick epithelial layer	Thin epithelial layer
	Keratinized	Nonkeratinized
	Rete peg formation	No rete peg formation
Texture	Stippled surface (like an orange peel)	Smooth
Color	Light pink	Red to bright red
Fiber	Collagenous fibers	Collagenous fibers and elastic fibers

comes even more so in the adult gingiva. The attached gingiva is highly keratinized and is covered by **stratified squamous epithelium** in which **rete peg formation** is evident. The dimple effect is caused by the rete peg formation, which is simply the irregular binding of the epithelium to the bone by collagen fibers. This causes depressions, or dimples, where the epithelium is pulled tight to the bone. The color of the gingiva varies from light to dark pink and may contain pigment, correlating to the skin pigmentation of the person. The darker a person's skin color is, the more likely the gingiva will be darker and contain **melanin pigment.**

Attached Gingiva

The gingiva is connected to the tooth by a meshwork of collagenous fibers. These fibers are formed by **fibroblasts,** which are the principal cells of connective tissue. All fibers embedded in the cementum are known as **Sharpey's fibers;** they extend from the cementum to the papillary area of the gingiva. These fibers pass outward from the cementum in groups of small bundles.

Some of the fibers (Fig. 27-2) curve toward the mucosa of the free gingiva. They interlace with one another as a meshwork of fiber bundles. Other fibers (B) pass directly across from the cementum to the gingiva. Still further apically, other fibers (C) pass from the cementum over the alveolar crest and turn apically between the outer periosteum of the alveolar process and the outer epithelial covering of the attached gingiva. These bundles of fibers hold the free gingiva firmly against the tooth. They prevent the free gingiva from being peeled away from the tooth, and the attached gingiva is held closely and firmly to the bone.

On the proximal side, the connective-tissue fibers arise from a higher level on the cementum because of the curvature of the cementoenamel junction on the interproximal surfaces of the teeth. This curvature allows more room for the cementum to attach to the gingiva. Attachment is made possible by groups of connective tissue fibers. The most occlusal group travels to the papillary layer of the epithelium of the interdental papilla. The next layer of fibers passes occlusally

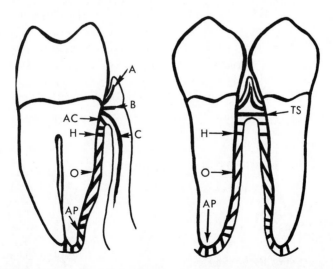

Fig. 27-2   Principal fiber groups of gingival unit and attachment unit. *Left,* Gingival fibers: groups *A, B,* and *C* are seen in buccolingual sketch. *Right,* Transseptal fibers *(TS)* are seen in mesiodistal sketch. Periodontal ligament fibers: alveolar crest fibers *(AC),* horizontal fibers *(H),* oblique fibers *(O),* and apical fibers *(AP).* (Kraus et al.)

into the interproximal gingiva. The next layer of fibers, the transseptal *(TS)* group, travels completely across the interproximal space and attaches to the adjacent tooth. These transseptal fiber bundles, formed from transseptal fibers, bind one tooth to another. In addition to these fibers, circular bands of connective tissue fibers surround the teeth, tying them together (Fig. 27-3).

The function of these gingival fibers is to keep the gingiva closely attached to the tooth surface. These fibers prevent the free gingiva from being peeled away from the tooth and keep the attached gingiva firmly attached. They also prevent the apical migration of the epithelial attachment and resist gingival recession.

The blood supply of the gingival tissue is derived from the **supraperiosteal** vessels. These in turn originate from the lingual, mental, buccal, infraorbital, and palatine arteries. The gingiva is quite rich in capillary vascularity. The alveolar mucosa is equally **vascular.** Its redder color can be directly attributed to numerous shallow blood vessels.

Alveolar Mucosa

The alveolar mucosa joins the attached gingiva at the mucogingival junction and is continuous with the rest of the tissues of the **vestibule.** This tissue is thin and soft and rather loosely attached to the underlying bone. The alveolar mucosa is composed of lining mucosa and has a deeper red color than the gingiva has. Its **submucosa** contains loose connective tissue and fat. The epithelium is smooth, thin, and nonkeratinized.

ATTACHMENT UNIT

The attachment unit consists of the cementum, the periodontal ligament, and the alveolar bone. Cementum is hard, bonelike tissue covering the roots of the teeth. The **periodontal ligament** is the tissue that surrounds the roots of the teeth and connects them to alveolar bone. The alveolar bone is the thin covering of compact bone that surrounds the teeth; when viewed radiographically it is called the **lamina dura** (Figs. 27-4 and 27-5). The function of the attachment apparatus is

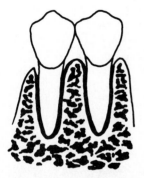

Fig. 27-3   Circular fibers of gingival unit.

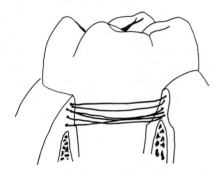

Fig. 27-4   Sketch of radiograph shows that periodontal ligament separates lamina dura from tooth. Notice width of periodontal ligament and direction of bone trabeculae. Black space around root of teeth is periodontal ligament.

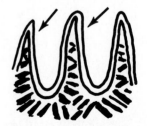

Fig. 27-5   Overview of Fig. 27-4 depicting lamina dura and direction of bone trabeculae. Arrows point to lamina dura.

not only supportive, but nutritive, formative, and sensory. The supportive function is to maintain the support of the tooth in the bone and to prevent its movement. The nutritive and sensory functions are fulfilled by the blood vessels and nerves. The nerves act as an indicator of pressure or pain around the tooth. The formative function is to replace cementum, periodontal ligament, and alveolar bone, which is accomplished by specialized cells called **cementoblasts,** fibroblasts, and osteoblasts. In addition to these functions, the periodontal ligament acts as a suspensory mechanism that keeps the root and bone from abrading each other. The periodontal ligament also acts as a hammock of live tissue, whose fibers cushion the impact of tooth and bone on the exertion of pressure. The fibers themselves become taut, thus dissipating the pressure and, at the same time, allowing the nerves associated with these fibers a method of measuring and equating the amount of pressure.

Cementum

Cementum, a hard, bonelike tissue that covers the root of the tooth, can be cellular or acellular. Both types are formed by cementoblasts that become embedded in the cellular type. The acellular type is free of embedded cementoblasts and is clear and structureless.

Acellular cementum always covers the cervical third of the root and sometimes extends over almost all of the root except the apical portion. Cellular cementum covers the apical portion of the root, and sometimes it may form over the acellular type. Cellular cementum is like bone in character and in the way it can be resorbed and added to. Like bone, cementum grows by the **apposition** (addition) of new layers, one on another. Changes in function and pressure will influence the growth activity of cementum.

Cellular and acellular cementum have collagen fibers embedded in them. These fibers, known as Sharpey's fibers, are the embedded ends of connective tissue fibers of the periodontal membrane. Some are embedded in cementum and, as we shall see, some are embedded in bone.

Alveolar Bone

The type of bone that lines the sockets in which the roots of the teeth are held is called alveolar bone proper. The socket in which the tooth rests is called an alveolus. These alveoli (plural of alveolus) are a part of the alveolar process that surrounds and supports the teeth in the maxilla and mandible. Alveolar bone proper is thin and compact, with many small openings through which blood vessels, nerves, and lymphatic vessels pass. The alveolar bone that forms the alveolus around a tooth's bony socket contains Sharpey's fibers. What other hard tissue has Sharpey's fibers? Sharpey's fibers are part of what membrane?

Bone tissue is continually undergoing change. The architectural arrangement of the **trabeculae** is directly related to the demands of function. Even bone apposition and resorption are related to the functional demands placed on the bone. Compared with cementum, bone is an extremely active tissue.

Very slow apposition of cementum occurs, whereas the alveolar bone undergoes changes readily. The extreme difference between these two tissues in their ability to undergo remodeling poses a significant problem. The two tissues are tied together by the periodontal ligament, which must make adjustments for the variation in their abilities.

Bone, like cementum, consists of an **organic matrix** and **inorganic matter.** The organic matrix is composed of collagen and intercellular substance; the inorganic matter is composed of **apatite crystals** of calcium, phosphate, and carbonates. Under normal conditions bone is constantly in flux, undergoing tissue growth (apposition) and resorption in a finely coordinated way. Bone may be laid down on one end and resorbed on the other.

Alveolar bone is deposited next to the periodontal ligament and supported by a more compact bone. The bone forming the alveoli is dependent on the functional demands of the tooth. If a tooth undergoes long-standing loss of function, as when the antagonists in the opposite arch are lost, the alveolar bone undergoes changes. If the teeth are subjected to **occlusal stress,** the supporting bone will be composed of thicker and more numerous trabeculae. The bone itself undergoes resorption when pressure is exerted on it and opposition when tension is placed on it. Sharpey's fibers, embedded in the bone at one end and in the cementum at the other, are capable of expressing such tension. The term **bundle bone** applies when numerous layers of bone are added to the socket wall. Bundle bone forms the immediate attachment of the periodontal ligament.

Periodontal Ligament

The fibers of the periodontal ligament attach to the alveolar bone and cementum. They are arranged in the following five groups:

1. **Alveolar crest group**—Fibers extending from the cervical area of the tooth to the alveolar crest
2. **Horizontal group**—Fibers running horizontally from the tooth to the alveolar bone
3. **Oblique group**—Fibers running obliquely from the cementum to the bone
4. **Apical group**—Fibers radiating apically from the tooth to the bone (Fig. 27-2)
5. **Interradicular**—Periodontal fibers between roots of multirooted teeth

This arrangement of fibers provides a hammock of tissue bundles that support the tooth within the bone. They not only tie the tooth to the bone but also prevent it from being pushed into the bone. Acting as a hammock of strings that allows the tooth to float in a bony cavity, they insulate the tooth and bone, thereby minimizing the trauma of being pushed together. Because fibers are constantly subjected to a variety of pressures exerted on the tooth, the periodontal ligament is constantly undergoing functional change. The main portion of the periodontal ligament is composed of bundles of white collagenous connective tissue fibers. These fibers extend from, and are embedded in, the cementum of the tooth and the alveolar bone and are bundled together like the many strands of a rope.

In addition to the collagen fibers, the periodontal ligament is composed of fibroblasts, one of the cellular elements of the periodontal ligament. They are found in alignment with the collagen fibers, arranged in groups. The periodontal ligament also contains small blood and lymph vessels and nerves. Loose connective tissue surrounds these vessels and nerves.

The tooth itself is actually suspended by this periodontal ligament in such a way that the tooth is allowed some degree of movement within the bony cavity. For instance, if pressure is exerted on the mesial surface, the periodontal fibers on the distal surface are compressed, and allow more space between the tooth and the bone.

This ability of the periodontal ligament to expand by becoming taut allows limited movement of the tooth, and the tooth therefore is able to tip, rotate, or be compressed within the bony cavity. Even total bodily movement is possible because of the periodontal ligament. An example of this is the constant abrading of neighboring teeth, not only occlusally but also interproximally. This causes wear on the contact areas and occlusal surfaces. Two forces that are active within the mouth allow for movement of the tooth. The first is mesial drift, which allows the tooth to move forward within the oral cavity, thus closing the spaces lost from interproximal wear. The second is an active eruption force of the tooth, which causes the tooth to migrate occlusally until it occludes with an antagonist. Both forces can be activated fairly rapidly because of the periodontal ligament's ability to tense and compress and the bone's ability to change the shape and size of the socket.

In addition to the periodontal ligament's ability to allow minor movement of the tooth, it also functions as a suspension system to absorb shocks. This protects the bone and the tooth from trauma imposed on the tooth that would be transferred to the bone. The periodontal ligament functions as a shock absorber because of three factors:

1. The principal fiber apparatus of the periodontal ligament is interwoven so that slip-

page between the periodontal fibers helps to dissipate traumatic forces.

2. The shape and size of the roots of the teeth help to dissipate occlusal stresses in a lateral and apical direction; also, in multirooted teeth the forces can be distributed between the roots of the same tooth.

3. The fluids contained within the periodontal ligament act as a hydraulic pressure system on the walls of the alveolus.

CLINICAL CONSIDERATIONS

There are several clinical situations that should be discussed. The first of these concerns how a tooth can move within a bony alveolus. Such movement is accomplished by several mechanisms already discussed.

For a tooth to move through bone, a force of some type must be acting on it. This force causes pressure on the root, periodontal ligament, and bone. It compresses the periodontal ligament and the alveolar bone on one side of the root. If this force continues for a long enough time, a biomechanical system of osteoclastic cells (bone-destroying cells) is initiated. The osteoclasts destroy bone to make room for the compressed tissues. If the pressure is extreme, the osteoclastic cells may even resorb portions of the root of the tooth.

On the other side of this same tooth root, the periodontal ligament is pulled taut. This results in a pulling force on the alveolar bone on that side of the socket. This constant tension causes an opposite biomechanical system. Osteoblastic cells (bone-forming cells) start laying down bone. These osteoblasts produce bone as a response to tension. This aids in relieving the tension on the periodontal ligament. The net affect is that the tooth moves away from the force exerted on it by remodeling bone. On one side bone is destroyed, and on the other side bone is formed.

The following are some of the forces that exert pressure on the teeth:

1. Active eruption—Tooth eruption into the

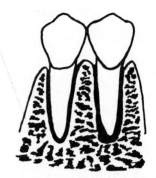

Fig. 27-6 Tooth on right shows widening of periodontal ligament, indicating tooth mobility.

oral cavity and eruption to compensate for occlusal **abrasion**

2. Mesial drift—The mesial movement of molars to compensate for proximal abrasion

3. Masticatory occlusal forces—Tooth occlusion during chewing

4. Orthodontic corrective forces—A dentist or orthodontist placing pressure-causing appliances on the teeth to correct malocclusion

5. Traumatic occlusal forces—Teeth being subjected to premature contact during occlusion

The first four of these forces can tip, rotate, or move the tooth because of the bone-remodeling system just mentioned. These forces must be relatively constant for the bone-remodeling mechanisms, osteoclasts and osteoblasts, to be activated.

The last of these forces, occlusal trauma, is not a consistent, constant force. It is usually intermittent and consequently does not result in tooth movement as much as tooth mobility. Although some osteoclastic activity occurs, it may be the result of constant pressure from inflammation caused by trauma more than the external force of the occlusion. In general the periodontal ligament is tensed and torn. The space between the cementum and the lamina dura is enlarged and widened. The lamina dura is compressed, and the tooth becomes loose and mobile within the socket (Fig. 27-6).

REVIEW QUESTIONS

1. Which of the following are true of attached gingiva?
   a. The tissue is soft and movable.
   b. The epithelial layer is thick and keratinized.
   c. The tissue can have a stippled texture.
   d. The tissue is fixed and firmly attached to the bone and cementum.
2. Which is most true of cementum?
   a. Sharpey's fibers are embedded in it.
   b. It is always smooth.
   c. Acellular cementum covers the apical end of the tooth.
   d. It is resorbed like bone.
3. Which is true of Sharpey's fibers?
   a. They can embed in bone only.
   b. They can embed in cementum only.
   c. They can embed in either bone or cementum.
   d. The same fiber embeds in bone at one end and cementum at the other.
4. When the tooth is subjected to occlusal stress, it relieves this stress by which of the following?
   a. The periodontal ligament tenses.
   b. The fluids in the periodontal ligament absorb some force.
   c. The walls of the alveolus spread the force out and divide it over a wider area.
5. Define the following by researching the glossary:
   a. rete peg formation
   b. stratified squamous epithelium
6. Which statements are true about fibers *A, B,* and *C* in Fig. 27-7?
   a. They are called Sharpey's fibers.
   b. They attach only the free gingiva to the cementum.
   c. They are called transseptal fibers.
   d. They are embedded in the cementum.
7. Draw and label the periodontal ligament fibers in Fig. 27-8 (a mandibular first molar).

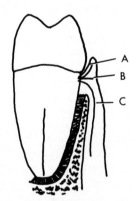

Fig. 27-7   Mesial view of permanent mandibular first molar.

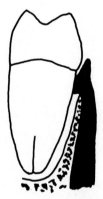

Fig. 27-8   Mesial view.

28

Clinical Considerations

OBJECTIVES

- To understand how clinical experience is related to the theory and lecture portion of dental anatomy
- To understand how preventive clinical situations are related to tooth form and supportive dental structures
- To understand how occlusal trauma and the natural shape and contour of the teeth can contribute to dental disease
- To understand how the placement of a restoration can contribute to the disease of the supporting tissues
- To evaluate the reliability of dental pain as a diagnostic aid
- To understand how tooth migration can affect the success of treatment or necessitate different treatment

When studying clinical considerations of an existing dental condition, we arrive at two alternatives: either the circumstances are preventive in nature, enhancing the ability of the oral tissues to protect themselves, or they are potentially pathological. It is important to recognize the difference. It is bad enough not to recognize a potentially pathological situation, but it is worse to be the cause of it because of ignorance in therapeutic treatment. It is for this reason that a study of preventive clinical situations is important.

PREVENTIVE CLINICAL CONSIDERATIONS

Preventive clinical considerations include the form, shape, and arrangement of the teeth that aid in the prevention of dental disease. Such preventive clinical considerations would be those that help prevent decay, occlusal trauma, and periodontal disease.

Remember that the teeth are encased in a hard, smooth outer covering, the enamel, which offers protection from the accumulation of bacteria and debris. (Together these are sometimes called plaque.) The smoothness of the enamel makes the adherence of plaque more difficult. This self-cleaning ability of the enamel therefore helps resist decay, since decay is caused by bacterially produced acids that etch away the tooth surface. If the bacteria cannot accumulate and adhere to the tooth surface, decay cannot occur.

Likewise, some prevention of periodontal disease is attributable to the very smoothness of this enamel, since bacteria that destroy gum and bone tissue are also prevented from accumulating on the tooth. It is important to remember, however, that not all periodontal disease is caused by bacteria.

If the tooth has rough pits, grooves, and fissures, these areas will allow debris to accumulate and provide a breeding ground for bacteria. The same is true if the tooth has rough margins on its restorations or if interproximally the tooth has an overhanging restoration, that is, a restoration that does not stay within the confines of the tooth form but leaves an excess part of the restoration sticking into the gingival tissue. This kind of restoration is called an overhang. An overhanging restoration will cause bacteria to adhere around the margins of the excess material, and such adherence leads to disease within the gum and tooth tissues. Restoration of any tooth must follow the normal anatomy of that tooth. A restoration must be polished smooth so that the tooth can resume normal function and the jaw its normal anatomy—anything less is doomed to failure. The dental personnel provide a valuable service in preventive dentistry by polishing dental restorations. It is much more comfortable for patients to undergo the polishing of their restorations than their replacement (Fig. 28-1).

Plaque that builds up because of improperly fitting restorations not only can lead to decay but can also cause the breakdown of the periodontal tissues. Rough surfaces on the roots of the tooth and extra projections of cementum and calculus can also lead to the same type of pathological conditions previously mentioned.

It therefore becomes extremely important for the health professional not only to remove calculus and stain from the roots of the teeth but also to smooth any rough areas on the root that may be formed from irregularities in the cementum or defects within the root formation. Any rough defect permitted to remain on the root acts as calculus does—it allows bacteria to adhere and multiply.

Since it is not uncommon for the roots of the teeth to have excess buildup of cementum or rough defects on the root surface, it is therefore extremely important for the health professional to clean these areas. Thus the cleaning can prevent disease by destroying any plaque-trapping areas that could harbor bacteria. This process is sometimes called **root planing.** The health professional must always remember how thin the

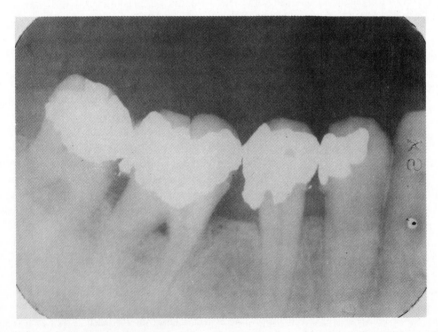

Fig. 28-1 Radiograph showing periodontal disease caused by bacteria, which are harbored by overextended restoration.

envelope of cementum is that wraps around the root. A painful situation occurs when the bare dentin is exposed because the cementum is stripped away from a part of the root of a tooth.

Trauma

The hardness of the enamel helps prevent occlusal wear *(attrition)*. But this same hardness allows the full impact of trauma to be transferred from tooth to tooth to bone. If a tooth prematurely contacts another, only two teeth will bear the initial brunt of forces when the jaws are closed. A more ideal situation is to have all the teeth hit equally on closure of the jaw, without any teeth hitting prematurely. This allows for the forces exerted on closing the jaws to be dissipated over all the teeth. Should one tooth hit with a greater force than the rest of the teeth, it would be traumatized by this excess force. Such a situation is known as **occlusal trauma** and results in disease of the periodontal tissue, crack-

ing of the enamel of the tooth, and possible fracture of the tooth (Fig. 28-2).

Occlusal trauma can also result during eating. When food is placed between the teeth, it is necessary to have spillways between the teeth to allow for the dissipation of forces. This dissipation of occlusal forces occurs because the spillways allow the food to escape from between the teeth.

Contours of Teeth

The contours of the teeth, buccally and lingually, determine the angle at which food is deflected off the teeth and onto the gingiva. If the buccal or lingual contours are underdeveloped (undercontoured), food and debris are pushed into the gingival crevice. If the buccal and lingual contours are overdeveloped (overcontoured), the food and debris pass off the tooth and onto the gingiva at a poor angle. This results in gingival inflammation because the gum tissue is denied proper frictional massage. (See Fig. 22-6.)

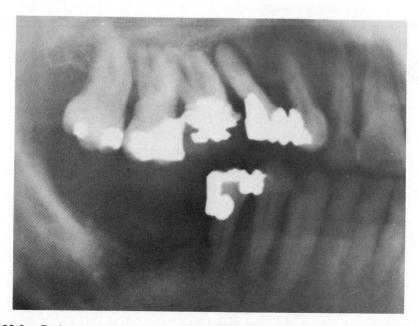

Fig. 28-2   Dark area around root of upper premolar indicates bone loss caused by occlusal trauma.

The amount of contour of the teeth buccally and lingually is important. An excess of contour, such as more than 1 mm of lingual contour on mandibular molars, creates an oral hygiene problem. If the tooth contour presents extreme undercuts, the natural cleaning action of the tongue and friction of the food and cheeks become ineffective. Special oral hygiene devices and instructions must be given to the patient.

THERAPEUTIC CONSIDERATIONS

Since it is very important in the restoration of teeth to reconstruct a tooth in its anatomical form, it is apparent that we need to know the anatomical shape of each individual tooth. We also need to know contact areas and buccal and lingual contours. For instance, it is evident that an overhanging restoration or an open interproximal contact is undesirable in restoring a tooth in the interproximal area. Measures should be taken to keep the filling material from impinging on the tissue. Thus to keep the overflow of any restoration from impinging on the tissue, a metal band is placed around the tooth and wedged into position (Fig. 28-3). The **matrix band** retains the material being packed against the tooth, and the **wedge** forces the inside of the matrix band against the tooth so that no excess of filling material can overflow into the gingiva. The wedge also forces the teeth apart so that a tight interproximal contact can be made. It also becomes apparent that there should be no rough margins or excesses on the marginal line of the filling

and the tooth. In other words, we want the margins and the filling of the tooth to be as smooth as possible, with the tooth restored to its proper form and function. Also, deep pits and fissures should not be recreated in the teeth to be restored because there is no point in doing so. The deep pits and grooves only become plaque traps. The buccal and lingual contours, however, should be restored in the best possible manner so that the gingiva is carefully protected. The restoration should not infringe on the pulp tissue of the tooth. In restoring the tooth an attempt should be made to protect the pulp. Any trauma to the pulp tissue of a tooth creates serious complications.

For example, if one were to hit his finger with a hammer, an inflammation process would ensue. The finger would immediately be painful, and soon blood would rush to the injured area. The finger would swell, and heat from the increased vascularity (blood flow) would be felt. The increased blood flow would cause edema (swelling), which in turn would cause pain.

The same factors exist for inflammation within the pulp cavity. If trauma occurs, the pulpal tissues become inflamed. An increase in the blood flow (vascularity) can be felt. The only problem is that, unlike the finger, the pulpal tissue cannot swell. It is encased in hard tooth structures. The pulp cavity walls are formed from dentin (Fig. 28-3). This hard material makes it virtually impossible for the pulpal tissue to expand, or swell. As the pressure from the increased vascularity builds up within the pulp cavity walls, the veins

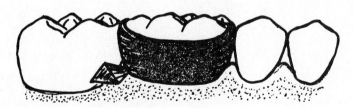

Fig. 28-3 Matrix band wedged interproximally with wooden wedge to prevent overhanging restoration.

within the pulp tissue begin to close. Since the arteries have thicker walls than the veins do, and they are affected less by pressure, they maintain the blood supply, but the veins, with thinner walls, collapse. Since the only opening into the pulp cavity is the small **apical foramen** at the root apex, not too much internal pressure is required to close this opening. As soon as the apical foramen is obstructed because the venous blood flow is stopped, the tooth literally chokes itself off from fresh blood. The result is that the tooth's pulpal tissues die from lack of blood (Fig. 28-4).

The dentist and auxiliary check the patient's bite after the restoration is in place by having the patient bite on articulating (ink) paper. This is done to ensure that no part of the restoration is hitting prematurely. This would result in occlusal trauma to the tooth, and such occlusal trauma could lead to the fracture of the restoration or even the tooth itself. Even if the tooth hits with just slightly more contact than the rest of the teeth, the result is extreme trauma. First, the tooth, by hitting prematurely, becomes sore be-

cause it is carrying more than its share of the burden of occlusal stress. Second, the soreness of the tooth leads to inflammation of the periodontal and other supporting tissues. Third, with inflammation, edema occurs; pressure and swelling within these tissues push the tooth out of its bony socket in an attempt to relieve some of these stresses. Fourth, the tooth now extends further from the bony socket than it did before it was inflamed. Because it extends farther from the bony socket, it hits the opposing teeth sooner and harder. Thus the tooth undergoes more severe occlusal trauma, resulting in more inflammation, swelling, and pain. The tooth is forced to extend even farther from the bony socket to relieve this new pressure from the inflammation and edema. If untreated, the cycle could be irreversible. Therefore the dentist must make sure that any new dental restorations fit properly according to the patient's bite.

Pain

When diagnosing dental pain, it is important to remember that the nerve centers within the tooth are not the only nerve centers capable of eliciting pain around the tooth. If a tooth is severely damaged so that the nerve of the tooth has degenerated or even been obliterated, the tooth could still cause pain. Even an endodontically treated tooth, whose pulp cavity has been completely **debrided** of all traces of nerve tissue and filled with root canal filling material, can respond to pain if the tooth is touched. Why? The answer is simply that the nerve tissues in the periodontal ligament and surrounding bone tissue are still alive. If trauma or infection from any source, such as periapical involvement or periodontal abscess, were present, the nerves in the supporting structures around the tooth would respond to the pain. It is important to realize that the nerve within the pulp cavity can give only a response to pain, whereas nerves within the periodontal tissue can give either a pain response or a pressure response. A patient who reports feeling pain from within a tooth may be experienc-

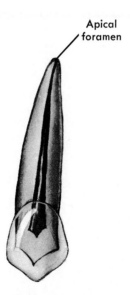

Apical foramen

Fig. 28-4 Pulp tissue of tooth is encased by hard dentin. Only pathway for blood's vital support is through apical foramen. (Massler and Schour.)

ing pain from the periodontal tissues or surrounding bone. A careful clinical examination is therefore absolutely necessary, since false and referred pains are common.

Tooth Migration

If a tooth were fractured so that it no longer hit its antagonist in the opposite arch, within 24 hours the tooth would begin to erupt to meet this antagonist.

The same thing would happen if a dentist cut a tooth for a crown preparation and the occlusal surface were cut away—the tooth would not hit its opposing antagonist. The tooth therefore would erupt to try to meet the antagonist. If an impression had been taken of the tooth preparation at that time so that the crown could be made, then when the crown was ready 2 weeks later, the tooth would have moved. (This **tooth migration** occurs as a result of the tooth trying to meet its opposite antagonist and also the existence of mesial drift.) The crown then might not fit. To avert this problem, a well-placed temporary restoration is made to fit the crown preparation. This temporary must not only replace the interproximal areas (to prevent mesial drift) but also restore the cut preparation to a functional occlusion (to prevent the tooth from erupting to meet its antagonist).

If a tooth were removed and not replaced, the tooth in the opposite arch might **supraerupt** (erupt past the occlusal plane in an attempt to meet its antagonist). This would destroy the effectiveness of the contact areas between this tooth and its neighboring teeth. With the contact areas changed, food impaction occurs. In the opposite arch mesial drift begins to cause any teeth immediately posterior to the extraction site to move in a mesial direction. This usually results in the tooth becoming mesially tipped as well. In Fig. 28-5 notice what has happened to the interproximal spaces and contact areas. All this resulted because a tooth was removed and not replaced.

Let us look at the dental tissue collapse initiated by the loss of a single tooth, a mandibular first molar (Fig. 28-5). The maxillary first molar supraerupts to meet its missing mandibular antagonist. Notice the relocation of the mesial and distal contact areas of the maxillary first molar. This causes food impaction between the maxillary teeth interproximally. Plaque adheres to these poor contact areas, which results in decay. Food debris and plaque cause gingival irritation and periodontal breakdown. Finally, premature occlusal contact occurs in centric occlusion because the distal area of the maxillary first molar prematurely hits the mesial area of the mandibular second molar. When the mandible goes into protrusive movement, the distal area of the maxillary first molar hits the mesial area of the mandibular second molar. (In protrusive movement only the anterior teeth should occlude; the posterior teeth disengage.)

This occlusal trauma results in mobility of the affected teeth and finally migration and tipping of these teeth. The mandibular second premolar migrates and tips distally. This results in an open contact between the mandibular premolars. This open contact can cause a periodontal pocket with loss of the lamina dura and formation of infraosseous periodontal pockets.

The teeth are not the only structures traumatized. The temporomandibular joint and especially the lateral pterygoid muscles suffer from trauma caused by premature occlusal contacts.

The combination of occlusal trauma and mesial drift cause the mandibular second molar to move mesially and tip gingivally. This in turn causes a poor contact area between the distal mandibular second molar and the mandibular third molar. This results in a periodontal pocket between these two molars. This malpositioned contact area allows the buildup of bacteria to initiate dental decay of the interproximal surfaces of these two molars. The mesial drift of the mandibular third molar causes the second molar to move into the decay area on the second molars. This causes a poor occlusal relationship between the two third molars.

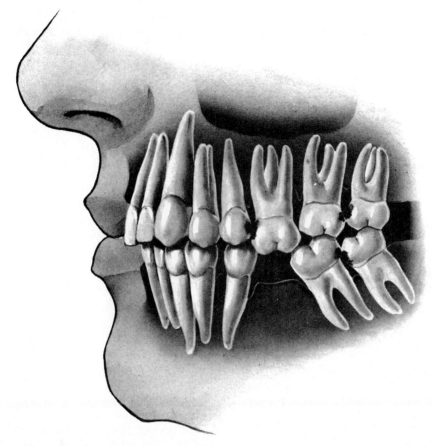

Fig. 28-5   Dental tissues collapse because of failure to replace missing mandibular first molar. (Massler and Schour.)

■ ■ ■

All this helps to illustrate the importance of good preventive dentistry and the interrelationships that exist within the oral cavity. All of the dental structures interrelate in a marvelous biomechanical system. Each mechanism protects and supports the others in some way. The breakdown of any one of these systems destroys the circle of mutual protection. If the contour of teeth is destroyed, sooner or later the gingiva and bone tissue are destroyed. If the occlusal relationship is destroyed, there is damage to the bone, teeth, gums, and temporomandibular joint.

Even the muscles responsible for movement of the jaw become traumatized and spasmodic. When an occlusal prematurity exists, the patient subconsciously tries to avoid this occlusal discrepancy. To do this, the patient overexerts the lateral pterygoid muscle. The muscle affected is usually the lateral pterygoid muscle on the opposite side from the occlusal prematurity. This muscle becomes overworked trying to protrude the jaw to avoid the premature contact. This is only one example among numerous possibilities.

It is important to understand that all the oral structures are mutually protective of each other.

A circle of natural prevention exists as long as all the oral tissues remain intact and in perfect harmony. An orthodontic malocclusion, for example, might occur naturally, but that would not allow the tissues to exist in perfect harmony. The best dentistry is preventive dentistry. Preventive dentistry maintains the oral structures in their most mutually protective harmony. It intercepts disease at the earliest possible circumstance so that the most natural, self-protective, functional, and preventive balances can be restored and maintained by these tissues.

The clinical considerations are endless but here it is intended that the student of dental anatomy merely have an example of how to apply the basic principles of dental anatomy to the clinical experience. Never cease to be alert and observant. Your reward will be the comfort of patients, pride in your work, and the progress of the dental profession.

REVIEW QUESTIONS

1. If a dentist restores a tooth in such a way that it is the first tooth to touch its antagonist when the patient closes his mouth, which of the following clinical problems could result?
   a. inflammation of the nerve of the tooth
   b. occlusal trauma
   c. tooth mobility
   d. tooth migration
   e. pain
   f. nerve involvement
   g. fracture of the restoration or the tooth
   h. inflammation of the supporting structures of the tooth
   i. all of the above

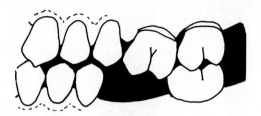

Fig. 28-6

2. If a dentist cuts a crown preparation but does not place a temporary restoration properly, which of the following could occur?
   a. gingival inflammation of the supporting structures because of bacteria buildup around the margins of the temporary restoration
   b. occlusal trauma to the tooth and temporary restoration
   c. tooth migration to avoid occlusal trauma
   d. supraeruption of the tooth to meet its antagonist
   e. pain caused by trauma, inflammation, or bacterial involvement
   f. sensitivity from hot or cold fluids
   g. tipping or mesial drifting of the tooth
3. What could happen to the nerve of a tooth if the tooth became inflamed because of occlusal traumatization?
4. Name all the possible pathological situations present in Fig. 28-6.

29

Tooth Identification

It would be rare to find a full set of teeth in which every tooth met all the anatomical criteria of what a perfect tooth should be; there is too much variation between individual teeth. When studying tooth identification, it is very important to remember the extreme amounts of variation possible. The individual tooth you are trying to identify may meet most of the criteria of a maxillary central incisor, may be missing certain criteria for a maxillary central incisor, and may even meet some of the criteria of a maxillary canine or lateral incisor, yet it may still be a maxillary central incisor. It is only after compiling all the characteristics that this tooth in question seems to possess and categorizing these characteristics that one can identify the individual tooth—and then only after it becomes apparent that the tooth meets more of the characteristics of one type of tooth than another.

Following is a description of general characteristics of each of the teeth by their respective groupings—incisors, canines, premolars, and molars.* In identifying teeth it is necessary to be able to differentiate between the left and right teeth in any particular group.

INCISORS

Incisal two thirds appear flattened on labial and lingual sides (Fig. 29-1).

Incisal "biting" edge, not a cusp (Fig. 29-2).

*Recently the term "facial" has been used as being synonymous with "labial" and "buccal." In general, "labial" and "buccal" will be used, since they are most commonly accepted, but "facial" will also be used. Keep in mind that "facial" can be substituted for "labial" and "buccal" and vice versa.

Maxillary

Crown wider mesiodistally than faciolingually (Figs. 29-3 and 29-4).

Root has triangular cross section, being broader on facial side. *tapers to a point on lingual*

Central

1. Greater crown-to-root ratio (crown larger, root about same as or smaller than lateral) (Figs. 29-5 and 29-6).
2. Mesioincisal angle relatively sharp (90-degree angle), with contact area in incisal third.
3. Broad smooth lingual fossa with well-developed cingulum.

Lateral

1. Lesser crown-to-root ratio (crown smaller, root about same as or larger than central).
2. Mesioincisal angle more rounded, with contact area at junction of middle and incisal thirds.
3. Small cingulum, often with a lingual pit (Figs. 29-7 and 29-8).

Right-left

1. Mesioincisal angles more square than distoincisal angles (Figs. 29-9 and 29-10).
2. Crest of cervical line more often displaced toward distal from labial or lingual view.
3. Mesiocervical line curves more incisally than distocervical line (Figs. 29-11 and 29-12).

Mandibular

Smaller than maxillary central or lateral incisor (Figs. 29-13 and 29-14).

Crown wider faciolingually than mesiodistally. Root has oval cross section.

Incisal edge wears on labial surface (Fig. 29-15). *Text continued on p. 317.*

Average permanent teeth dimensions as recorded by Dr. Russell C. Wheeler

	Length of crown	Length of root	Mesio-distal diameter of crown*	Mesio-distal diameter at cervix	Labio- or bucco-lingual diameter	Labio- or bucco-lingual diameter at cervix	Curvature of cervical line-mesial	Curvature of cervical line-distal
Maxillary teeth								
Central incisor	10.5	13.0	8.5	7.0	7.0	6.0	3.5	2.5
Lateral incisor	9.0	13.0	6.5	5.0	6.0	5.0	3.0	2.0
Canine	10.0	17.0	7.5	5.5	8.0	7.0	2.5	1.5
First premolar	8.5	14.0	7.0	5.0	9.0	8.0	1.0	0.0
Second pre-molar	8.5	14.0	7.0	5.0	9.0	8.0	1.0	0.0
First molar	7.5	b 1 12 13	10.0	8.0	11.0	10.0	1.0	0.0
Second molar	7.0	b 1 11 12	9.0	7.0	11.0	10.0	1.0	0.0
Third molar	6.5	11.0	8.5	6.5	10.0	9.5	1.0	0.0
Mandibular teeth								
Central incisor	9.0†	12.5	5.0	3.5	6.0	5.3	3.0	2.0
Lateral incisor	9.5†	14.0	5.5	4.0	6.5	5.8	3.0	2.0
Canine	11.0	16.0	7.0	5.5	7.5	7.0	2.5	1.0
First premolar	8.5	14.0	7.0	5.0	7.5	6.5	1.0	0.0
Second pre-molar	8.0	14.5	7.0	5.0	8.0	7.0	1.0	0.0
First molar	7.5	14.0	11.0	9.0	10.5	9.0	1.0	0.0
Second molar	7.0	13.0	10.5	8.0	10.0	9.0	1.0	0.0
Third molar	7.0	11.0	10.0	7.5	9.5	9.0	1.0	0.0

Wheeler, R.C.: A Textbook of dental anatomy and physiology, ed. 4, Philadelphia, 1965, W.B. Saunders Co.
*The sum of the mesiodistal diameters, both right and left, which gives the arch length, is maxillary 128 mm, mandibular 126 mm.
†Lingual measurement is approximately 0.5 mm longer.

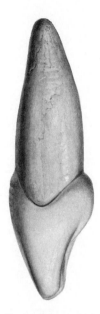

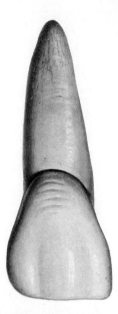

Fig. 29-1 Maxillary right central incisor, mesial view. (Zeisz and Nuckolls.)

Fig. 29-2 Maxillary right central incisor, labial view. (Zeisz and Nuckolls.)

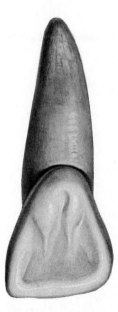

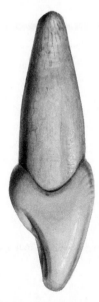

Fig. 29-3 Maxillary right central incisor, lingual view. (Zeisz and Nuckolls.)

Fig. 29-4 Maxillary right central incisor, distal view. (Zeisz and Nuckolls.)

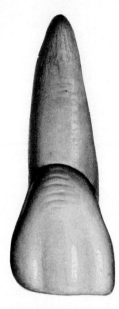

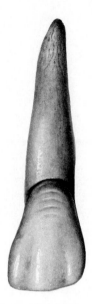

Fig. 29-5 Maxillary right central incisor, labial view. (Zeisz and Nuckolls.)

Fig. 29-6 Maxillary left lateral incisor, labial view. (Zeisz and Nuckolls.)

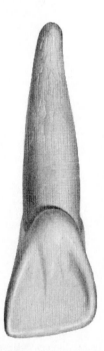

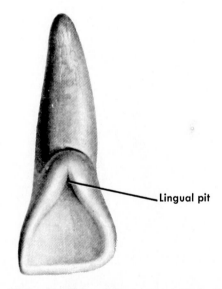

Lingual pit

Fig. 29-7 Maxillary right lateral incisor, lingual view. (Zeisz and Nuckolls.)

Fig. 29-8 Maxillary right lateral incisor, lingual view. (Zeisz and Nuckolls.)

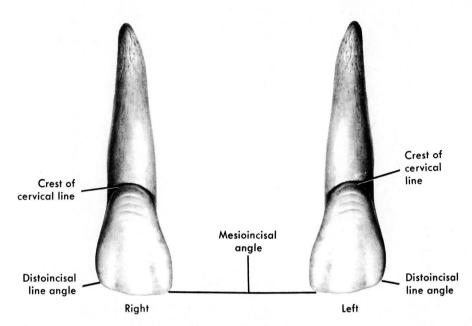

Crest of cervical line

Crest of cervical line

Mesioincisal angle

Distoincisal line angle

Distoincisal line angle

Right

Left

Fig. 29-9   Maxillary right lateral incisor. (Zeisz and Nuckolls.)

Fig. 29-10   Maxillary left lateral incisor. (Zeisz and Nuckolls.)

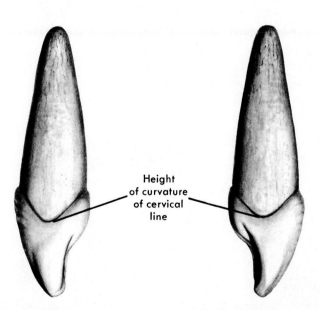

Height of curvature of cervical line

Fig. 29-11   Maxillary right lateral incisor, mesial view. (Zeisz and Nuckolls.)

Fig. 29-12   Maxillary right lateral incisor, distal view. (Zeisz and Nuckolls.)

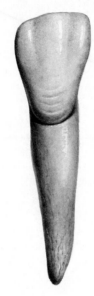

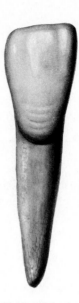

Fig. 29-13 Maxillary left lateral incisor. (Zeisz and Nuckolls.)

Fig. 29-14 Mandibular right lateral incisor. (Zeisz and Nuckolls.)

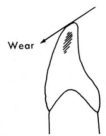

Wear

Fig. 29-15 Mandibular right lateral incisor, mesial view.

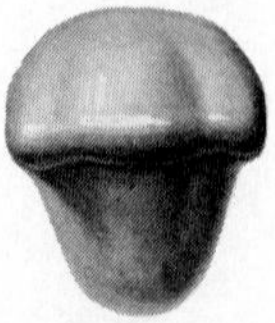

Fig. 29-16 Mandibular right central incisor, incisal view. (Zeisz and Nuckolls.)

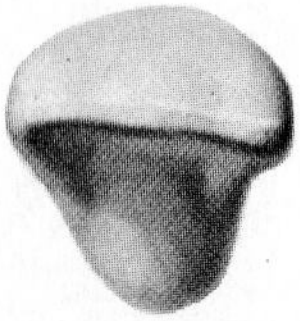

Fig. 29-17 Mandibular right lateral incisor, incisal view. (Zeisz and Nuckolls.)

Central

1. Incisal view—incisal edge perpendicular to faciolingual axis of tooth.
2. Mesial and distal lobes appear identical (Fig. 29-16).

Right-left

1. Cervical line curves more incisally on mesial than on distal surface.
2. Height of curvature of cervical line on mesial greater than on distal surface.
3. Root tip may have slight distal curve.
4. Incisal edge is worn wider on distal surface.

Lateral

1. Incisal view—distoincisal edge angled toward lingual side.
2. Distal lobe appears larger than mesial lobe (Fig. 29-17).

Right-left

1. Cervical line curves more incisally on mesial than on distal surface.

2. Incisal view—distal half of incisal edge rotated toward lingual side.
3. Incisal edge is worn wider and longer on distal surface.

CANINES

Single conical cusp with a well-developed mesiofacial lobe.

Lingual cusp ridge from cusp tip to lingual fossa.

Maxillary

Lingual surface has well-developed marginal ridges, cingulum, and fossa (Fig. 29-18).

Larger and bulkier crown than the incisors and lower canines.

More distal convexity (Fig. 29-19).

Cusp tip directly midcenter over root.

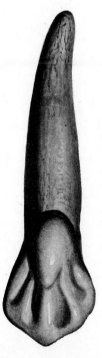

Fig. 29-18 Maxillary right canine, lingual view. (Zeisz and Nuckolls.)

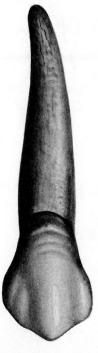

Fig. 29-19 Maxillary right canine, labial view. (Zeisz and Nuckolls.)

Right-left

1. Cervical line curves more incisally on mesial than on distal surface (Figs. 29-20 and 29-21).
2. Incisal view—distofacial lobe elongated, or "pulled out."
3. Facial view—distal surface more rounded, and contact area located more cervically.

Mandibular

Lingual surface is almost smooth and has poorly developed ridges, cingulum, and fossa (Fig. 29-22).

Smaller mesiodistal width than the maxillary.

More wear on facial (labial) surface (Fig. 29-23) when compared with the maxillary canine.

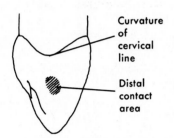

Fig. 29-20 Maxillary right canine, distal view.

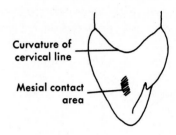

Fig. 29-21 Maxillary right canine, mesial view.

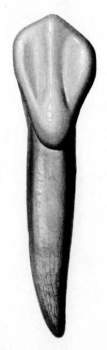

Fig. 29-22 Mandibular right canine, lingual view. (Zeisz and Nuckolls.)

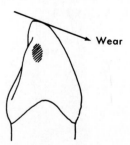

Fig. 29-23 Mandibular right canine, mesial view. (Zeisz and Nuckolls.)

PREMOLARS

At least two cusps, one a single facial cusp, with one or two lingual cusps.

Maxillary

higher occlusion

Two major cusps, one buccal and one lingual, approximately equal in size.

Distinctly wider faciolingually than mesiodistally.

Proximal view—facial and lingual cusps nearly same height and both located over root trunk (Fig. 29-24). *Buccal usually higher*

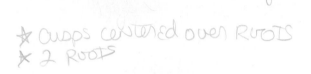

★ *Cusps centered over ROOTS*
★ *2 ROOTS*

First premolar

1. Facial cusp slightly longer than lingual cusp (Fig. 29-25).
2. Frequently has two roots, buccal and lingual.
3. Occlusal surface has well-developed central groove, with little supplemental grooving.
4. Mesial surface has depression above contact area starting below cervical line and usually extending onto root. *fluted*

Right-left

1. Mesial marginal groove. *continuation of*
2. Cervical line on mesial surface curves more occlusally than on distal surface.

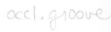

occl. groove

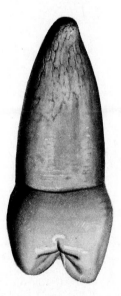

Fig. 29-24 Maxillary right second premolar, distal view. (Zeisz and Nuckolls.)

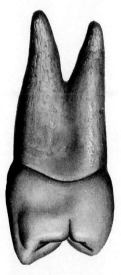

Fig. 29-25 Maxillary right first premolar, mesial view. (Zeisz and Nuckolls.)

3. Occlusal view—mesiofacial cusp ridge forms 90-degree angle with mesial marginal ridge; the distofacial cusp ridge forms a more rounded angle with distal marginal ridge (Fig. 29-26).

Second premolar

1. Facial and lingual cusps nearly same height *(slightly higher)* (Fig. 29-27).
2. Usually single rooted.
3. Central groove short, with frequent and numerous supplemental grooves.
4. No depression on mesial or distal crown surfaces. *(LESS)*

Right-left *Leans slightly mesially*

1. Lingual cusp displaced slightly toward mesial side (Fig. 29-28).

Mandibular

Prominent facial cusp with one or two much smaller lingual cusps. *usually on 2nd pre.*

Nearly equal faciolingual and mesiodistal widths.

Proximal view—facial cusp much larger. Facial cusp tip at or near midaxis of root. Lingual cusp(s) extend lingually past lingual border of root (Fig. 29-29).

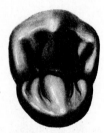

Fig. 29-26   Maxillary right first premolar, occlusal view. (Zeisz and Nuckolls.)

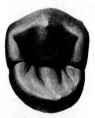

Fig. 29-28   Maxillary right second premolar, occlusal view. (Zeisz and Nuckolls.)

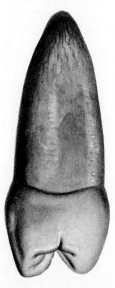

Fig. 29-27   Maxillary right second premolar, mesial view. (Zeisz and Nuckolls.)

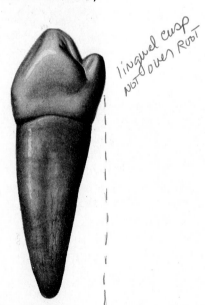

lingual cusp not over root

Fig. 29-29   Mandibular right first premolar, mesial view. (Zeisz and Nuckolls.)

First premolar

1. Occlusal view—oval outline with strong trans-verse ridge and no central pit (Fig. 29-30).
2. Proximal view—occlusal surface tilted strongly toward lingual side (Fig. 29-31). *1st pul,*

Right-left

1. Cervical line on mesial surface curves more occlusally than on distal surface.

mostly on 1st pul,

2. Frequently a depression or groove where mesial marginal ridge joins lingual cusp ridge (Fig. 29-32).
3. Distal marginal ridge more prominent.

Second premolar

1. Occlusal view—pentagonal outline, with a central pit and no transverse ridge (Fig. 29-33).

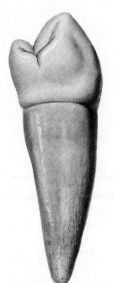

Fig. 29-30   Mandibular right first premolar, occlusal view. (Zeisz and Nuckolls.)

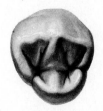

Fig. 29-31   Mandibular right first premolar, distal view. (Zeisz and Nuckolls.)

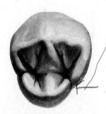

Fig. 29-32   Mandibular left first premolar, occlusal view. (Zeisz and Nuckolls.)

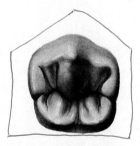

Fig. 29-33   Mandibular right second premolar, occlusal view. (Zeisz and Nuckolls.) *PENTAGONAL*

2. Proximal view—occlusal surface less tilted lingually (Fig. 29-34).
3. May have two lingual cusps. *more likely than 1st pre.*

Right-left

1. Proximal view—more of occlusal surface visible from distal than from mesial because of distal inclination of crown axis to root axis.

MOLARS

Three to five cusps, at least two facial.

Maxillary

Crowns wider faciolingually than mesiodistally. Three roots, two on facial and one on lingual side.

First molar

1. Occlusal view—strong **oblique ridge** less likely to be crossed by a groove (Fig. 29-35).
2. Three roots widely separated. *1 Ling. 2 Buccal*
3. Frequently has a fifth cusp (Carabelli's) on mesiolingual cusp (Fig. 29-36).

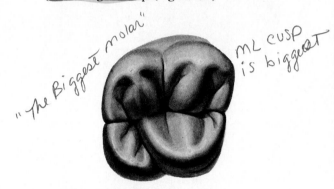

"The Biggest molar"

ML cusp is biggest

Fig. 29-35 Maxillary right first molar, occlusal view. (Zeisz and Nuckolls.)

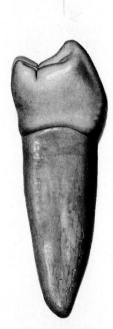

Fig. 29-34 Mandibular right second premolar, distal view. (Zeisz and Nuckolls.)

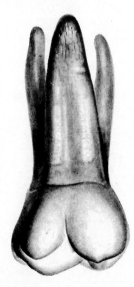

Fig. 29-36 Maxillary right first molar, lingual view. (Zeisz and Nuckolls.)

Right-left

1. Mesiolingual cusp always much larger than distolingual cusp.

Second molar

1. Occlusal view—smaller oblique ridge usually interrupted by a groove (Fig. 29-37).
2. Roots closer together (Fig. 29-38).
3. No fifth cusp.
4. Distolingual cusp smaller than on first molar.

Right-left

1. Mesiolingual cusp always much larger than distolingual cusp.

Third molar

1. Distolingual cusp progressively smaller or missing entirely (Fig. 29-39).
2. Roots either fused or very close together and much shorter.
3. No oblique ridge (Fig. 29-40).

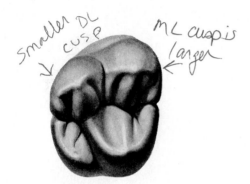

Smaller DL ↓ cusp   *ML cusp is larger ←*

Fig. 29-37   Maxillary right second molar, occlusal view. (Zeisz and Nuckolls.)

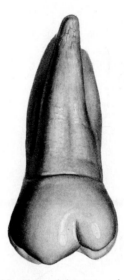

Fig. 29-38   Maxillary right second molar, lingual view. (Zeisz and Nuckolls.)

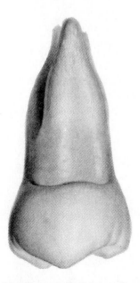

Fig. 29-39   Maxillary right third molar, lingual view. (Zeisz and Nuckolls.)

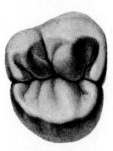

Fig. 29-40   Maxillary right third molar, occlusal view. (Zeisz and Nuckolls.)

Right-left
1. Distofacial cusp much shorter.
2. Roots curved distally.

Mandibular

Crowns wider mesiodistally than faciolingually. Two roots, one mesial and one distal.

First molar
1. Three facial cusps and two facial grooves (Fig. 29-41).
2. Roots widely separated and relatively vertical.

Right-left
1. Distal cusp smallest facial cusp (Fig. 29-42).

Second molar
1. Only two facial cusps and one facial groove (Fig. 29-43).
2. Occlusal groove well defined but travels straight mesial to distal, and forms a cross (+) with facial and lingual grooves (Fig. 29-44).
3. Roots close together.

Right-left
1. Buccal height of contour in cervical third; lin-

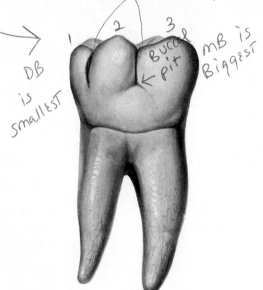

Handwritten annotations: DB is smallest; 1 2 3; Buccal pit; MB is Biggest

Fig. 29-41 Mandibular right first molar, buccal view. (Zeisz and Nuckolls.)

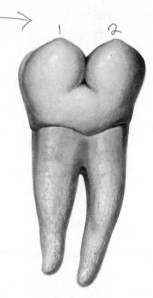

Handwritten annotations: 1 2

Fig. 29-43 Mandibular right second molar, buccal view. (Zeisz and Nuckolls.)

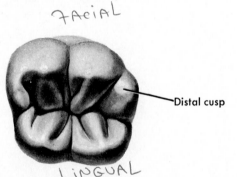

Handwritten annotations: FACIAL; LINGUAL

Distal cusp

Fig. 29-42 Mandibular right first molar, occlusal view. (Zeisz and Nuckolls.)

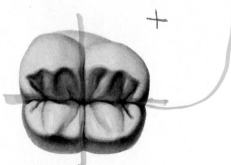

Handwritten annotation: +

Fig. 29-44 Mandibular right second molar, occlusal view. (Zeisz and Nuckolls.)

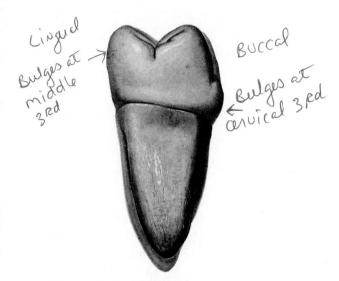

Lingual
Bulges at middle 3rd

Buccal
Bulges at cervical 3rd

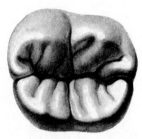

Fig. 29-45   Mandibular right second molar, distal view. (Zeisz and Nuckolls.)

Fig. 29-46   Mandibular right third molar, occlusal view. (Zeisz and Nuckolls.)

gual height of contour in middle third (Fig. 29-45).

Third molar
1. Secondary and tertiary anatomy (Fig. 29-46).
2. 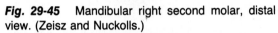Roots—short, often fused, and curved distally.

Right-left
1. Crown tapers distally so it is wider faciolingually on mesial than on distal surface. (This is also true of the mandibular first and second molars.)

30

Incisors

OBJECTIVES

- To identify the particular anatomical features of incisor teeth
- To compare maxillary central incisors with maxillary lateral incisors
- To compare maxillary incisors with their mandibular incisor counterparts
- To identify an extracted incisor
- To recognize the normal and the deviated anatomical forms of incisor teeth

There are eight permanent incisors, four maxillary (upper) and four mandibular (lower). The maxillary consist of two central and two lateral incisors, as do the mandibular group (Fig. 30-1).

Our discussion begins with a comparison of maxillary incisors, the shearing, or cutting, teeth. The maxillary central incisors are larger than the lateral incisors. These teeth complement each other in form and function. The central incisors erupt about the seventh to eighth year, the lateral incisors a year or so later.

Maxillary incisors

CENTRAL INCISORS

Evidence of calcification	3 months
Eruption	7-8 years
Root completed	10 years

The most prominent teeth in the mouth are the maxillary incisors. A maxillary central incisor (Fig. 30-2) is the widest mesiodistally of any of the anterior teeth. Its labial appearance is less rounded than that of a maxillary lateral incisor or canine.

The crown usually looks symmetrical and normally formed, having a nearly straight incisal edge, a mesial side with a straight outline, and the distal side more curved. The mesioincisal angle is relatively sharp and the distoincisal angle rounded.

Maxillary central incisors usually develop normally. Two anomalies that sometimes occur are a short root or an unusually long crown.

Labial Aspect (Figs. 30-3 and 30-8, A)

The labial surface of the crown is slightly convex, bulging out from the cervical portion of the crown. The enamel surface is very smooth. When the tooth first erupts, mamelons will be seen on the incisal ridge. These mamelons are rounded portions of the incisal ridge of newly erupted teeth. Each mamelon forms the incisal ridge portion of one of the labial primary lobes.

Developmental lines on the labial face divide the surface into three parts, each developmental line separating a primary lobe.

The distal outline of the crown is more rounded, or convex, than the mesial outline, the height of curvature being higher toward the cervical line. The cervical line crests slightly distal to the center of the tooth.

The incisal outline is usually regular and straight across the incisal ridge after the tooth has been in function long enough to wear down the mamelons. When an incisor first erupts, the incisal portion of the crown is rounded and the mamelons are quite distinct and clear. This ridge

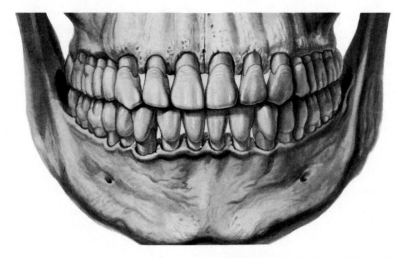

Fig. 30-1   Anterior view of lower portion of adult skull. (Zeisz and Nuckolls.)

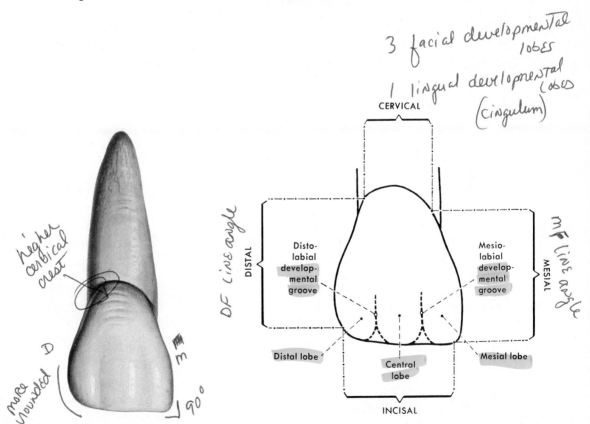

higher cervical crest

more rounded   D

m

90°

Fig. 30-2   Maxillary right central incisor. (Zeisz and Nuckolls.)

3 facial developmental lobes

1 lingual developmental lobes (cingulum)

CERVICAL

DF line angle

DISTAL

Disto-labial developmental groove

Mesio-labial developmental groove

mF line angle

MESIAL

Distal lobe

Central lobe

Mesial lobe

INCISAL

Fig. 30-3   Labial surface of maxillary right central incisor. (Zeisz and Nuckolls.)

portion is then called the incisal ridge. However, normal use eventually wears down the rounded ridge into a flat edge, and therefore the term "incisal edge" is more appropriate than "ridge."

The root of a central incisor from the labial aspect is cone shaped, in most instances with a blunt apex. The root is usually 2 to 3 mm longer than the crown, though the root-crown ratio varies considerably.

Lingual Aspect (Figs. 30-4 and 30-8, *B*)

The lingual outline of a maxillary central incisor is the reverse of that found on the labial or facial aspect. The facial surface of the crown is smooth, whereas the lingual surface is bordered by rounded convexities and a concavity. The outline of the cervical line is similar, but immediately below the cervical line is a smooth convexity, called the cingulum.

Mesially and distally confluent with the cingulum is a shallow concavity, called the lingual fossa. The marginal and incisal ridges, which are rounded convexities, border the lingual fossa. Usually there are developmental grooves extending from the cingulum into the lingual fossa.

The crown and root taper lingually. The lingual portion of the root is narrower than the labial portion.

Mesial Aspect (Figs. 30-5 and 30-8, *D*)

The crown is triangular, with the base of the triangle at the cervix and the apex at the incisal ridge.

The incisal ridge of the crown is centered over the middle of the root. This alignment is *characteristic* of maxillary central and lateral incisors.

The labial outline of the crown from the crest of curvature to the incisal edge is very slightly convex, with the height of curvature about one third of the way down from the cervical line.

The cervical curvature is greater on the mesial surface of these teeth than on any surface of *any other* teeth in the mouth.

From the mesial aspect the root of a maxillary central incisor is cone shaped, with apex blunted.

Distal Aspect (Figs. 30-6 and 30-8, *E*)

There is a little difference between the distal and mesial outlines of these teeth. The curvature of the cervical line indicating the cementoenamel junction is less on the distal than on the mesial surface. It is generally true that if there is a difference in the curvatures of the mesial and distal cervical lines of the same tooth, the mesial curvature will be greater. If mesial curvature is 2.5 mm, the distal might be 1.5 mm.

Incisal Aspect (Figs. 30-7 and 30-8, *C*)

The incisal ridge may be seen clearly, sloping lingually. The crown shows a triangular shape, with its apex on the lingual surface.

LATERAL INCISORS

Evidence of calcification	1 year
Eruption	8-9 years
Root completed	11 years

Maxillary lateral incisors complement the central incisors in function and resemble each other in form. Lateral incisors are small in all dimensions except root length. The features—curvatures, concavities, and convexities—of the lateral incisors are more prominent and show more distinction and contrast than those of the central incisors. These teeth differ from the central incisors in that their individual development may vary considerably. Maxillary lateral incisors vary in form more than any other teeth in the mouth except the third molars. If the variation is too great, it is considered a developmental anomaly. A not uncommon situation is to find maxillary lateral incisors that have a nondescript, pointed form; such teeth are called **peg-shaped** lateral incisors. In some persons the lateral incisors are missing entirely.

One type of malformed maxillary lateral incisor displays a large, pointed tubercle as part of the cingulum; some have deep developmental grooves that extend down the root lingually with a deep fold in the cingulum. Other maxillary lateral incisors show twisted roots or distorted crowns.

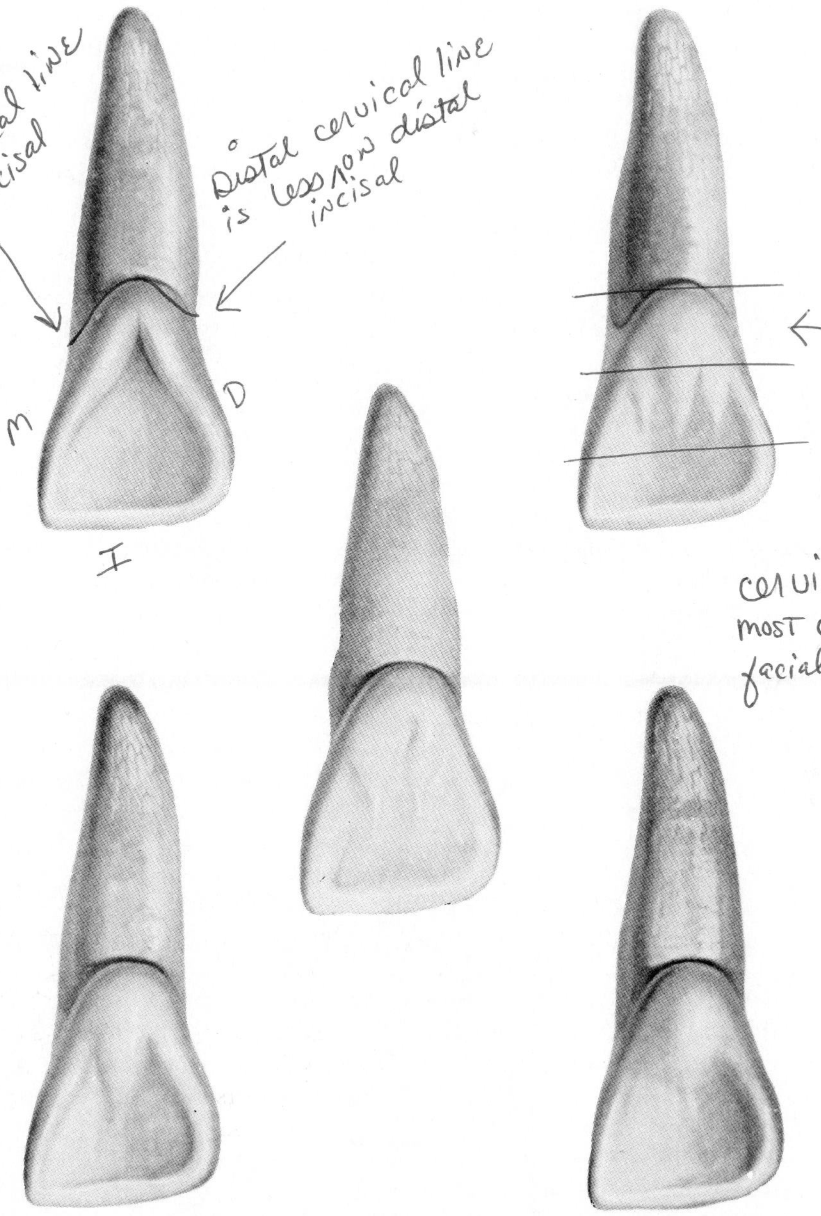

infrequently deformed

root of central is same size of lateral

root is triangular △

mesial cervical line is more incisal

Distal cervical line is less on distal incisal

M

D

I

cervical ⅓ has most curvature faciolingually

Fig. 30-4   Lingual views of five maxillary central incisors. (Zeisz and Nuckolls.)

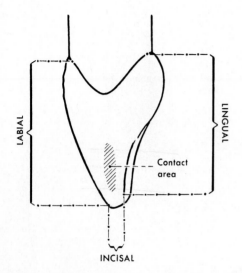

Fig. 30-5 Mesial surface of maxillary right central incisor. (Zeisz and Nuckolls.)

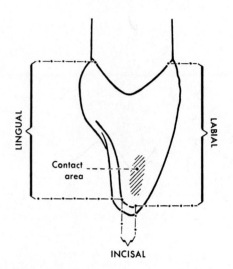

Fig. 30-6 Distal surface of maxillary right central incisor. (Zeisz and Nuckolls.)

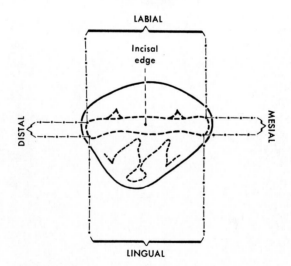

Fig. 30-7 Incisal edge of maxillary right central incisor. (Zeisz and Nuckolls.)

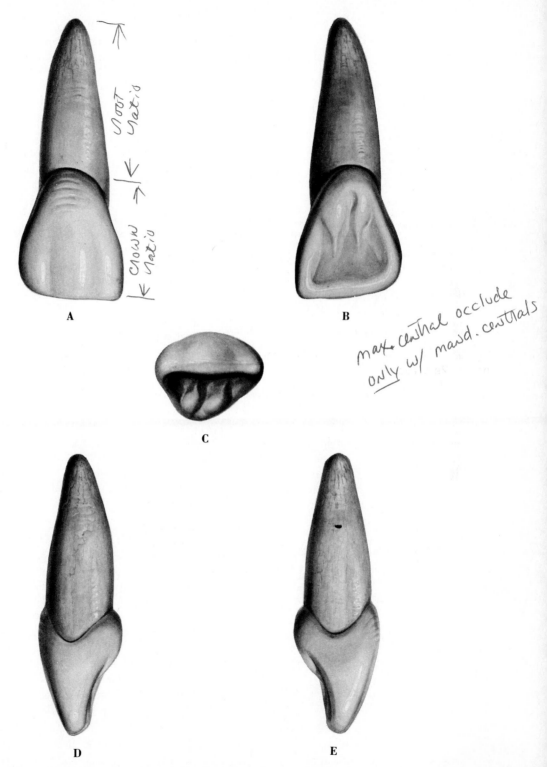

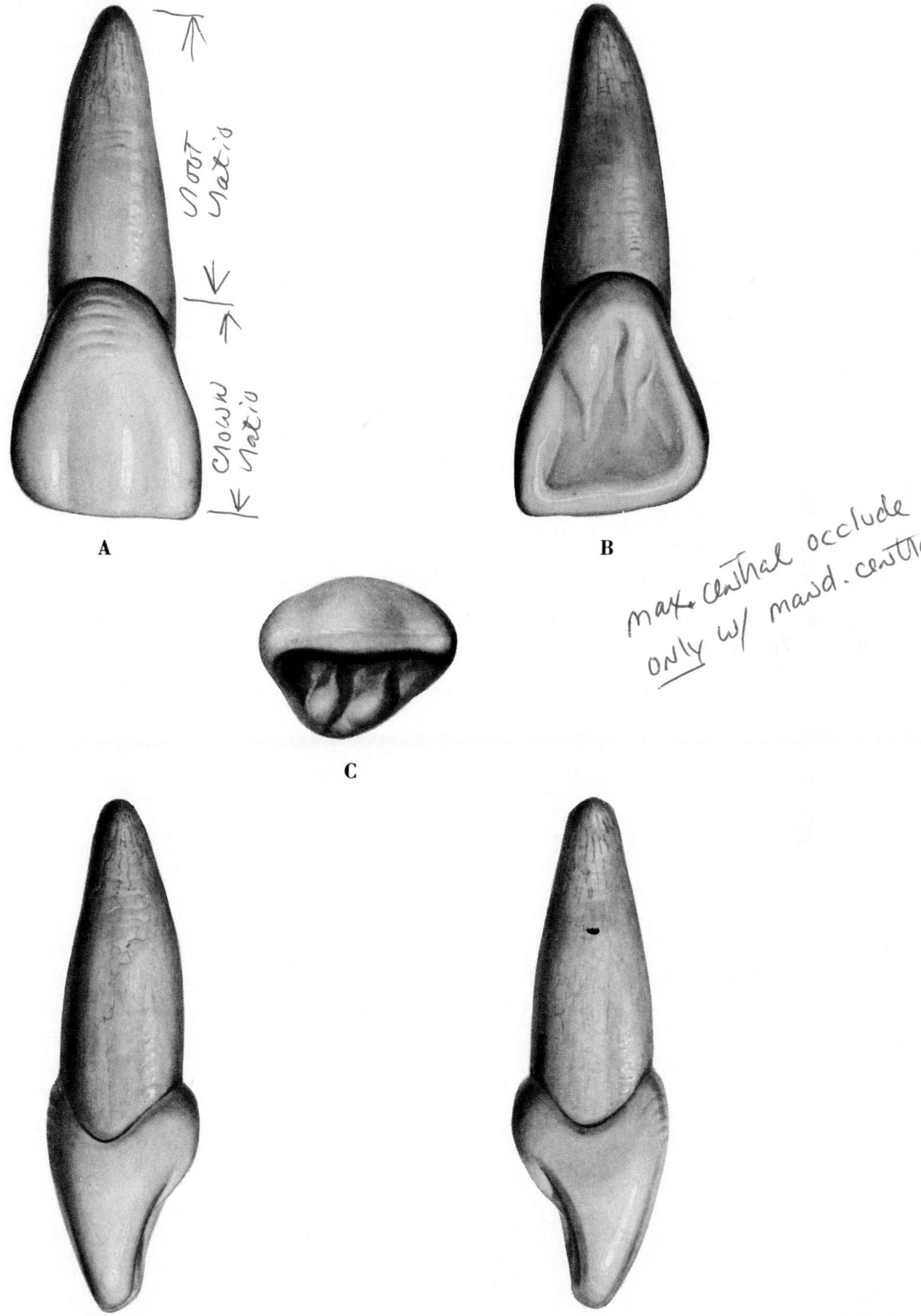
root ratio
crown ratio
A
B
max. central occlude only w/ mand. centrals
C
D
E

Fig. 30-8 Maxillary right central incisor. **A,** Labial view. **B,** Lingual view. **C,** Incisal view. **D,** Mesial view. **E,** Distal view. (Zeisz and Nuckolls.)

Labial Aspect (Fig. 30-9, *A*)

Although the labial aspect of a maxillary lateral incisor may appear to resemble that of a central incisor, it usually has more curvature, with rounded incisal ridge and angles mesially and distally.

The distal outline is always more rounded and the height of contour more cervical, usually in the center of the middle third.

The labial surface of the crown is more convex than that of a central incisor.

As a rule, the root length is greater in proportion to the crown length than that of a central incisor. The root is often about one and one-half times the length of the crown.

Lingual Aspect (Fig. 30-9, *B*)

The lingual view of a lateral incisor shows more contrast than does the central. Mesial and distal marginal ridges are pronounced and the cingulum is usually prominent, with a tendency toward deep developmental grooves within the lingual fossa, where it joins the cingulum. The linguoincisal ridge is better developed, and the lingual fossa is more concave and circumscribed than that of the central incisor.

Mesial Aspect (Fig. 30-9, *D*)

The mesial aspect of a maxillary lateral incisor is similar to that of a small central incisor, except the root appears longer.

Distal Aspect (Fig. 30-9, *E*)

The distal aspect of the maxillary lateral incisor is the same as the mesial aspect except for less curvature of the cervical line.

Incisal Aspect (Fig. 30-9, *C*)

The incisal aspect of these teeth sometimes resembles that of the central incisors, or it may resemble that of a small canine. The cingulum and the incisal ridge, however, may be large; the labiolingual dimension may be greater than usual in comparison with the mesiodistal dimension. If these variations are present, the teeth show a strong resemblance to the canines.

All maxillary lateral incisors exhibit more convexity labially and lingually from the incisal aspect than do the maxillary central incisors.

ROOT

The maxillary central incisor usually has a straight, thick, cylindrically shaped root. The maxillary lateral incisor has a narrower root mesiodistally. The root is as long as that of the central incisor but appears thinner. The apical portion of the lateral incisor's root often curves distally, and ends in a sharp apex, rather than a blunt, straight one as in the central incisor.

Neither maxillary central nor lateral shows evidence of a division, bifurcation, indentation, or proximal groove.

PULP CAVITY

The pulp cavity varies in size with the age of the tooth. When the tooth first erupts, it is very large and the root is incompletely formed, so the canal becomes somewhat funnel shaped in the region of the apical foramen. As the tooth develops completely, the entire pulp cavity to the apex of the root becomes smaller and the dentin becomes thicker in both crown and root. The apical foramen is then very small. This process continues throughout the life of the tooth. It is not unusual to find in very elderly persons that the entire pulp cavity has become calcified and there is solid dentin filling the entire root canal. This variation in the size of the pulp cavity with aging is common to all of the permanent teeth.

The pulp cavity of the maxillary central incisor (Fig. 30-10) mirrors the configuration of the tooth. There is only one root canal, which is rather large. The pulp chamber lies in the coronal portion of the tooth and presents three sharp elongations, the mesial, distal, and central pulp horns. The central is usually shorter than the other two and more rounded.

The pulp cavity of the maxillary lateral incisor is quite simple, consisting of a pulp chamber and a single pulp canal. The chamber is quite similar

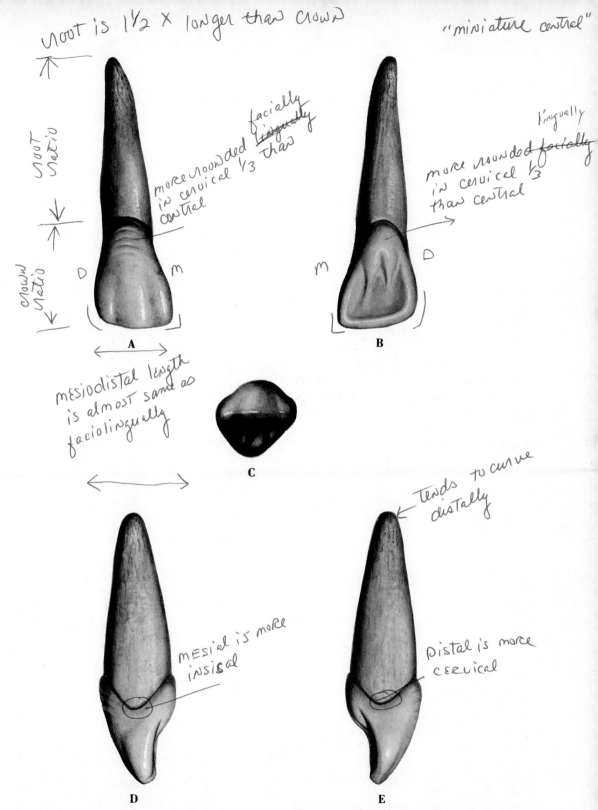

root is 1½ × longer than crown

"miniature central"

root ratio

crown ratio

more rounded facially ~~lingually~~ in cervical ⅓ than central

lingually

more rounded ~~facially~~ in cervical ⅓ than central

mesiodistal length is almost same as faciolingually

Tends to curve distally

mesial is more insisal

Distal is more cervical

Fig. 30-9   Maxillary right lateral incisor. **A,** Labial view. **B,** Lingual view. **C,** Incisal view. **D,** Mesial view. **E,** Distal view. (Zeisz and Nuckolls.)

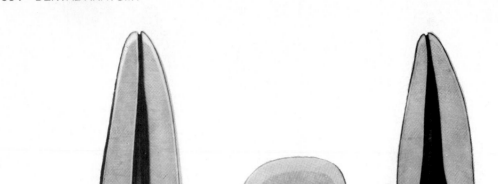

3 pulp horns always

Fig. 30-10 Pulp cavity of maxillary right central incisor. **A,** Distomesial section, lingual view. **B,** Cross section, incisal view. **C,** Linguolabial section, mesial view. (Zeisz and Nuckolls.)

to that of the maxillary central incisor, but the lateral usually does not have three sharp pulp horns. More often the pulp chamber ends incisally as one rounded form or two less sharp pulp horns, a mesial and distal (Fig. 30-11).

PERTINENT DATA
Maxillary Central Incisors

	Right	Left
Universal Code	8	9
International Code	11	21
Palmer notation	1⌋	⌊1
Number of roots	1	
Number of pulp horns	3	
Number of developmental lobes	4	

Location of proximal contact areas
MESIAL: Incisal third
DISTAL: Junction of incisal and middle thirds

Height of contour
FACIAL: Cervical third, 0.5 mm
LINGUAL: Cervical third, 0.5 mm

Identifying characteristics
These incisors are the largest and most prominent incisors. The distoincisal is more rounded than the mesioincisal angle. The lingual surface has a prominent cingulum, broad lingual fossa, and distinct marginal ridges. The pulp cavity is one large single chamber and root canal.

Maxillary Lateral Incisors

	Right	Left
Universal Code	7	10
International Code	12	22
Palmer notation	2⌋	⌊2
Number of roots	1	
Number of pulp horns	1 to 3	
Number of developmental lobes	4	

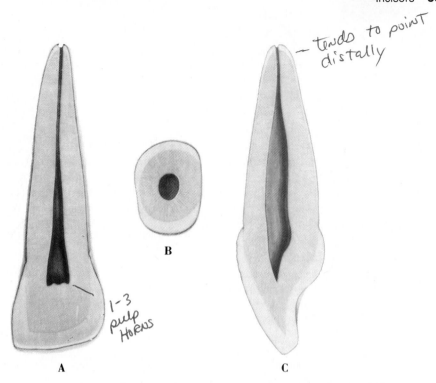

— tends to point distally

1-3 pulp HORNS

Fig. 30-11 Pulp cavity of maxillary right lateral incisor. **A,** Distomesial section, lingual view. **B,** Cross section, incisal view. **C,** Linguolabial section, mesial view. (Zeisz and Nuckolls.)

Location of proximal contact areas
MESIAL: Junction of incisal and middle thirds
DISTAL: Middle third
Height of contour
FACIAL: Cervical third, 0.5 mm
LINGUAL: Cervical third, 0.5 mm
Identifying characteristics
The lingual anatomical features are similar to those of the central incisors but are more highly developed and have more prominent marginal ridges and deeper lingual fossae. Lateral incisors are more likely to have a lingual pit. The cingulum may be smaller, almost absent. The labial surface resembles that of a central incisor except that the labial surface is more convex. The crown-root ratio is less than in a central incisor because the crown is usually smaller, whereas the root is almost as long. In all other ways the lateral incisors appear as smaller, more rounded versions of the central incisors.

Mandibular incisors
CENTRAL INCISORS

Evidence of calcification	3 months
Eruption	6-7 years
Root completed	9 years

The smallest teeth in the mouth are the mandibular central incisors—smaller than the mandibular lateral incisors. How does this differ from the maxillary teeth? Which are the larger, the maxillary central or lateral incisors?

A mandibular central incisor occludes only with one opposing tooth, a maxillary central incisor (Fig. 30-1).

Similar to other anterior teeth, a mandibular

central incisor is derived from four lobes, three labial and one lingual. When mandibular incisors erupt, mamelons can be seen on the incisal ridges.

Of all the teeth, mandibular central incisors are the most difficult to identify as either right or left. They are bilaterally symmetrical and very difficult to differentiate. The following features will not always be obvious, but, if present, they may support a good guess.

1. The distoincisal angle is just slightly greater than the mesioincisal.
2. The distofacial line angle is more rounded than the mesiofacial (Fig. 30-12).
3. The cervical line crests slightly toward the distal side (Fig. 30-13).
4. A straight line drawn between the end points of the distofacial line angle *(y)* to the end points of the mesiofacial line angle *(x)* is shorter (Fig. 30-14).

Labial Aspect (Figs. 30-15 and 30-19, *A*)

The labial aspect exhibits a very smooth facial surface. The gingivoincisal outline is almost straight up and down. On both the mesial and distal surfaces the height of contour is at the incisal third.

Lingual Aspect (Figs. 30-16 and 30-19, *B*)

The lingual view presents a cingulum much smaller than that of the maxillary anteriors. There are no tubercle extensions or lingual pits, and the fossa is very shallow.

Mesial and Distal Aspects (Figs. 30-17 and 30-19, *D* and *E*)

The proximal views reveal that the incisal edge tends toward the lingual half of the tooth and slants labially from this edge.

The height of contour at the cervical third is about 0.5 mm on the labial and lingual surfaces.

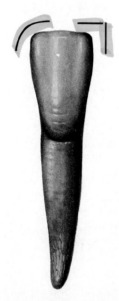

Fig. 30-12 Distofacial line angle of mandibular-right central incisor is more convex than mesiofacial line angle. (Zeisz and Nuckolls.)

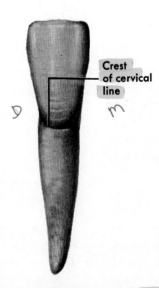

Crest of cervical line

Fig. 30-13 Cervical line of mandibular right central incisor has its crest slightly toward distal surface. (Zeisz and Nuckolls.)

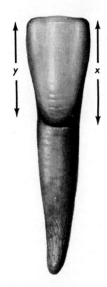

Fig. 30-14   Line *x* is longer than line *y*. (Zeisz and Nuckolls.)

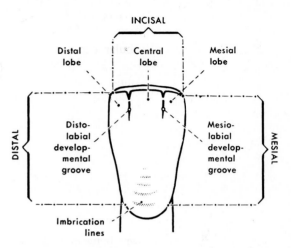

Fig. 30-15   Labial surface of mandibular right central incisor. (Zeisz and Nuckolls.)

3 labial lobe
1. lingual lobe

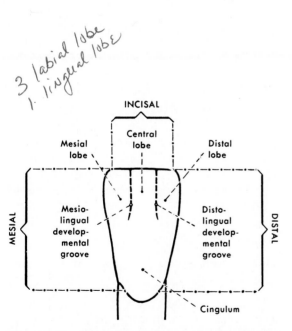

Fig. 30-16   Lingual surface of mandibular right central incisor. Notice that there are no pits or tubercles. (Zeisz and Nuckolls.)

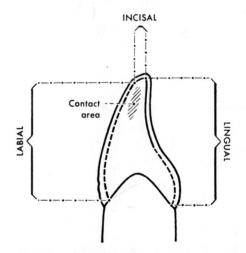

Fig. 30-17   Mesial surface of mandibular right central incisor. (Zeisz and Nuckolls.)

Is the cervical curvature greater mesially or distally? There is not always a difference between the amount of cervical curvature on the mesial and distal sides, but if there is a difference, the mesial will show more curvature.

Incisal Aspect (Figs. 30-18 and 30-19, *C*)

The incisal view shows wear on the incisal ridge. Notice that incisal wear occurs toward the facial aspect. In what way do the maxillary central incisors wear?

When the upper teeth touch the lower teeth, the lower incisors touch the lingual surface of the upper incisors. Therefore the upper incisors wear down the lingual part of their incisal ridges, and the lower incisors wear down the labial portion of their incisal ridges.

LATERAL INCISORS

Evidence of calcification	4 months
Eruption	7-8 years
Root completed	10 years

The mandibular lateral incisors appear to have nearly the same form as the mandibular central

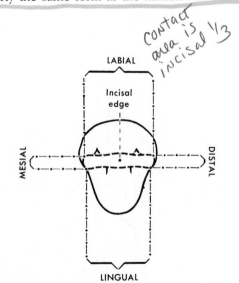

Contact area is incisal 1/3

Fig. 30-18 Incisal surface of mandibular right central incisor. (Zeisz and Nuckolls.)

incisors. Indeed, it is very difficult to tell them apart.

In general, the following principles help differentiate between the mandibular lateral and the mandibular central incisors in the same mouth. Mandibular lateral incisors are bigger, wider, and longer than the mandibular centrals. This situation is different from that of the maxillary incisors. The laterals are wider because their distal developmental lobe is larger than the distal lobe of mandibular centrals. Lateral incisors have more prominent anatomical features on the lingual aspect than the central incisors have. In mandibular teeth the difference is not so extreme as in the maxillary. But the lateral incisors are still slightly more convex and concave than their counterparts, the central incisors, in the *same* mouth.

The laterals have greater facial curvature than the central incisors have. The end points of the mesiofacial line angle are longer than those of the distofacial line angle (Fig. 30-20).

Compared with the central incisors, the lateral incisors are larger versions of the same thing but are wider mesiodistally and longer gingivoincisally.

Labial Aspect (Figs. 30-21 and 30-25, *A*)

The facial view shows a more rounded appearance mesially and distally. The developmental grooves on the labial surface are all deeper on the lateral incisors as compared with the central incisors. The height of contour at the contact areas is at the incisal third on the mesial and distal aspects. The distal contact area is slightly more gingival than mesial. As a general rule, this is usually true of all teeth.

Lingual Aspect (Figs. 30-22 and 30-25, *B*)

When compared with the central incisors, the lingual view shows more prominent features. The ridges are more developed, the fossa appears, and often enamel tubercles extend into the fossa. A lingual pit is also more often, but still rarely, present.

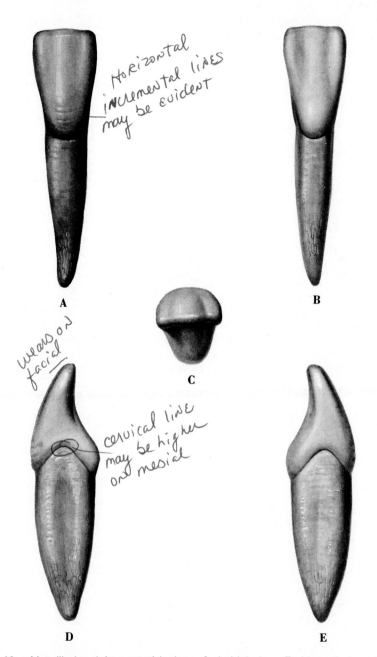

Horizontal incremental lines may be evident

wears on facial

cervical line may be higher on mesial

Fig. 30-19   Mandibular right central incisor. **A,** Labial view. **B,** Lingual view. **C,** Incisal view. **D,** Mesial view. **E,** Distal view. (Zeisz and Nuckolls.)

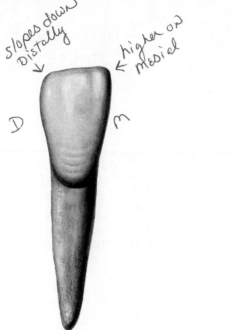

slopes down Distally ↓

← higher on Mesial

D   M

Fig. 30-20   Distal lobe of mandibular right lateral incisor is larger than distal lobe of central incisor. (Zeisz and Nuckolls.)

INCISAL

Distal lobe

Central lobe

Mesial lobe

DISTAL

Disto-labial develop-mental groove

Mesio-labial develop-mental groove

MESIAL

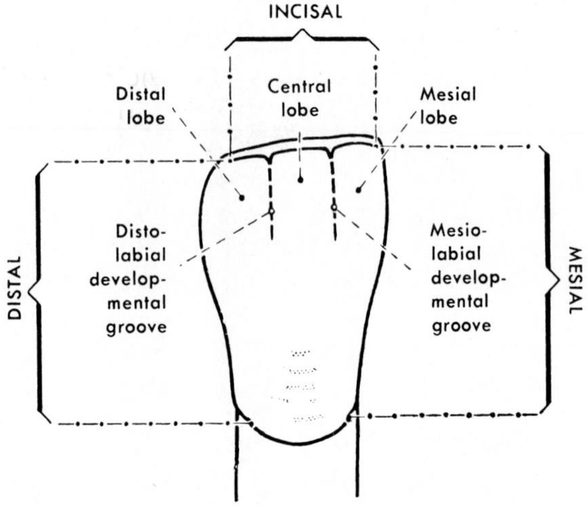

Fig. 30-21   Labial surface of mandibular right lateral incisor. (Zeisz and Nuckolls.)

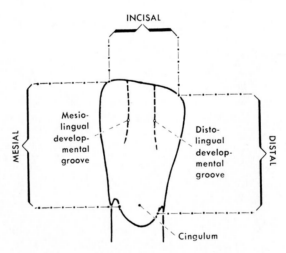

INCISAL

MESIAL

Mesio-lingual develop-mental groove

Disto-lingual develop-mental groove

DISTAL

Cingulum

Fig. 30-22   Lingual surface of mandibular right lateral incisor. (Zeisz and Nuckolls.)

There is much more deviation in the form of a lateral incisor. All features are usually more prominent if present.

Mesial and Distal Aspects (Figs. 30-23 and 30-25, *D* and *E*)

The proximal views reveal that the height of contour on the labial and lingual surfaces is at the gingival third. Notice that a lateral incisor is thicker than a central at the linguoincisal ridge.

A lateral incisor is narrower labiolingually, thus making an already thicker linguoincisal ridge appear much thicker in comparison. Once again the cervical curvature is greater on the mesial than on the distal side. This is generally true for all teeth.

Incisal Aspect (Figs. 30-24 and 30-25, *C*)

The incisal view depicts a more rounded general appearance for the lateral incisors, and the developmental grooves appear deeper.

The lateral incisors appear to be rotated on their root axis because the distal developmental lobe of the mandibular lateral incisors is larger and located more lingually than its mesial lobe.

The reason for this extra bulk and lingual location is that the laterals have to curve distally to fit into the mandibular arch. Remember that the mandibular arch curves more than the maxillary because it has to fit inside the maxillary arch.

ROOT

The root of the mandibular incisor is usually straight. The root of the lateral incisor is slightly wider, thicker, and longer than that of the central incisor. The apex of the lateral incisor's root may point toward the labial or distal. Proximal grooves are commonly found on the root surface, giving the appearance of a double root (Fig. 30-25.)

PULP CAVITY

The pulp cavities of the mandibular central and lateral incisors are simple. They usually have three pulp horns and a single root canal.

The root canals of all four mandibular incisors are similar to their maxillary counterparts. They are straight and narrow and present very little

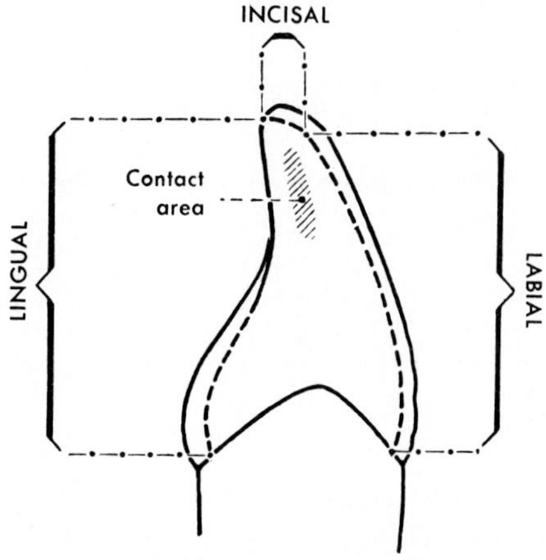

Fig. 30-23   Distal surface of mandibular right lateral incisor. (Zeisz and Nuckolls.)

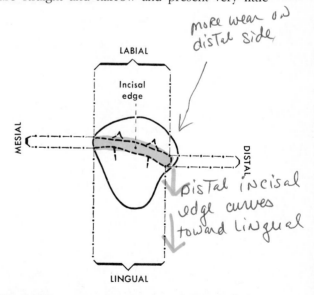

more wear on distal side

Distal incisal edge curves toward lingual

Fig. 30-24   Incisal surface of mandibular right lateral incisor. (Zeisz and Nuckolls.)

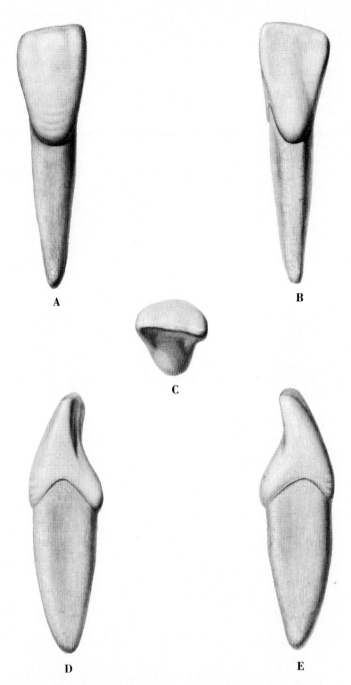

Fig. 30-25 Mandibular right lateral incisor. **A,** Labial view. **B,** Lingual view. **C,** Incisal view. **D,** Mesial view. **E,** Distal view. (Zeisz and Nuckolls.)

variation. The mandibular lateral pulp canal is larger and may show more variation than the central. It is a rare occurrence for either to have two root canals (Fig. 30-26.)

PERTINENT DATA

Mandibular Central Incisors

	Right	Left
Universal Code	25	24
International Code	41	31
Palmer notation	1⌋	⌊1
Number of roots	1	
Number of pulp horns	3	
Number of developmental lobes	4	

Location of proximal contact areas
MESIAL: Incisal third
DISTAL: Incisal third
Height of contour
FACIAL: Cervical third, less than 0.5 mm
LINGUAL: Cervical third, less than 0.5 mm
Identifying characteristics

The distoincisal and mesioincisal angles are nearly identical. The lingual surface is shallow, with no prominent features. The crown is wider faciolingually than mesiodistally. The root is oval shaped in cross section. The incisal edge shows wear on the facioincisal edge. From a proximal view the incisal edge appears to be tilted toward the lingual side.

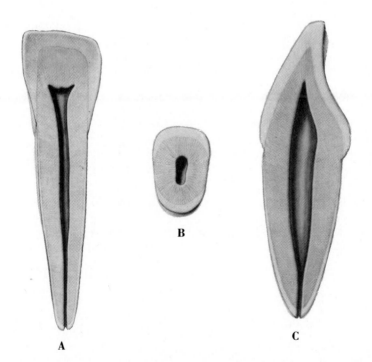

A

B

C

Fig. 30-26   Pulp cavity of mandibular right lateral incisor. **A,** Mesiodistal section, lingual view. **B,** Cross section, incisal view. **C,** Labiolingual section, mesial view. (Zeisz and Nuckolls.)

Mandibular Lateral Incisors

	Right	Left
Universal Code	26	23
International Code	42	32
Palmer notation	2⌐	⌐2
Number of roots	1	
Number of pulp horns	3	
Number of developmental lobes	4	

Location of proximal contact areas
MESIAL: Incisal third
DISTAL: Incisal third
Height of contour
FACIAL: Cervical third, less than 0.5 mm
LINGUAL: Cervical third, less than 0.5 mm
Identifying characteristics
The crown is similar to that of the mandibular central incisors. The distal lobe is more highly developed than the mesial. The distal incisal ridge angles toward the lingual as if rotating on the root axis. The crown and the root are slightly larger than those of the central incisors.

REVIEW QUESTIONS

1. A permanent maxillary central incisor, as compared with a maxillary lateral incisor in a proximal view, is
   a. thicker at the incisal edge.
   b. identical at the incisal edge.
   c. thinner at the incisal edge.
   d. similar but smaller overall.
2. Which one of the following is not characteristic of the maxillary central incisors?
   a. distal line angle that is shorter in the facial view
   b. more rounded distoincisal angle
   c. mesial line angle that is more nearly straight
   d. more rounded mesioincisal line angle
3. With normal wear, the incisal edge of the maxillary incisors
   a. slopes upward toward the facial side.
   b. flattens.
   c. slopes upward toward the lingual side.
   d. becomes more rounded.
4. The mesiofacial line angle of the maxillary central incisors differs from the distal in that it is
   a. less rounded.
   b. longer.
   c. sharper.
   d. all of the above.
5. In contrast to the maxillary lateral incisors, the maxillary central incisors usually have how many pulp horns?
   a. 1
   b. 2
   c. 3
   d. 4
6. Which of the following anatomical features of the mandibular incisors provide evidence of the four developmental lobes of these teeth?
   a. mamelons and faint developmental lines at eruption
   b. lingual pit, marginal ridges, and incisal edge
   c. mamelons, faint developmental lines at eruption, and cingulum
   d. incisal edge and lingual concavity
7. The proximal contact area on the distal surface of a mandibular lateral incisor is located incisocervically
   a. in the incisal third.
   b. at the junction of the incisal and middle thirds.
   c. just cervical to the junction of the incisal and middle thirds.
   d. in the middle third.
8. The structure of the mandibular lateral incisors, when compared with the mandibular centrals, is
   a. identical but larger.
   b. almost identical but smaller.
   c. almost identical but larger.
   d. the same.
9. The mesiodistal crown width of the maxillary lateral incisors, when compared with the central incisors, is
   a. greater.
   b. smaller.

c. about equal.

d. sometimes smaller but more often greater.

10. The distofacial line angle of maxillary lateral incisors, when compared with the maxillary central incisors, is

   a. the same.

   b. more rounded.

   c. less rounded.

   d. very straight.

11. Which is the more acute incisal angle on the maxillary central incisors?

   a. facial

   b. mesial

   c. distal

   d. lingual

12. In contrast to a mandibular incisor, a maxillary incisor can be identified by which of these?

   a. its rotated incisal edge

   b. central location of its cingulum

   c. prominent longitudinal grooves on the root

   d. prominent lingual features of the crown

13. Where does the height of contour of the facial and lingual surfaces of the anterior teeth occur?

   a. mesial third

   b. incisal third

   c. middle third

   d. cervical third

14. Which anterior teeth have the most prominent and widest crowns in the permanent dentition?

   a. maxillary canines

   b. mandibular lateral incisors

   c. mandibular canines

   d. maxillary central incisors

15. A more prominent cingulum is found on which tooth?

   a. maxillary central

   b. mandibular central

   c. mandibular lateral

   d. maxillary lateral

31

Canines

The four maxillary and mandibular permanent canines, one on each side of each jaw, are the longest teeth in the mouth. Located at the corners of the mouth, they are well anchored in the bone by their extremely long roots. Their location in this area requires extra anchorage, which is furnished by the length and the shape of their roots, as well as a special projection of bone called the **canine eminence.** The term "canine" recalls the fanglike teeth of our canine friends, the dogs, and it is from the animal family Canidae that they derive their name, canines.

In function the canines act as holding and tearing tools and assist both the incisors and premolars. In addition, their V shape at the corner of the mouth allows for dissipation of pressures that can force the premolars to protrude out of the mouth or the incisors back into the mouth. The self-cleaning qualities of the canines, their smooth, pointed shape, the thickness of their crowns, and their anchorage by an extremely long root embedded in a heavy bony eminence make the canines the most stable teeth in the mouth.

MAXILLARY CANINES

Evidence of calcification	4 months
Enamel completed	6-7 years
Eruption	11-12 years
Root completed	13-15 years

A maxillary canine resembles an incisor in its composition of four developmental lobes, three facial and one lingual. The three facial lobes resemble the incisors, except that the middle facial lobe extends further incisally when the tooth is viewed from the labial or lingual aspect. This middle lobe extension results in the formation of a single cusp. The cusp tip is formed by the junction of four ridges. One of the ridges extends along the middle lobe of the tooth on its most facial part; another extends along the lingual part. The other two ridges run from the mesioincisal corner of the tooth to the cusp and from the distoincisal corner to the cusp tip. All four ridges converge to form the cusp tip.

The lingual lobe of a canine is much larger and thicker than the lingual lobe of an incisor. This results in a canine being a much wider tooth labiolingually than a maxillary incisor is. The cingulum of a maxillary canine shows greater development in that it is larger and bulkier than on any of the other anterior teeth.

Labial Aspect (Figs. 31-1 and 31-6, *A*)

The crown and root are more narrow mesiodistally than those of a maxillary central incisor. The cervicoincisal length of the crown is much larger on a maxillary canine than any other anterior tooth, except the maxillary central incisor and the mandibular canine. Each of these sometimes has a longer crown than a maxillary canine has, but the roots of the maxillary canines are longer and thus make them the longest teeth in the mouth.

Mesially the outline of the crown is straighter, with a slight convexity at the contact area. The center of the mesial contact area is approximately at the junction of the middle and incisal thirds of the crown.

Distally the outline of the crown is more rounded in appearance. The reason is that the distal contact area is usually at the center of the middle third of the crown. This position makes the distal convexity appear larger and more uniform. How does this differ from the location of the mesial contact area? Which contact area is located more incisally, the mesial or the distal?

The labial surface of the crown is smooth. The developmental lines are two shallow depressions dividing the three labial lobes. The middle lobe is much larger and has greater development than the other lobes, resulting in a ridge on the labial surface of the crown. This ridge ends incisally at the cusp tip, which is centered in the middle of the tooth.

The cervical line crests slightly mesial to the center of the tooth.

The root of a maxillary canine is more slender in comparison with the crown and is conical in shape, with a blunt root apex. It is not uncommon for the root to turn sharply to the distal or mesial side in the apical third. A general rule is that most roots, if they do have an apical curvature, will point toward the distal side. Although this rule applies to almost all single-rooted teeth, it is not uncommon to find exceptions. If an apical curvature is not present, the root itself will have a tendency to point more often toward the distal than to the mesial side.

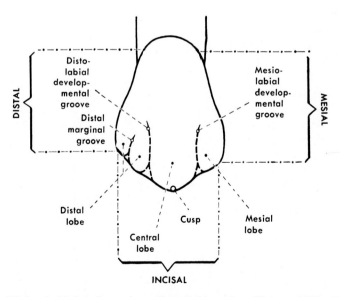

Fig. 31-1 Labial surface of maxillary right canine. (Zeisz and Nuckolls.)

Lingual Aspect (Figs. 31-2 and 31-6, *B*)

The root of a maxillary canine tapers toward the lingual surface. The lingual sides of both the crown and root are narrower than the labial.

The cervical line shows a more even curvature, and the crest is straighter and centered over the middle of the tooth.

The most obvious structure on the lingual surface of a maxillary canine is the well-developed cingulum. It is huge in comparison with those of all the other anterior teeth.

Confluent to the cingulum and running from the cusp tip is a well-developed lingual ridge. This ridge runs from the cusp tip on the lingual side to the cingulum. Unlike other anterior teeth that have a lingual fossa, this area on a maxillary canine is occupied by the lingual ridge. This ridge divides the lingual side of the three facial lobes, creating two separate lingual fossae, one on the mesial and one on the distal side of the lingual ridge. These fossae are bordered by a mesial and a distal marginal ridge, respectively. When present, these fossae are called the mesial and distal lingual fossae.

The borders of the lingual fossae are the incisal ridge, the lingual ridge (dividing the lingual fossae into mesial and distal sides), and the mesial or distal marginal ridge (the mesial marginal ridge bordering the mesial lingual fossa and the distal marginal ridge bordering the distal fossa).

Sometimes the lingual surface of a canine crown is so smooth that no concavities or fossae are present. Usually the cingulum and marginal ridges are less developed in these instances, with little evidence of developmental grooves.

The lingual side of the root is narrower than the labial. A cross-sectional view of the root appears to be triangular in shape, with the lingual portion more tapered than the labial.

Mesial Aspect (Figs. 31-3 and 31-6, *D*)

The functional form of a maxillary canine is well emphasized on the mesial view. When one looks at the wedge-shaped outline of the crown, it becomes apparent that a canine shows greater labiolingual bulk than any other anterior tooth. The greatest measurement labiolingually is at the cervical third. This is because of the huge cingu-

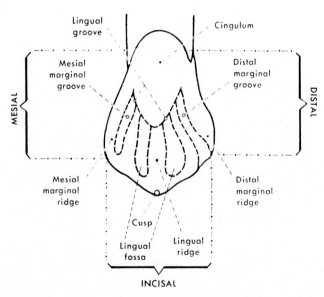

Fig. 31-2 Lingual surface of maxillary right canine. (Zeisz and Nuckolls.)

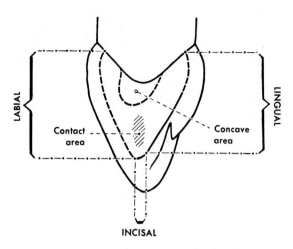

Fig. 31-3 Mesial surface of maxillary right canine. (Zeisz and Nuckolls.)

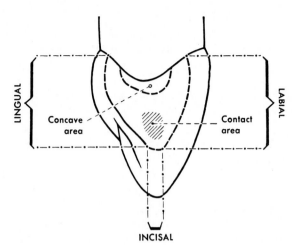

Fig. 31-4 Distal surface of maxillary right canine. (Zeisz and Nuckolls.)

lum of the lingual side and the more convex labial outline of the canine. The entire labial surface is more convex from the cervical line to the cusp tip than any other maxillary anterior tooth.

The cervical line curves toward the cusp an average of 2.5 mm.

The root of a canine is broad labiolingually and usually extremely long. The end of the root apex is blunt and may often curve to the lingual or distal lingual.

The mesial surface of a canine crown is convex throughout, except for a small area between the contact area and the cervical line, which may be flat.

The mesial surface of the root shows much labiolingual development, with a shallow developmental depression extending from the cervical line halfway to the apex of the root. This developmental depression appears to divide the single root into two roots. In extremely well developed roots it helps anchor a canine in the bone and prevents root rotation.

Distal Aspect (Figs. 31-4 and 31-6, *E*)

The distal aspect of a maxillary canine shows the same form and outline as the mesial does. However, the cervical line shows less curvature toward the cusp tip. The distal marginal ridge is more developed and heavier in outline than the mesial marginal ridge. Although both the mesial and the distal surfaces show a slightly flat or concave area above the contact area, the distal surface displays much more concavity. The root surface on the distal aspect may show a more pronounced developmental depression than that on the mesial.

Incisal Aspect (Figs. 31-5 and 31-6, *C*)

An incisal view of a maxillary canine shows that the tooth is not only rather wide mesiodistally but also has the thickest labiolingual measurement of any anterior tooth. Although these two measurements are about equal, the crown is usually larger in a labiolingual direction. The cusp tip is labial to the center of the crown labiolingually and mesial to the center mesiodistally.

The distal aspect of the crown appears thinner than the mesial. Indeed, it seems to stretch out to make contact with the first premolars (Fig. 31-6).

Root

The root of the upper canine is usually the longest of any tooth in the mouth. It is very strong and firmly embedded in the maxilla.

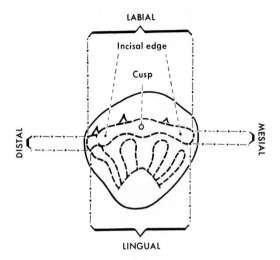

Fig. 31-5 Incisal edge of maxillary right canine. (Zeisz and Nuckolls.)

In a cross-sectional view it appears to taper from the labial toward the lingual areas. From a proximal view a longitudinal groove may be seen. The apical portion will often point distally but seldom mesially.

Pulp Cavity

The pulp cavity of the maxillary canine consists of a large pulp chamber and a single root canal. The pulp chamber has one single pulp horn, which extends toward the tip of the cusp. The root canal is usually straight but can be tortuous when the root is curved (Fig. 31-7).

PERTINENT DATA
Maxillary Canines

	Right	Left
Universal Code	6	11
International Code	13	23
Palmer notation	3⌋	⌊3
Number of roots	1	
Number of pulp horns	1	
Number of cusps	1	
Number of developmental lobes	4	

Location of proximal contact areas
MESIAL: Junction of incisal and middle thirds
DISTAL: Middle third
Height of contour
FACIAL: Cervical third, 0.5 mm
LINGUAL: Cervical third, 0.5 mm
Identifying characteristics

The maxillary canines are the longest teeth in the mouth. They have a single cusp with mesial and distal ridges forming an incisal edge. A prominent facial ridge is off-center toward the mesial. The cingulum is prominent. The prominent mesiofacial lobe forms this facial ridge of the cusp. The centrofacial lobe also forms the lingual ridge of the cusp. This lingual ridge divides the mesial and distal fossae. The distofacial ridge is longer and more rounded than the mesiofacial.

Mandibular canines

Evidence of calcification	4 months
Enamel completed	7 years
Eruption	9-10 years
Root completed	13 years

The mandibular canines resemble the maxillary canines in that they have the same wedge-shaped outline, long crown and root, and well-developed cingulum. They differ from the maxillary canines, however, in the following ways.

1. A mandibular canine crown is narrower mesiodistally by about 0.5 mm.
2. A mandibular canine crown length is as long as that of a maxillary canine and sometimes longer.
3. The root may be as long as that of a maxillary canine but more often is shorter.
4. The labiolingual measurement of the crown and the root is usually a fraction of a millimeter less than for a maxillary. How then does the total length of a mandibular tooth—crown and root—compare with the other teeth?
5. The lingual surface of a mandibular canine is smoother, the cingulum less developed,

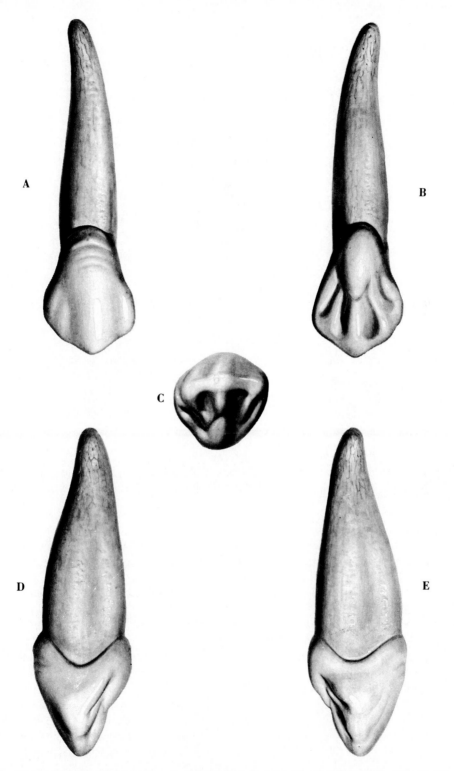

Fig. 31-6   Maxillary right canine. **A,** Labial view. **B,** Lingual view. **C,** Incisal view. **D,** Mesial view. **E,** Distal view. (Zeisz and Nuckolls.)

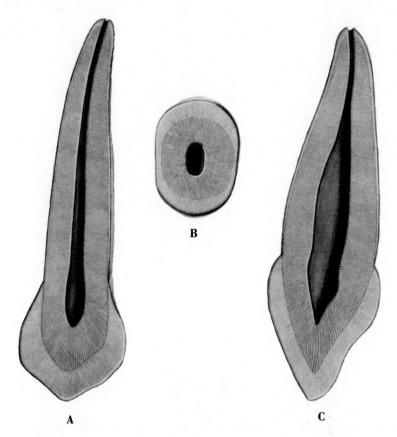

Fig. 31-7 Pulp cavity of maxillary right canine. **A,** Distomesial section, lingual view. **B,** Cross section, incisal view, **C,** Linguolabial section, mesial view. (Zeisz and Nuckolls.)

and the marginal ridges less prominent than those of a maxillary canine. The lingual surface of a mandibular canine resembles the lingual surface of the other mandibular anterior teeth.

6. The cusp tip of a mandibular canine is not so well developed as that of a maxillary, and the cusp ridges are thinner labiolingually than those of a maxillary.
7. The cusp tip of a mandibular canine may be centered more lingually than a maxillary canine cusp tip.
8. An anomaly (a variation or deviation from the ordinary or normal form) of a mandib-

ular canine is bifurcated roots. In this variation a mandibular canine has two roots, one buccal and one lingual. Usually only the apical third of the root is the bifurcated part.

Labial Aspect (Figs. 31-8 and 31-14, *A*)

From the facial view, a mandibular canine shows a straighter mesial outline than does a maxillary. The distal outline resembles that of a maxillary, which means that the mesial outline of a mandibular canine is less convex than its distal outline. Which surface, mesial or distal, shows the greater convexity on a maxillary canine? Is it the same for a mandibular canine?

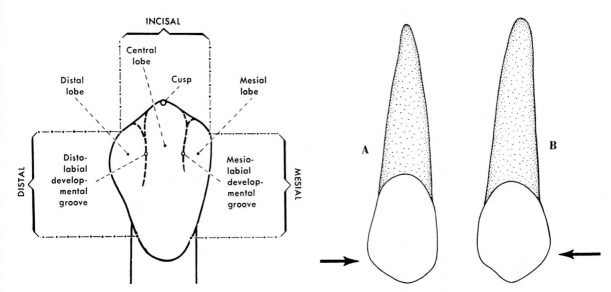

Fig. 31-8   Labial surface of mandibular right canine. (Zeisz and Nuckolls.)

Fig. 31-9   Comparison of mandibular, **A,** and maxillary, **B,** left canine.

The distal contact area is more incisal on a mandibular canine than the same contact area on its maxillary counterpart and is located somewhat cervical to the junction of its incisal and middle thirds (Fig. 31-9). Where is the distal contact on a maxillary canine?

The mesial contact area of a mandibular canine is nearer the mesioincisal point angle than its maxillary counterpart, at the incisal third of the tooth. Where is the mesial contact area of a maxillary canine?

Facially the cervical line of a mandibular canine is more symmetrically contoured than the cervical line of a maxillary canine. The cervical line of a maxillary canine is less uniform, cresting slightly mesial to the midline of the tooth (facial view).

Lingual Aspect (Figs. 31-10 and 31-14, *B*)

The lingual surface of the crown of a mandibular canine is flatter than that of a maxillary canine. Lingual features are less prominent—the

cingulum is relatively smooth, the marginal ridges are less distinct, and the lingual fossae and ridge are less pronounced.

The lingual surface of a mandibular canine resembles the other mandibular anterior teeth but has a larger cingulum and a pronounced lingual ridge. The cingulum is larger and more developed than those on the other mandibular anterior teeth. In comparison to a maxillary canine, a mandibular canine's cingulum tapers more lingually and is less developed.

The lingual ridge of a mandibular canine is less distinct than the same ridge on a maxillary canine, except toward the cusp tip where it is raised. There are no lingual pits present on the mandibular canines.

A mandibular canine resembles the other mandibular teeth from a lingual view in that the marginal ridges and lingual fossae are flatter. In fact, the lingual surfaces of all the mandibular teeth are smoother and more hollowed out than those of their maxillary counterparts.

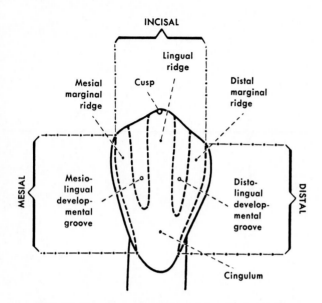

Fig. 31-10 Lingual surface of mandibular right canine. (Zeisz and Nuckolls.)

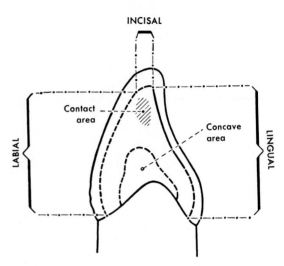

Fig. 31-11 Mesial surface of mandibular right canine. (Zeisz and Nuckolls.)

Mesial Aspect (Figs. 31-11 and 31-14, *D*)

A mandibular canine resembles its maxillary counterpart from a mesial view, with the same wedge shape and pointed cusp. It differs from a maxillary canine in that it has a less developed cingulum, as well as thinner marginal ridges. The cusp tip of a mandibular is more lingually inclined, whereas the cusp tip of a maxillary is centered slightly labially. As the canines become more abraded with wear, this discrepancy in the centering of a canine cusp tip becomes more apparent. If one considers the position of a mandibular canine in relation to a maxillary canine when the two are touching, the reason becomes apparent.

The cervical line curves more toward the incisal portion than does the cervical line on a maxillary canine.

The roots of the teeth are similar except that a mandibular canine's root may be more pointed at the apex. The developmental depression on the root of a mandibular canine is more pronounced and sometimes the root is bifurcated.

Distal Aspect (Figs. 31-12 and 31-14, *E*)

The distal aspect of a mandibular canine resembles a maxillary canine except for those features mentioned in the discussion of the mesial aspects.

Incisal Aspect (Figs. 31-13 and 31-14, *C*)

From an incisal view, the incisal edge of a mandibular canine slants toward the lingual side, with the distal incisal ridge slanting more lingually than the mesial. The cusp tip is located more lingually on a mandibular canine than on a maxillary. In all other ways the mandibular canines resemble the maxillary canines.

Root

The root of the mandibular canine is the longest mandibular root, and of all the teeth it is sec-

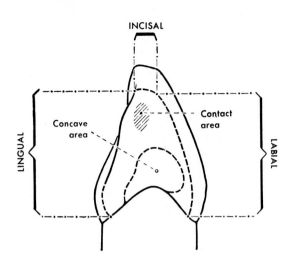

Fig. 31-12 Distal surface of mandibular right canine. (Zeisz and Nuckolls.)

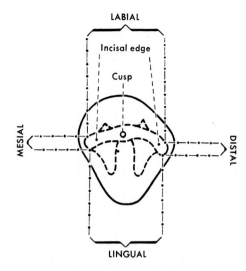

Fig. 31-13 Incisal edge of mandibular right canine. (Zeisz and Nuckolls.)

ond only to the maxillary canine. It is wide labiolingually and narrow mesiodistally. Some specimens show a bifurcated root in the apical third. It is the *anterior tooth most likely to be bifurcated*. When the root is bifurcated, one branch is labial and the other lingual. The single-rooted form is much more common, and if deep longitudinal grooves are present on the proximal surfaces of the root, then there is a tendency for two root canals even if these join together at the apex.

Pulp Cavity

The pulp cavity of the mandibular canine resembles that of the maxillary canine in that they both have a large pulp chamber and usually a single root canal. There is also only one pulp horn present.

The major difference between the two teeth is that the mandibular canine may have two separate root canals. When this happens, one canal is to the labial and the other is to the lingual side.

The canals may join at the apex or have separate apical foramina. When the root is bifurcated, there are almost always two canals, each with its own apical foramen (Fig. 31-15).

PERTINENT DATA
Mandibular Canines

	Right	Left
Universal Code	27	22
International Code	43	33
Palmer notation	3⌋	⌊3
Number of roots	1 or 2	
Number of pulp horns	1	
Number of cusps	1	
Number of developmental lobes	4	

Location of proximal contact areas
MESIAL: Incisal third
DISTAL: Just cervical to the junction of incisal and middle thirds

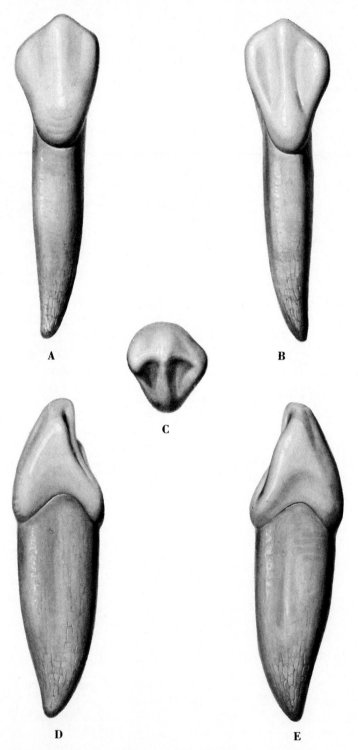

Fig. 31-14 Mandibular right canine. **A,** Labial view. **B,** Lingual view. **C,** Incisal view. **D,** Mesial view. **E,** Distal view. (Zeisz and Nuckolls.)

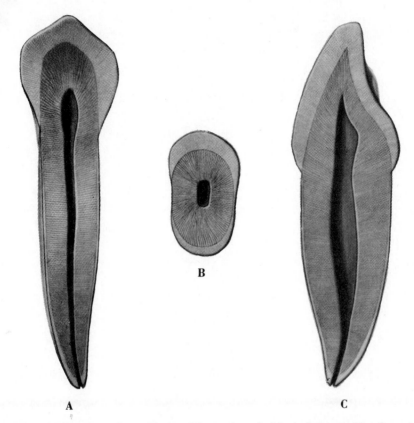

Fig. 31-15 Pulp cavity of mandibular right canine. **A,** Mesiodistal section, lingual view. **B,** Cross section, incisal view. **C,** Labiolingual section, mesial view. (Zeisz and Nuckolls.)

Height of contour
FACIAL: Cervical third, less than 0.5 mm
LINGUAL: Cervical third, less than 0.5 mm
Identifying characteristics
The crown is similar to the crown of the maxillary canines but narrower and smoother. It has less prominent lingual features. From a proximal view, the cusp tip is inclined to the lingual. From an incisal view, the distal end of the incisal edge is rotated to the lingual. They have the longest roots in the mandibular arch, with longitudinal grooves on the root.

REVIEW QUESTIONS

1. A maxillary canine can be distinguished from a mandibular canine by which of the following characteristics?
   a. A mandibular canine has a less prominent cingulum.
   b. The mesial side of a mandibular canine crown and root is relatively straight.
   c. The incisal edge of a mandibular canine is located lingual to the center of the tooth.
   d. all of the above

2. Which of the following is characteristic of the root of a mandibular canine?
   a. It is longer than the root of a maxillary canine.
   b. The root is never bifurcated.
   c. It is flattened or slightly concave on the mesial and distal surfaces.
   d. all of the above
3. Generally, on the lingual surface of a maxillary canine there is (are)
   a. one fossa.
   b. two fossae.
   c. three fossae.
   d. four fossae.
4. Compared with other anterior teeth a mandibular canine is the most likely to have
   a. longitudinal grooves.

b. a root that is narrow mesiodistally.
c. two root canals.
d. accessory canals.
5. A mandibular canine root sometimes bifurcates into a
   a. mesiofacial and distolingual root.
   b. facial and lingual root.
   c. mesial and distal root.
   d. none of the above. The mandibular canine root does not bifurcate.
6. Canine teeth exhibit
   a. a facial ridge.
   b. a lingual ridge.
   c. a mesial marginal ridge.
   d. all of the above.

32

Premolars

OBJECTIVES

- To identify an extracted premolar as maxillary or mandibular, first or second, right or left
- To recognize and name the pertinent dental anatomical form of each tooth—cusps, ridges, developmental grooves, triangular grooves, pits, and developmental depressions
- To make comparisons between maxillary and mandibular premolars
- To discuss the major differences and similarities between the maxillary first and second premolars
- To describe briefly the various occlusal forms possible for a mandibular second premolar
- To compare the mandibular first premolars with the mandibular second premolars (development, shape, and diversities of anatomical form)
- To understand how development occurs through the formation and fusion of the lobes
- To understand how the form of a tooth relates to its ultimate function

The premolars succeed the deciduous molars. There are eight premolar teeth—two in each quadrant. How many maxillary and how many mandibular premolars are there? The term "premolar" implies that these are the teeth that will be located immediately anterior to the permanent molars. In the study of human dentition the term "bicuspid" is often used in place of "premolar." This is inaccurate, since "bicuspid" presupposes that a tooth has only two cusps. In human dentition, however, mandibular premolars show a variation in the number of cusps from one to three. Thus the use of the term "bicuspid" is discouraged in favor of the term "premolar."

The maxillary first and second premolars, as well as the mandibular first premolars, are developed from the same number of lobes as the anterior teeth. The mandibular second premolars usually develop from five lobes, three buccal and two lingual.

The buccal cusp of a premolar is developed from three labial lobes, as in the anterior teeth. The primary difference in development is the fact that the lingual cusp, which is extremely well formed, develops from the single lingual lobe. In anterior teeth the lingual lobe forms the cingulum of the incisors and canines. In premolars this single lingual lobe forms an extremely well-developed lingual cusp.

In the case of the three-cusp form (mandibular second premolar) there are two lingual lobes, each of which forms a separate small lingual cusp. It should be noted that there is also a two-cusp form of the mandibular second premolar, which develops from just four lobes. How many lingual lobes would it have? The lingual cusps of the mandibular premolars are small and **afunctional** when compared with the larger lingual cusps of the maxillary premolars.

The premolar crowns and roots are shorter than those of the canines.

Maxillary premolars

FIRST PREMOLARS

Evidence of calcification	1½ years
Enamel completed	5-6 years
Eruption	10-11 years
Root completed	12-13 years

359

Maxillary first premolars have two cusps, a buccal and a lingual. The buccal cusp is usually 1 mm or more longer than the lingual cusp. These teeth are also the only premolars that normally have two roots, a buccal and a lingual, though occasionally there is only a single root. *fused*

Most maxillary first premolars have two roots and two pulp canals. Even when only one root is present, two pulp canals can usually be found. It is not uncommon for maxillary second premolars to also have two roots; however, there is usually only one.

Facial (Buccal) Aspect (Figs. 32-1 and 32-7, *A*)

A maxillary first premolar is similar in appearance to a maxillary canine. However, the crown is shorter and narrower mesiodistally, and unlike a canine, the contact areas, mesially and distally, are at about the same level. The mesial and distal marginal ridges are also sharper than those of a canine.

The tip of the facial cusp is located distally to the midline and separates the occlusal border into a long, straight mesial ridge and a short, convex distal ridge. The mesial ridge may even have a slight indentation at the junction of the mesial and middle lobes. From the contact areas cervically, the distal border is straight, whereas the mesial border is more concave. Two developmental lines on the facial surface mark the coalescence of the developmental lobes. The facial surface of the crown is convex, and an extremely well-developed middle facial lobe is present.

Lingual Aspect (Figs. 32-2 and 32-7, *B*)

From the lingual view, the crown converges toward the lingual cusp, which is shorter than the facial cusp. The tip of the lingual cusp is located slightly toward the mesial side of the midline.

Mesial Aspect (Figs. 32-3 and 32-7, *D*)

On the mesial surface of the crown, a groove extends from the mesial marginal ridge cervically. This groove is called the **mesial marginal groove.** It crosses the mesial marginal ridge and runs from the occlusal to the middle third of the crown, lingual to the contact area. The mesial surface can also be identified by a **mesial developmental depression** located cervically to the

Buccal cusp leans Distally

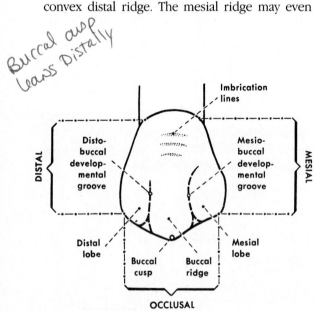

Fig. 32-1 Buccal surface of maxillary right first premolar. (Zeisz and Nuckolls.)

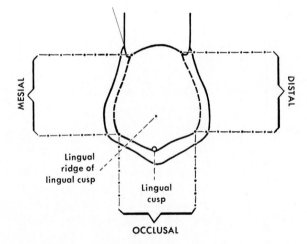

Fig. 32-2 Lingual surface of maxillary right first premolar. (Zeisz and Nuckolls.)

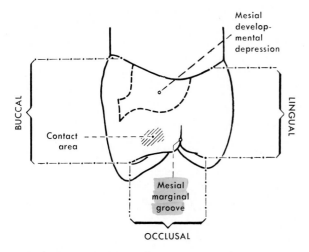

Fig. 32-3 Mesial surface of maxillary right first premolar. (Zeisz and Nuckolls.)

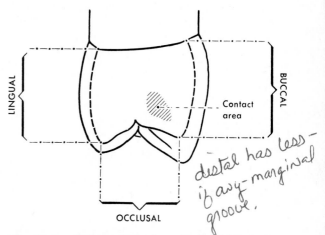

distal has less — if any — marginal groove.

Fig. 32-4 Distal surface of maxillary right first premolar. (Zeisz and Nuckolls.)

mesial contact area. The concavity continues cervically from above the contact area across the cervical line, where it joins a deep **developmental depression** between the roots. The mesial marginal groove is not always present, but the mesial developmental depression usually is. *fluted*

The facial outline is convex, with the crest of contour located within the cervical third of the crown. The lingual outline is also convex, with its crest of contour located within the middle third of the crown. The curvature of the cervical line is greater on the mesial surface than on the distal surface.

Distal Aspect (Figs. 32-4 and 32-7, *E*)

From the distal view, a maxillary first premolar is similar to the mesial view, except that there is usually no groove crossing the distal marginal ridge and no developmental depression is present. Fig. 32-7, *E*, illustrates a distal **marginal groove.** Some specimens show a distinct groove, but the mesial marginal groove is deeper and more obvious. The curvature of the cervical line is less on the distal surface. The crown also appears more rounded and smooth. Both the buccal and lingual cusp tips are centered over the

root. This is also true from the mesial view. *All maxillary* premolars have their cusp tips centered over their root.

Occlusal Aspect (Figs. 32-5 and 32-7, *C*)

The occlusal surface shows two well-developed cusps. The lingual cusp is more pointed than the facial cusp, but the buccal cusp is much larger and longer than the lingual. Each has four ridges emanating from it, named according to their location—facial, lingual, distal, and mesial ridges.

On the facial cusp, the facial ridge descends from the cusp tip cervically onto the facial surface. The mesial and distal ridges descend from the cusp tip to their respective point angles. They are called the mesial and distal cusp ridges.

The lingual cusp ridge extends from the cusp tip lingually to the central area of the occlusal surface. Any ridge that runs from the cusp tip to the central groove of the occlusal surface is called a triangular ridge. Examples are the lingual cusp ridge of the buccal cusp and the buccal cusp ridge of the lingual cusp, which runs from the cusp tip of the lingual cusp to the central groove (Fig. 32-6).

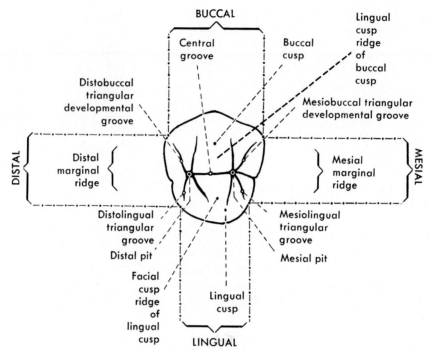

BUCCAL

Central groove

Buccal cusp

Lingual cusp ridge of buccal cusp

Distobuccal triangular developmental groove

Mesiobuccal triangular developmental groove

DISTAL

MESIAL

Distal marginal ridge

Mesial marginal ridge

Distolingual triangular groove

Mesiolingual triangular groove

Distal pit

Mesial pit

Facial cusp ridge of lingual cusp

Lingual cusp

LINGUAL

Fig. 32-5 Occlusal surface of maxillary right first premolar. (Zeisz and Nuckolls.)

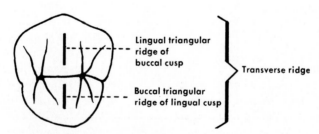

Lingual triangular ridge of buccal cusp

Transverse ridge

Buccal triangular ridge of lingual cusp

Fig. 32-6 Occlusal surface of maxillary right first premolar. (Zeisz and Nuckolls.)

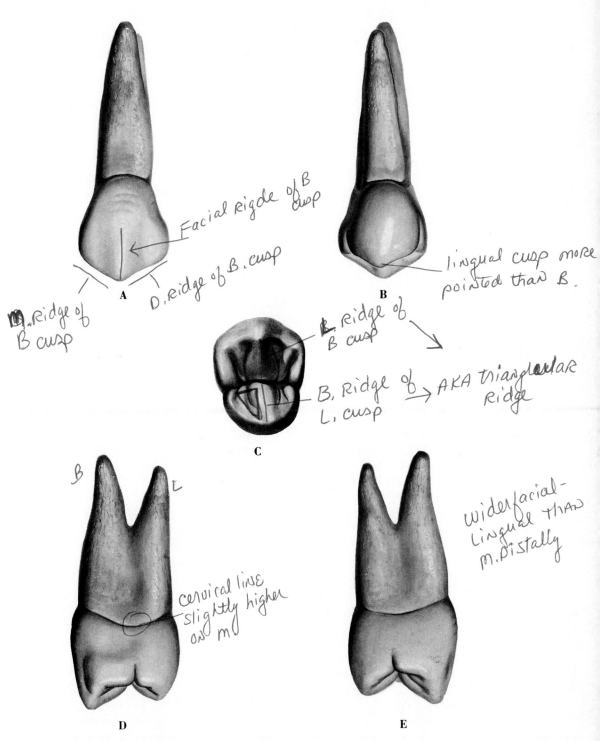

Facial Rigde of B cusp

D.Ridge of B.cusp

M.Ridge of B cusp

A

lingual cusp more pointed than B.

B

B. Ridge of B cusp

B. Ridge of L. cusp

AKA triangular Ridge

C

B   L

cervical line slightly higher on M

D

wider facial- lingual than M.Distally

E

Fig. 32-7 Maxillary right first premolar. **A,** Buccal view. **B,** Lingual view. **C,** Occlusal view. **D,** Mesial view. **E,** Distal view. (Zeisz and Nuckolls.)

The lingual cusp has four ridges, like its counterpart the buccal cusp. The lingual cusp ridge of the lingual cusp extends onto the lingual surface. The mesial and distal cusp ridges extend from the cusp tip to their respective point angles and fuse into the mesial and distal marginal ridges.

When two triangular ridges join, after traversing the tooth buccolingually, they form a transverse ridge. Thus a transverse ridge exists on the occlusal surface of a maxillary first premolar. It is formed by the union of the two triangular ridges—the lingual cusp ridge (triangular ridge) of the buccal cusp and the facial cusp ridge (triangular ridge) of the lingual cusp. In Fig. 32-6, notice the transverse ridge formed by the two joining triangular ridges.

From the occlusal aspect, close observation reveals that the crown is wider on the buccal than on the lingual surface. Notice also that the buccolingual dimension of the crown is much greater than the mesiodistal dimension.

At this point it is important to mention that primary anatomical features are composed of the major structures, grooves, and pits that are pertinent to the teeth. They must occur regularly with uniformity in shape and size.

Thus primary grooves are sharp, deep, and V shaped. They occur consistently and mark the junction of major anatomical boundaries. All developmental grooves are primary grooves because they occur routinely and are of major importance to anatomical development. Developmental grooves mark the union of what structures?

Secondary grooves are of lesser importance. They differ from primary grooves in that they usually are shallower and more irregular in shape, giving the tooth a more wrinkled appearance. They are not always present.

As a general rule, first premolars and first molars will have fewer secondary anatomical features. Second premolars and second molars will have more secondary grooves and pits. Third molars will have even more secondary anatomical grooves, pits, and fissures. Therefore the third molars will appear more wrinkled because of the more numerous and shallow anatomical features.

Few secondary grooves are seen on the occlusal side of a maxillary first premolar. In most instances the surface is relatively smooth. A well-defined **central developmental groove** divides the tooth buccolingually. A **mesial marginal developmental groove** extends from the central developmental groove, across the mesial marginal ridge, and onto the mesial surface of the tooth.

Two developmental grooves connect to the central groove just inside the mesial and distal marginal ridges. These grooves are the **mesiobuccal developmental groove** and the **distobuccal developmental groove.** Each can connect at opposite ends of the central developmental groove, at which point they usually end in a deep depression in the occlusal surface called the mesial and distal developmental pits.

The triangular depression that harbors the mesiobuccal developmental groove is called the mesial triangular fossa. Likewise, the depression in which the distobuccal developmental groove lies is called the distal triangular fossa. *Note:* The terms "mesiobuccal developmental groove" and "mesiobuccal triangular groove" are synonymous.

Root

The root of a maxillary first premolar may be either single or bifurcated. The bifurcated root form is far more common, but even in the single root form two root canals are usually present. The number of pulp horns corresponds to the number of cusps—in this case, two.

On the bifurcated root form there is one buccal (facial) and one **palatal** (lingual) **root.** The facial root is larger and longer than the lingual (Fig. 32-7, *D* and *E*).

On the single-rooted form grooves are usually present lengthwise in the middle of the root, giving the appearance of a root trying to divide itself. The mesial root surface will have the more highly developed root groove.

Pulp Cavity

The pulp cavity of the maxillary first premolar has two pulp horns, one for each cusp, and two root canals, one for each root.

Sometimes there is only one undivided root. When this occurs, there are still usually two root canals, though often they combine to form one apical foramen. In some specimens with only one root there may be only one single root canal (Fig. 32-8).

■ ■ ■

The maxillary first premolars exemplify some characteristics that are common to all posterior teeth when compared to anterior teeth.

1. The posterior teeth have a greater faciolingual measurement in relation to their mesiodistal measurements.

2. The mesial and distal contact areas are broader and closer to the same level on the tooth.
3. The mesial and distal curvature of the cervical line is less.
4. The crown measurements cervico-occlusally are less, giving the appearance of shorter crown length.

SECOND PREMOLARS

Evidence of calcification	2 years
Enamel completed	6-7 years
Eruption	10-12 years
Root completed	12-14 years

Maxillary second premolars resemble the maxillary first premolars in both form and function. The crown, however, has a less angular and

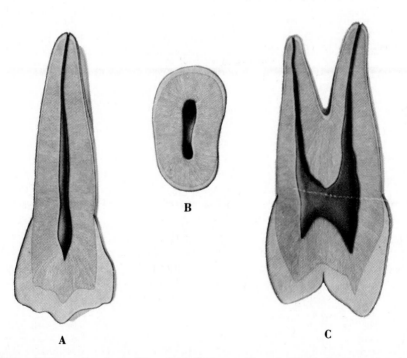

Fig. 32-8 Pulp cavity of maxillary right first premolar. **A,** Mesiodistal section, buccal view. **B,** Cross section, occlusal view. **C,** Buccolingual section, distal view. (Zeisz and Nuckolls.)

more rounded appearance. The second premolars also vary from the first in that they usually have only one root. How many roots do the maxillary first premolars have?

Second premolars vary individually more than first premolars. A maxillary second premolar may have a crown that is noticeably smaller cervicoocclusally and mesiodistally. On the other hand, it may be larger in those dimensions and usually is.

Generally the root of a second premolar is longer than that of a first premolar. Although a second premolar usually has only one root, it is common to find these premolars with two roots.

Facial (Buccal) Aspect (Figs. 32-9 and 32-13, *A*)

From the buccal view, it is evident that the buccal cusp of a second premolar is not so long as that of a first premolar, and it appears less pointed.

A second premolar has the same general markings as the first, but they are not so well defined.

Lingual Aspect (Figs. 32-10 and 32-13, *B*)

Little variation can be seen from the lingual view except that the lingual cusp is almost the same length as the buccal cusp.

Mesial Aspect (Figs. 32-11 and 32-13, *D*)

The mesial view shows the difference in cusp length between the maxillary first and second premolars. The buccal cusp of a second premolar is shorter, and the lingual cusp is almost as long; thus the buccal and lingual cusps are nearly the same length.

There is no deep developmental groove crossing the mesial marginal ridge, just as there is no deep developmental depression on the mesial surface of the crown; instead, the crown surface is convex. A shallow developmental groove bisects the single root form, giving the appearance of two roots fused into one.

Distal Aspect (Fig. 32-13, *E*)

The distal view shows that the features of the first and second premolars are the same, except that the buccal and lingual cusps of a second premolar are more even in length.

Occlusal Aspect (Figs. 32-12 and 32-13, *C*)

The occlusal outline is more rounded than that of a first premolar, and the second premolar is ovoid rather than hexagonal.

There appears to be more distance between the cusp tips buccolingually, and the lingual cusp

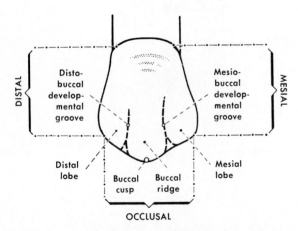

Fig. 32-9 Buccal surface of maxillary right second premolar. (Zeisz and Nuckolls.)

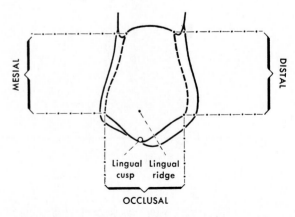

Fig. 32-10 Lingual surface of maxillary right second premolar. (Zeisz and Nuckolls.)

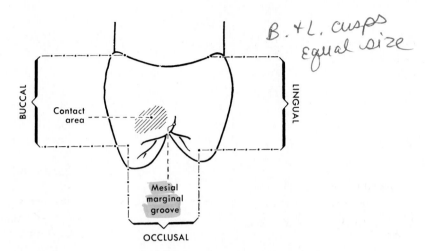

B. + L. cusps equal size

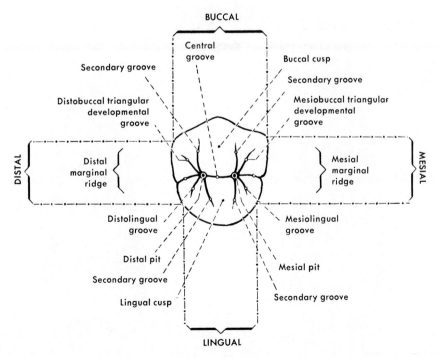

Fig. 32-11 Mesial surface of maxillary right second premolar. *Note:* Although mesial and distal marginal grooves are present in all maxillary second premolar drawings, one should understand that these grooves are shallower than mesial marginal groove of maxillary first premolar. (Zeisz and Nuckolls.)

Fig. 32-12 Occlusal surface of maxillary right second premolar. (Zeisz and Nuckolls.)

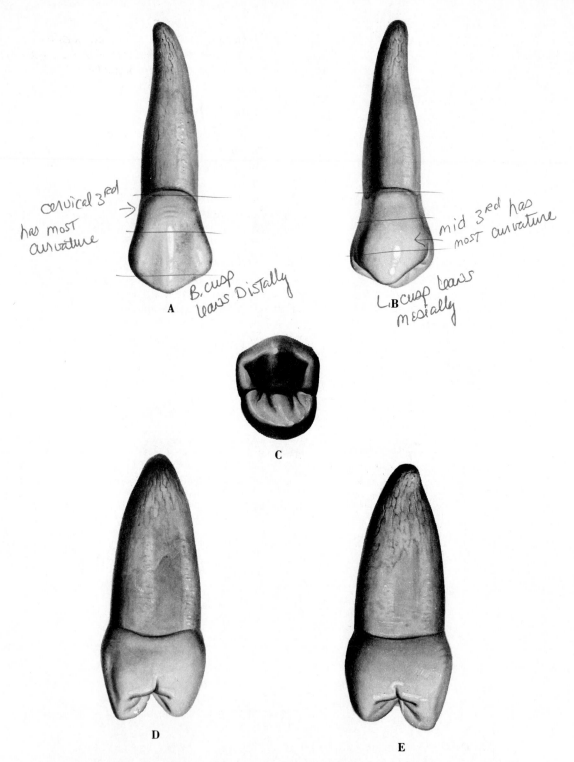

Handwritten annotations:

cervical 3rd has most curvature →

B. cusp leans Distally

A

mid 3rd has most curvature ←

L.B cusp leans mesially

B

C

D

E

Fig. 32-13 Maxillary right second premolar. **A,** Buccal view. **B,** Lingual view. **C,** Occlusal view. **D,** Mesial view. **E,** Distal view. (Zeisz and Nuckolls.)

is almost as wide as the buccal. Is this true of a first premolar?

The groove pattern is less distinct, and the grooves are shorter, shallower, and more irregular. The central developmental groove is shorter and more irregular, with numerous supplemental grooves radiating from it. This gives the occlusal surface a more wrinkled appearance.

Root

The root of a maxillary second premolar is usually single with a longitudinal groove on the mesial and distal surfaces. This groove gives the appearance of trying to divide the root into two, buccally and lingually. Usually there is only one root canal, but often a divided canal occurs in at least a portion of the root. A bifurcated root similar to that of a first premolar is common; this form has two root canals.

Pulp Cavity

The pulp cavity of the maxillary second premolar has two pulp horns and one single root canal. The single-rooted form is more common; it is also more common to have one root canal. If two canals are present, they usually join to form one single apical foramen, though it is not rare to find two apical foramens. In the bifurcated root there are two canals and two apical foramens. (Fig. 32-14).

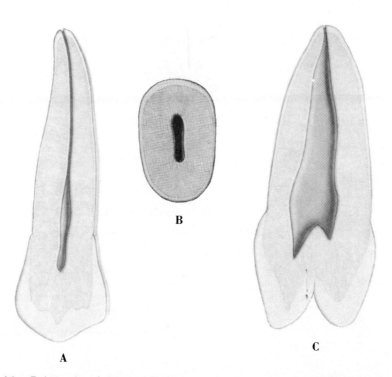

Fig. 32-14   Pulp cavity of right maxillary second premolar. **A,** Mesiodistal section, buccal view. **B,** Cross section, occlusal view. **C,** Linguobuccal section, mesial view. (Zeisz and Nuckolls.)

PERTINENT DATA
Maxillary First Premolars

	Right	Left
Universal Code	5	12
International Code	14	24
Palmer notation	4⌋	⌊4
Number of roots		2
Number of pulp horns		2
Number of cusps		2
Number of developmental lobes		4

Location of proximal contact areas
MESIAL AND DISTAL: Just cervical to the junction of occlusal and middle thirds
Height of contour
FACIAL: Cervical third, 0.5 mm
LINGUAL: Middle third, 0.5 mm
Identifying characteristics
These premolars have bifurcated roots. A longitudinal groove is present on the root. The mesial surface shows a developmental fossa. The mesial marginal groove crosses the mesial marginal ridge and extends onto the mesial surface. The facial cusp is wider and longer than the lingual cusp. The mesial ridge of the facial cusp may have a slight concavity.

Maxillary Second Premolars

	Right	Left
Universal Code	4	13
International Code	15	25
Palmer notation	5⌋	⌊5
Number of roots	1	
Number of pulp horns	2	
Number of cusps	2	
Number of developmental lobes	4	

Location of proximal contact areas
MESIAL AND DISTAL: Just cervical to the junction of occlusal and middle thirds
Height of contour
FACIAL: Cervical third, 0.5 mm
LINGUAL: Middle third, 0.5 mm
Identifying characteristics
These premolars usually have a single root. About 40% have two root canals. The buccal and lingual cusps are nearly equal in length. The buccal cusp is shorter than that of a first premolar. The entire crown, especially the occlusal outline, is less angular and more rounded. The occlusal surface has more supplemental grooves. The occlusal developmental grooves are shorter, shallower, and more irregular.

REVIEW QUESTIONS
Which of the following features are more true for a maxillary first premolar than for a maxillary second premolar?
1. It usually has two roots.
2. It usually has two root canals, even if it has only one root.
3. It has a mesial developmental fossa.
4. Its mesial marginal ridge is crossed by a mesial marginal developmental groove.
5. The lingual and buccal cusps are nearly the same height.
6. The occlusal outline is more rounded.
7. The facial contour is less angular.
8. The occlusal grooves are shorter, shallower, and more irregular.
9. It has more secondary anatomical features and more supplemental grooves.
10. It has a shorter buccal cusp.

Mandibular premolars
smaller than 2nd premolar
FIRST PREMOLARS

Evidence of calcification	2 years
Enamel completed	5-6 years
Eruption	10-12 years
Root completed	12-13 years

The mandibular first premolars have many of the characteristics of the mandibular canines. They have a short buccal cusp, which is the only part that occludes with the maxillary teeth. Their function and appearance are therefore similar to those of the mandibular canine.

As a rule, the mandibular first premolars are always smaller than the mandibular second premolars. In most cases this is not true of the maxillary premolars.

The mandibular first premolars develop from four lobes, just as the maxillary first and second premolars. The three facial lobes form the large buccal cusp, and the single lingual lobe forms into a lingual cusp. This lingual cusp is much smaller than the lingual cusp of the maxillary premolars. It is so small in height and width that it does not occlude with any of the maxillary teeth. It is for this reason that the lingual cusp of the mandibular first premolars is considered afunctional. As in the case of the maxillary premolars, each cusp has its own pulp horn. How many pulp horns would the mandibular first premolars have?

Facial (Buccal) Aspect (Figs. 32-15 and 32-20, A)

A mandibular first premolar resembles a mandibular canine from the facial view. This premolar has nearly the same buccolingual measurement as a canine, and like the canine it has a sharp buccal cusp. The middle buccal lobe is well developed. The mesial cusp ridge is shorter than the distal cusp ridge, but the contact areas are almost at the same level mesially and distally.

They are located slightly occlusal to the midpoint of the tooth cervicoincisally. In what third of the tooth will the contact areas be located?

A mandibular premolar is more convex than a maxillary premolar at the cervical and middle thirds.

The root of this tooth is usually 3 mm or more shorter than that of a mandibular canine.

Developmental depressions are often seen between the three lobes. However, developmental lines are usually not present.

Lingual Aspect (Figs. 32-16 and 32-20, B)

The crown and root of a mandibular first premolar taper toward the lingual side. Like a canine, a first premolar is broader mesiodistally on the buccal cusp portion of the tooth than on the part developed from the lingual lobe. The lingual cusp is small in comparison to the buccal cusp.

The occlusal surface slopes toward the lingual side in a cervical direction.

On each side of the triangular ridge, mesial and distal occlusal pits can be seen within the fossae.

The most striking and characteristic identifying feature of this tooth is the **mesiolingual develop-**

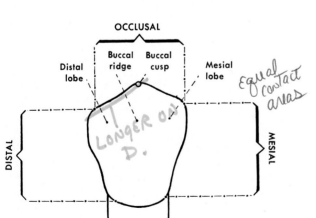

Fig. 32-15 Buccal surface of mandibular right first premolar. (Zeisz and Nuckolls.)

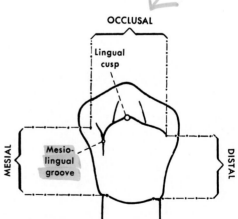

Fig. 32-16 Lingual surface of mandibular right first premolar. (Zeisz and Nuckolls.)

mental groove, which separates the mesial marginal ridge from the lingual cusp.

Mesial Aspect (Figs. 32-17 and 32-20, *D*)

From the mesial view, the buccal cusp overshadows the smaller lingual cusp. The tip of the buccal cusp is centered directly over the root, and the tip of the lingual cusp is centered lingually to the root. How does this differ from the maxillary premolars?

The buccal crest of curvature is located in the cervical third of the crown, the lingual crest near the middle third.

The mesiolingual developmental groove can be seen between the mesiobuccal and the lingual lobes.

Distal Aspect (Figs. 32-18 and 32-20, *E*)

The distal view resembles the mesial except for the following characteristics:

1. There is no mesiolingual developmental groove.
2. The distal marginal ridge is much more developed than the mesial, and its continuity is unbroken by any deep developmental lines.

3. The curvature of the cervical line is less than the 1 mm usually found on the mesial.
4. The distal contact area is broader than the mesial, though it is centered in the same relationship to the crown.
5. The root exhibits more convexity distally than mesially and rarely shows a developmental groove.
6. A shallow developmental depression, less prominent than on the mesial, is often found.

Occlusal Aspect (Figs. 32-19 and 32-20, *C*)

The occlusal aspect displays considerable individual variation. Much more variation exists on either mandibular first or second premolars than on their maxillary counterparts.

The crown converges sharply toward the lingual, the marginal ridges are well developed, and the lingual cusp is small.

The buccal cusp shows a heavy facial triangular ridge and a smaller lingual triangular ridge. Two depressions, the mesial and distal fossae, are apparent, one on each side of the lingual triangular ridge of the buccal cusp.

These are the only premolars, maxillary or

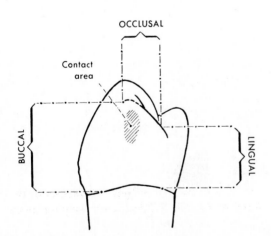

Fig. 32-17 Mesial surface of mandibular right first premolar. (Zeisz and Nuckolls.)

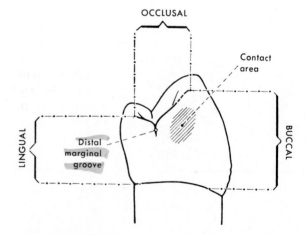

Fig. 32-18 Distal surface of mandibular right first premolar. (Zeisz and Nuckolls.)

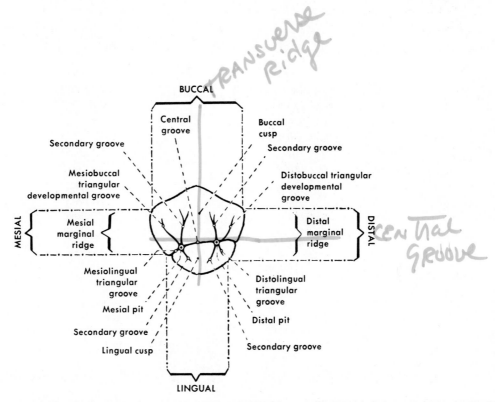

Fig. 32-19   Occlusal surface of mandibular right first premolar. Central groove is not always present. (Zeisz and Nuckolls.)

mandibular, that may have a transverse ridge that does not cross an occlusal developmental groove. The mesial developmental groove extends from the mesial fossa lingually, between the mesial marginal ridge and the lingual cusp, onto the lingual surface. Either fossa may contain a pit. What would the name of these pits be, should they occur? Does a mandibular first premolar always have a central developmental groove?

Root

A mandibular first premolar is normally single rooted. The mesial and distal surfaces are usually slightly convex. If a longitudinal groove is present, then the mesial and distal surfaces may be concave. Occasionally, there may be two roots, a buccal and a lingual. A deep longitudinal groove will separate the roots on the proximal sides.

Pulp Cavity

The mandibular first premolar consists of two pulp horns, a pulp chamber, and a single root canal. The buccal pulp horn is well accented, and the lingual pulp horn is small and insignificant. Each pulp horn is located within a cusp (Fig. 32-21).

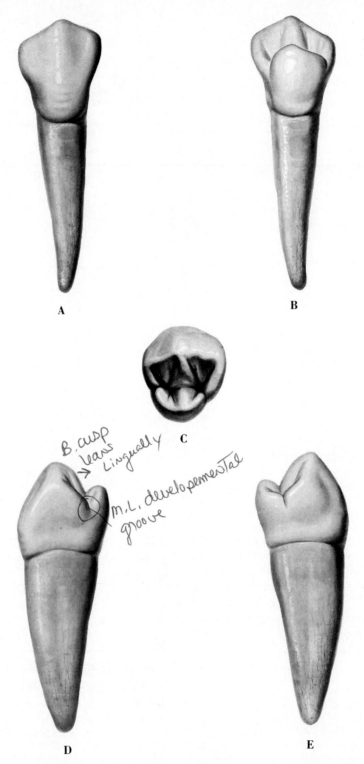

A

B

C

B. cusp leans Lingually →

m.L. developemental groove

D

E

Fig. 32-20 Mandibular right first premolar. **A,** Buccal view. **B,** Lingual view. **C,** Occlusal view. **D,** Mesial view. **E,** Distal view. (Zeisz and Nuckolls.)

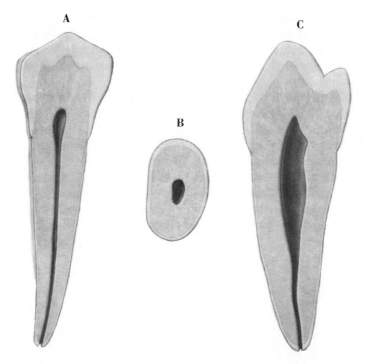

Fig. 32-21 Pulp cavity of mandibular right first premolar. **A,** Mesiodistal section, buccal view. **B,** Cross section, occlusal view. **C,** Buccolingual section, mesial view. (Zeisz and Nuckolls.)

SECOND PREMOLARS

Evidence of calcification	2½ years
Enamel completed	6-7 years
Eruption	11-12 years
Root completed	13-14 years

A mandibular second premolar is always larger than a mandibular first premolar. From a labial view, the crown resembles a first premolar in its general shape and in the fact that the contact areas, mesially and distally, are near the same level. The buccal cusp is shorter, however, and the root is longer.

The lingual cusps of a second premolar are much more developed, and both marginal ridges are higher. This produces a more efficient occlusion with its maxillary antagonist. Therefore a mandibular second premolar functions more like a molar than a canine. How does this differ from a mandibular first premolar?

There are two common forms of this tooth, the three-cusp and the two-cusp types, with one pulp horn in each cusp. The three-cusp form has how many lingual pulp horns? How many pulp horns does the two-cusp form have?

The three-cusp form resembles the molars in the following ways: (1) it has two lingual cusps; (2) it has two lingual pulp canals; (3) it has afunctional lingual cusps; (4) it has higher mesial and distal marginal ridges; and (5) the marginal ridges function in occlusion, offering more efficient contact and intercuspation of the teeth, despite the fact that lingual cusps are afunctional (unlike the lingual cusps of mandibular molars).

The single root of a second premolar is larger and longer than that of the first. It is sometimes bifurcated, but this is rare.

Facial (Buccal) Aspect (Figs. 32-22 and 32-30, A)

From the buccal view, a mandibular second premolar appears to have a shorter buccal cusp than that of a first premolar. The mesiobuccal and distobuccal cusp ridges are more rounded. The contact areas, mesial and distal, are broad, and they are located just cervical to the junction of the middle cervical third of the crown.

The root is wider mesiodistally and slightly longer, with a more blunt apex.

Lingual Aspect (Figs. 32-23 and 32-30, B)

The lingual view of a second premolar shows much variation because there are two different cusp forms. In general, however, the following statements are true of a mandibular second premolar as compared with the first premolar.

1. The lingual lobes are developed to a greater degree. At least one lingual cusp will be longer than a lingual cusp of a first premolar.

2. In the three-cusp form there is a **mesiolingual** and a **distolingual cusp.** The mesiolingual is usually the wider and longer of the two cusps, which are divided by a lingual groove.

3. In the two-cusp form the single lingual lobe is higher than on a mandibular first premolar. There is no groove on the lingual, as in the three-cusp form, but a developmental depression can be seen distolingually where the lingual cusp ridge joins the distal marginal ridge.

4. The lingual surface of the root is wider than that of a first premolar. Thus the convergence of the root toward the lingual side is less. This is true even though the root is wider buccally, because the root is much wider lingually than on a first premolar. This results in less convergence toward the lingual.

The lingual portion of the crown and root is slightly convex.

Mesial Aspect (Figs. 32-24 and 32-30, D)

A second premolar differs mesially from a first premolar in the following ways:

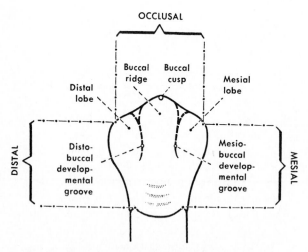

Fig. 32-22 Buccal surface of mandibular right second premolar. (Zeisz and Nuckolls.)

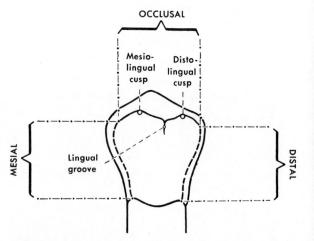

Fig. 32-23 Lingual surface of mandibular right second premolar. (Zeisz and Nuckolls.)

1. The buccal cusp is shorter and its tip is located more to the buccal side.
2. The crown and root are wider buccolingually.
3. The lingual lobe shows more development.
4. The marginal ridge is at a right angle to the long axis of the tooth.
5. There is no mesiolingual developmental groove.
6. The root is longer and the apex more blunt.

Distal Aspect (Figs. 32-25 and 32-30, *E*)

From the distal view, more of the occlusal surface can be seen because the distal marginal ridge is at a lower level than the mesial marginal ridge.

As a general rule, the crowns of all posterior teeth, maxillary or mandibular, are tipped distally to the long axis of the root. Thus, if a specimen is held vertically, more of the occlusal surface of a posterior tooth can be seen from the distal aspect.

Another general rule is that more roots of posterior teeth will tip toward the distal side. In other words, the apex of the root will curve distally.

Occlusal Aspect (Figs. 32-26 and 32-30, *C*)

In both the two- and three-cusp forms the buccal cusp is similar. In the three-cusp form the buccal cusp is the largest, the mesiolingual cusp the next largest, and the distolingual the smallest.

Each of the three cusps has well-developed triangular ridges separated by deep developmental grooves. These grooves form a wide pattern on the occlusal surface. The three developmental grooves are the mesial, the distal, and the lingual. Three pits may be present—a central, a mesial, and a distal. Of the three, the central pit is the most likely to be present. Mesial and distal **triangular fossae** are also present.

Supplemental grooves are more commonly found on a second premolar than on a first, and the developmental grooves are usually not so deep.

In the two-cusp type, as compared with the three-cusp type, the following observations can be noted:

1. The occlusal outline of the crown is more rounded.
2. The lingual surface of the crown is more convex and tapers toward the lingual side.
3. There is no lingual developmental groove.

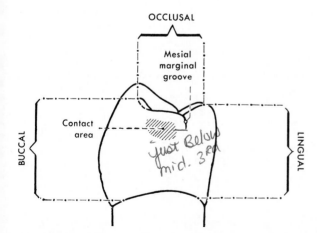

Fig. 32-24 Mesial surface of mandibular right second premolar. (Zeisz and Nuckolls.)

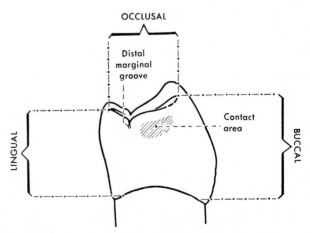

Fig. 32-25 Distal surface of mandibular right second premolar. (Zeisz and Nuckolls.)

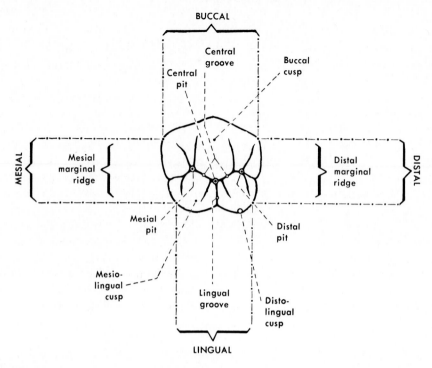

Fig. 32-26 Occlusal surface of mandibular right second premolar (three-cusp variety). (Zeisz and Nuckolls.)

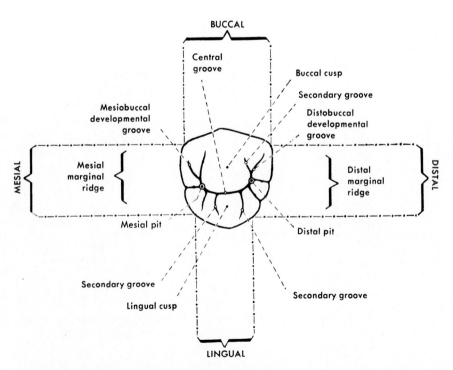

Fig. 32-27 Occlusal surface, U type (two-cusp variety). (Zeisz and Nuckolls.)

4. There is only one well-developed lingual cusp on the two-cusp form, and it is located directly opposite the buccal cusp in a lingual direction.
5. There is usually no central pit; a mesial or distal pit is much more likely.

In the three-cusp type, the groove pattern is commonly called a Y-groove pattern. In the two-cusp type, the groove pattern can be either a U- or H-groove pattern, depending on whether the central developmental groove is straight mesiodistally or curves buccally at its ends. The central groove of the two-cusp form terminates in mesial and distal fossae. If lingual triangular grooves radiate from these fossae, the H-groove pattern is present (Figs. 32-27 to 32-29).

As a general rule, second premolars and molars have shallower developmental grooves than first premolars and molars. They also have more secondary (supplemental) grooves. In general, the more posterior the tooth, the more wrinkled it appears.

Root

The root of the mandibular second premolar is similar to that of the first premolar. It is longer and wider buccolingually. There is no tendency for it to bifurcate as sometimes the mandibular first premolar does (Fig. 32-30).

Pulp Cavity

The pulp cavity of the mandibular second premolar shows two pointed pulp horns, three in the three-cusp variety. The pulp horns are more pointed than in the mandibular first premolar. One single root canal is present, with even less tendency to have divided root canals than in the first premolar (Fig. 32-31).

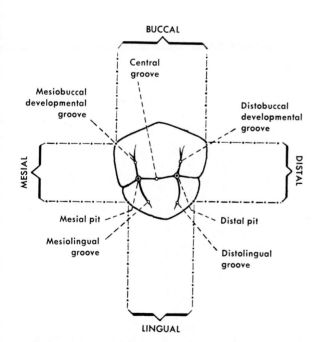

Fig. 32-28 Occlusal surface, H type (two-cusp variety). (Zeisz and Nuckolls.)

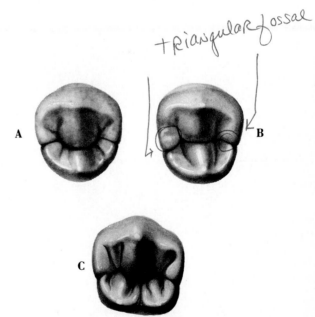

+triangular fossae

Fig. 32-29 Occlusal views. **A,** U type. **B,** H type. **C,** Y type. (Zeisz and Nuckolls.)

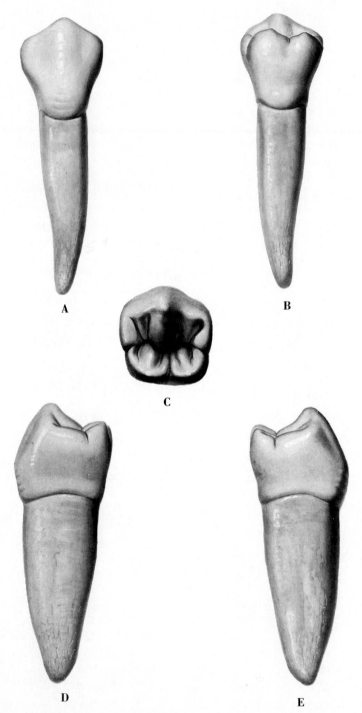

Fig. 32-30 Mandibular right second premolar. **A,** Buccal view. **B,** Lingual view. **C,** Occlusal view. **D,** Mesial view. **E,** Distal view.

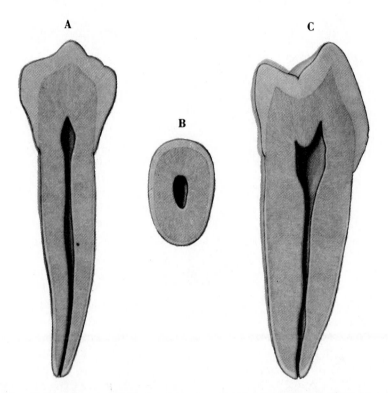

Fig. 32-31 Pulp cavity of mandibular right second premolar. **A,** Mesiodistal section, buccal view. **B,** Cross section, occlusal view. **C,** Linguobuccal section, mesial view. (Zeisz and Nuckolls.)

PERTINENT DATA
Mandibular First Premolars

	Right	Left
Universal Code	28	21
International Code	44	34
Palmer notation	4⏋	⌐4
Number of roots	1	
Number of pulp horns	1 or 2	
Number of cusps	2	
Number of developmental lobes	4	

Location of proximal contact areas
MESIAL AND DISTAL: Just cervical to junction of occlusal and middle thirds

Height of contour
FACIAL: Cervical third, 0.5 mm
LINGUAL: Middle third, 1 mm

Identifying characteristics
These premolars have two cusps, one large buccal and one small lingual. The buccal cusps are centered directly over the root. The lingual

cusps are centered lingual to the root and are afunctional and nonoccluding. The occlusal surface slopes sharply lingual in a cervical direction. The mesiobuccal cusp ridge is shorter than the distobuccal cusp ridge. It has a mesiolingual developmental groove and one root.

Mandibular Second Premolars

	Right	Left
Universal Code	29	20
International Code	45	35
Palmer notation	5⌉	⌈5
Number of roots		1
Number of pulp horns		2 or 3
Number of cusps		2 or 3
Number of developmental lobes		5 4 3 B / 2 L

Location of proximal contact areas
MESIAL AND DISTAL: Just cervical to junction of occlusal and middle thirds
Height of contour
FACIAL: Cervical third, 0.5 mm
LINGUAL: Middle third, 1 mm
Identifying characteristics
These premolars have two or three cusps. The buccal cusp is very large. If two lingual cusps are present, the mesiolingual is the larger. Although the lingual cusps are larger than on the first premolar, they are afunctional and do not occlude with the maxillary teeth. A second premolar has more secondary anatomical features and more variation than any other tooth except a third molar. The two-cusp form has a U- or H-groove pattern. A mesiolingual groove is rare and is poorly developed if present. The three-cusp form has a lingual developmental groove between the two lingual cusps. The single root is longer and larger than that of a first premolar.

REVIEW QUESTIONS

1. In which one of the following is a maxillary second premolar different from a maxillary first premolar?
   a. number of developmental lobes
   b. size of cusps and number of roots
   c. existence of a central groove
   d. location of proximal contacts
2. Which of the following best describes the functional cusp(s) of a mandibular first premolar?
   a. both facial and lingual
   b. facial
   c. lingual
   d. neither facial nor lingual
3. Which tooth in the human dentition is derived from five developmental lobes?
   a. maxillary right first premolar
   b. maxillary right second premolar
   c. mandibular left first premolar
   d. mandibular right second premolar
4. When comparing the mandibular and maxillary first premolars,
   a. the facial cusp of a mandibular premolar is more lingually located.
   b. the lingual cusp is more facially located.
   c. the occlusal surface of a mandibular first premolar is relatively large.
   d. the occlusal outline is wider mesiodistally in the lingual portion of the mandibular first premolar.
5. A maxillary first premolar may be identified by
   a. a noticeable mesial concavity in the cervical area.
   b. rounded cusps of nearly equal height.
   c. long supplemental grooves.
   d. a single root canal.
6. Which of the following best describes the location of the proximal contacts of a maxillary second premolar?
   a. just cervical to the junction of occlusal and middle thirds
   b. just occlusal to the junction of cervical and middle thirds
   c. just cervical to the junction of cervical and middle thirds
   d. just occlusal to the junction of occlusal and middle thirds
7. The mandibular first and second premolars are distinguished with respect to
   a. the number of developmental lobes.

b. the number of root canals.

c. the incisocervical location of proximal contacts.

d. the number of developmental lobes forming the facial portion.

8. A mandibular first premolar usually lacks which of the following grooves?

a. central

b. mesiolingual

c. faciolingual

d. mesial

9. Which are the three developmental grooves on the most common occlusal form of a mandibular second premolar?

a. distal, mesial, and central

b. mesial, distal, and lingual

c. centrofacial, mesiolingual, and distolingual

d. facial, lingual, and central

10. When the triangular ridge of the buccal cusp joins the triangular ridge of the lingual cusp, it is known as a

a. triangular ridge.

b. marginal ridge.

c. transverse ridge.

d. occlusal ridge.

11. One permanent premolar has the most pronounced cervical concavity of any of the premolars, which requires special consideration when a matrix band is adapted. The premolar and the proximal surface where the concavity is located is the

a. distal surface of a mandibular second premolar.

b. mesial surface of a maxillary first premolar.

c. distal surface of a maxillary second premolar.

d. mesial surface of a maxillary second premolar.

12. Which of the permanent premolars often has fewer pulp horns than the other premolars?

a. maxillary first premolar

b. maxillary second premolar

c. mandibular first premolar

d. mandibular second premolar

13. A cusp has how many ridges?

a. 2

b. 3

c. 4

d. 5

14. If you examined an extracted premolar tooth and found a single root, a symmetrical rounded effect of the crown in all aspects, and many secondary grooves arising from the central groove, you could assume it to be a

a. maxillary first premolar.

b. maxillary second premolar.

c. mandibular first premolar.

d. mandibular second premolar.

15. A premolar with a root that is most commonly bifurcated is a

a. maxillary first premolar.

b. mandibular first premolar.

c. maxillary second premolar.

d. mandibular second premolar.

33

Molars

The twelve permanent molars are the largest and strongest teeth in the mouth by virtue of their crown bulk size and their root anchorage in bone (Fig. 33-1).

The permanent molars erupt long after all the deciduous teeth have already erupted. The first permanent molars erupt distal to the primary second molars. In humans the first permanent teeth to erupt are the first molars. It is only after these molars have erupted that the permanent incisors begin replacing the deciduous incisors.

The following chart shows the approximate eruption time for molars. Bear in mind that there is much individual variation. Which teeth usually erupt first, the mandibular or the maxillary? Whose teeth usually erupt first, boys' or girls'? (Refer to Chapter 24.)

The molars are nonsuccedaneous teeth; that is, they do not replace any primary teeth. They are referrred to as **accessional,** or nonsuccedaneous, as opposed to succedaneous teeth, which do replace deciduous teeth.

Generally the first molars are formed from five lobes, but some second and third molars may have only four. The lobes in Fig. 33-2 are numbered in the order of their size, number 1 being the largest.

In general each cusp of a molar is formed from its own lobe. For instance, a maxillary first molar forms from five lobes, three of which form major cusps. These major cusps are large and well developed, characteristic of and usually present on all maxillary molars—first, second, or third. The fourth lobe on a maxillary first molar forms a minor cusp. A minor cusp has smaller proportions and less development. It is less functional than the major cusps and may not always be present on the second and third molars. The maxillary first molars have a fifth lobe, which develops into a supplementary cusp. A supplementary cusp is completely afunctional and is not usually present on either the second or third molars. First molars are the most highly developed and largest of the molars and are more likely to have minor and supplementary cusps in addition to their major cusp.

The maxillary molars have only three major cusps, one minor cusp, and sometimes one supplementary cusp. The mandibular molars usually have four major cusps and sometimes one minor cusp. (See Figs. 24-4 and 24-5.)

The minor cusps of the maxillary teeth are the distolingual cusps; those on the mandibular teeth are the distal cusps. The supplementary cusp, which is afunctional, occurs only on a maxillary

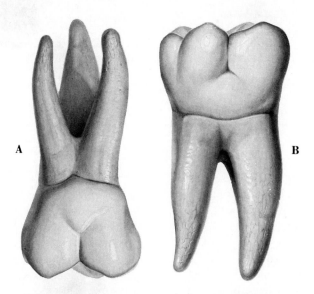

Fig. 33-1 **A,** Maxillary first molar. **B,** Mandibular first molar. (Zeisz and Nuckolls.)

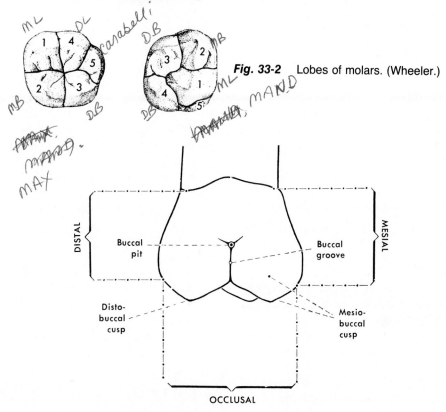

Fig. 33-2 Lobes of molars. (Wheeler.)

Fig. 33-3 Buccal surface of maxillary right first molar. (Zeisz and Nuckolls.)

Eruption times of molars

	Eruption	Enamel completion	Root completion
First molar	6 to 7 years	4 years	9-10 years
Second molar	11 to 13 years	7-8 years	14-16 years
Third molar	17-22 years	12-16 years	18-25 years

first molar. However, it may not be present at all.

In review, the most developed of the molars are the first molars, whether maxillary or mandibular. The second molars usually have no supplementary cusps, and the minor cusps will be even more minor in relation to the major cusps. Third molars may not develop minor cusps at all. A maxillary third molar may have only three major cusps, or a mandibular third molar may have four major cusps. (See Figs. 24-4 and 24-5.)

After studying the molar-cusp developmental relationships, it is easy to understand that the primary function of the molars is to grind up or crush food.

Maxillary molars
FIRST MOLARS

Evidence of calcification	Birth
Enamel completed	4 years
Eruption	6-7 years
Root completed	9-10 years

The maxillary first molars are normally the largest teeth in the maxillary arch. There are three molars on each side—the first, second, and third maxillary molars. Each has three well-developed major cusps and one minor cusp, all of which are functional. The fifth, or supplemental, cusp, which is afunctional, is called the cusp or tubercle of Carabelli. This fifth cusp, or the remnant of it, is usually found on all maxillary first molars.

The crown of a first molar is broad mesiodistally and buccolingually and just slightly wider buccolingually than mesiodistally. Of the four functional cusps, two are found on the buccal and two on the lingual side.

Facial (Buccal) Aspect (Figs. 33-3 and 33-8, *A*)

From the buccal view, four cusps can usually be seen—mesiobuccal, distobuccal, mesiolingual, and distolingual. The two lingual cusps are not located directly behind the buccal cusp but are distal and lingual to them. Although the mesiobuccal cusp is broader than the distobuccal cusp, the distobuccal is usually sharper and longer. The mesiobuccal cusp forms an obtuse angle (more than 90 degrees) where its mesial slope meets its distal slope at the cusp tip. The distobuccal cusp usually forms a less obtuse angle where the mesial slope meets the distal slope.

The buccal developmental groove divides the two buccal cusps. This groove runs in a line parallel to the long axis of the tooth, terminating halfway from its point of origin to the cervical line of the crown. Although not very deep at any point, at its terminal end it splits into a buccal pit with two small grooves radiating from it.

The cervical line is irregular and curved, generally toward the occlusal side at the mesial and distal ends.

The mesial outline is straight from the cervical line to the mesial contact area. Below the contact area it curves distally until it reaches the mesiobuccal cusp tip. The height of curvature is just cervical to the junction of the middle and occlusal thirds.

Distally the outline of the crown is convex, and the contact area is in the center of the middle third.

Lingual Aspect (Figs. 33-4 and 33-8, *B*)

The lingual cusps alone can be seen from the lingual aspect. The mesiolingual cusp is much

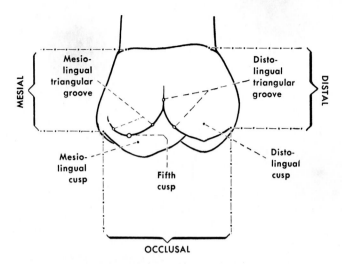

Fig. 33-4 Lingual surface of maxillary right first molar. (Zeisz and Nuckolls.)

longer and larger than either of the buccal cusps. Wider mesiodistally and buccolingually, the mesiofacial cusp is the next largest, though it is not so long as the distofacial. The distolingual cusp is the smallest and the shortest of the functional cusps. Of course, the cusp of Carabelli is the shortest and smallest of the five cusps, but it is afunctional. In fact, the cusp of Carabelli is not a cusp at all but rather a tubercle. A **fifth-cusp developmental groove,** called the **mesiolingual groove,** separates the cusp of Carabelli from the mesiolingual cusp.

The outline of the crown is as straight mesially as it is buccally. The distal outline is more convex because of the roundness of the distolingual cusp. The **lingual developmental groove** extends from the center of the lingual surface occlusally, between the two lingual cusps, where it curves sharply to the distal side and becomes the **distal oblique groove.** These two grooves (lingual and distal oblique grooves) are sometimes considered to be one, and they are then known as the **distolingual developmental groove.**

The distolingual cusp of a maxillary first molar is functional even though it is small. On a first molar the cusp occupies approximately 40% of

the lingual surface, and the mesiolingual cusp occupies the other 60%. It is interesting to note that the distolingual cusp is even progressively smaller on the maxillary second and third molars.

All three roots can be seen from the lingual aspect. On the average, the roots are about twice as long as the crown. The lingual root is usually longer than either of the two buccal roots, which are the same length.

As a general rule, the more posterior the molar, the smaller the crown. Thus a second molar has a smaller crown than a first molar. Theoretically a third molar should have an even smaller crown than a second molar. Third molars vary so much that it is necessary to preface any general rule about them by mentioning their variability.

Mesial Aspect (Figs. 33-5 and 33-8, *D*)

The mesial aspect of a maxillary first molar usually shows a clear profile of the cusp of Carabelli. The lingual crest of curvature is at the center of the middle third of the crown, the buccal crest at the cervical third. The cervical line is slightly convex mesially.

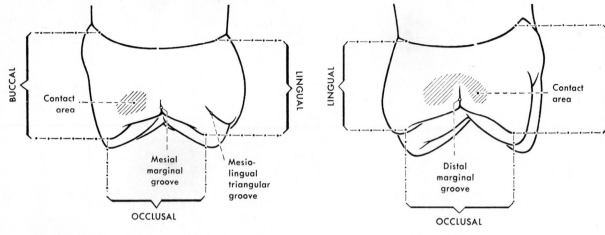

Fig. 33-5 Mesial surface of maxillary right first molar. (Zeisz and Nuckolls.)

Fig. 33-6 Distal surface of maxillary right first molar. (Zeisz and Nuckolls.)

Distal Aspect (Figs. 33-6 and 33-8, *E*)

The crown has the tendency to taper toward the distal side. The buccolingual measurement of the crown on the mesial side is greater than the same measurement distally. The cervical line is usually straighter and less curved than that on the mesial. Although the distal surface of the crown is rather convex and smooth, there is a slight concavity on the distal surface of the root trunk, from the cervical line to the distobuccal root.

The distal marginal ridge is shorter and less prominent than the mesial, and more of the occlusal surface in general can be seen from the distal view.

The distobuccal root is the narrowest of all three roots.

Occlusal Aspect (Figs. 33-7 and 33-8, *C*)

A maxillary first molar has a rhombiodal occlusal outline. The molar crown is wider mesially then distally; it is also wider lingually than buccally. This is the only tooth that is wider lingually than buccally. Is the occlusal outline of a maxillary first molar more like a square or more like a square that has been squashed sideways? What is the difference between a rhomboidal and a square form?

Notice the four functional cusps on the first molar and the one afunctional fifth cusp. A maxillary first molar has four major cusps. At least they are major in the sense that they are functional. In development, however, there are three primary developmental cusps—the two buccal cusps and the mesiolingual cusp. The distolingual and the fifth cusps are secondary. The fifth cusp is present only on a maxillary first molar as a rule and may not develop on the second and third molars. The distolingual cusp is considered a minor cusp on the second and third molars but a major cusp on the maxillary first molars. It is a minor cusp on the second and third molars because it becomes progressively smaller the more posterior the tooth. In fact, it may not be present at all on third molars.

The distolingual cusp is still a major cusp, however, on a maxillary first molar. On this tooth it is still as large as or larger than the distobuccal cusp and functions like any of the other three cusps.

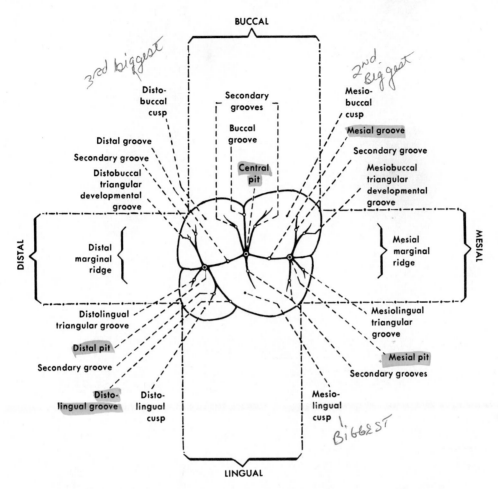

BUCCAL

3rd biggest

2nd Biggest

Disto-
buccal
cusp

Secondary
grooves

Buccal
groove

Mesio-
buccal
cusp

Mesial groove

Distal groove

Secondary groove

Secondary groove

Distobuccal
triangular
developmental
groove

Central
pit

Mesiobuccal
triangular
developmental
groove

DISTAL

Distal
marginal
ridge

Mesial
marginal
ridge

MESIAL

Distolingual
triangular groove

Mesiolingual
triangular
groove

Distal pit

Mesial pit

Secondary groove

Secondary grooves

Disto-
lingual groove

Disto-
lingual
cusp

Mesio-
lingual
cusp

BIGGEST

LINGUAL

Fig. 33-7 Occlusal surface of maxillary right first molar. (Zeisz and Nuckolls.)

There are two major fossae and two minor fossae. The major fossae are the **central fossa,** which is mesial to the oblique ridge, and the distal fossa, which is distal to the oblique ridge. The minor fossae are the mesial fossa and the distal triangular fossa, both of which are located on the inside of their respective marginal ridges.

The **central developmental pit** lies in the central fossa. The **buccal developmental groove** radiates from this pit buccally, between the two buccal cusps. The central developmental groove proceeds in a mesial direction, originating in the central developmental pit and terminating at the mesial triangular fossa. Here it is joined by the mesiofacial triangular and mesiolingual triangular grooves, which appear as branches of the **central groove.** The mesial marginal groove, a branch of the central groove, lies between these two triangular grooves and may cross the mesial marginal ridge of the crown. The **mesial pit** is found in the mesial triangular fossa.

Sometimes another developmental groove radiates from its central pit in a distal direction. If it crosses the oblique ridge, joining the central and

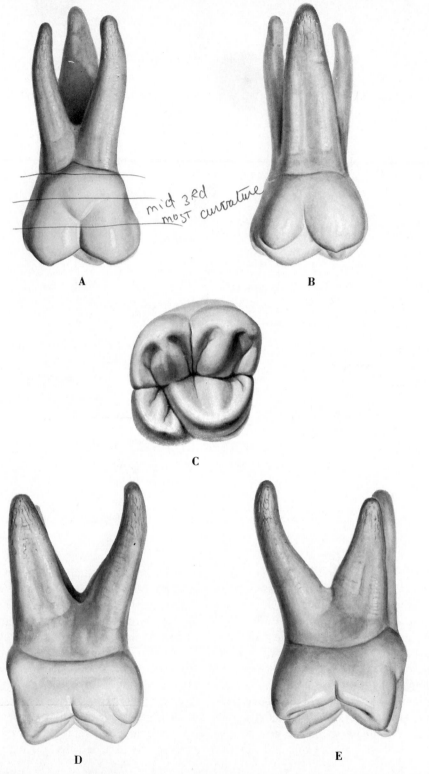

mid 3rd
most curvature

Fig. 33-8 Maxillary right first molar. **A,** Buccal view. **B,** Lingual view. **C,** Occlusal view. **D,** Mesial view. **E,** Distal view. (Zeisz and Nuckolls.)

distal fossae, it is called the **transverse groove of the oblique ridge,** or merely the distal part of the central developmental groove.

The **oblique ridge** is a transverse ridge and is peculiar to maxillary molars. A transverse ridge is formed by two triangular ridges joining together and crossing the surface of a posterior tooth diagonally rather than straight across buccolingually. In this case the triangular ridge of the mesiolingual cusp joins the triangular ridge of the distobuccal cusp. This cannot happen unless the ridges cross the tooth transversely, as opposed to buccolingually. Therefore the oblique ridge runs from the cusp tip of the mesiolingual cusp to the tip of the distobuccal cusp.

The distal fossa of a maxillary first molar runs along parallel with and distal to the oblique ridge. This fossa is linear rather than circular; it is long and narrow. In this fossa lies the distal oblique groove from which it takes its shape.

The **distal pit** is found in the distal fossa.

The distal triangular fossa is mesial to the distal marginal ridge. The distal oblique groove terminates in the distal triangular fossa, where the distal oblique groove gives off three branches, the distofacial triangular groove, the distolingual triangular groove, and the **distal marginal groove.**

It is important for you to realize that second and third molars have more secondary anatomical features than the first molars. The second molars have more secondary grooves with less well-defined cusps, less sharp ridges, and more rounded and less accentuated details. They also have more pits, not all of which occur in the usual locations.

Before we can study secondary anatomical features and grooves, it is important to know which grooves are primary.

The primary grooves of the maxillary first molars are as follows:

1. Facial groove
2. Central groove (two parts—mesial and distal)
3. Distolingual groove (two parts—lingual and distal oblique grooves)
4. Mesiolingual groove (cusp of Carabelli groove)
5. Mesial marginal groove
6. Distal marginal groove
7. Mesiofacial triangular groove
8. Mesiolingual triangular groove
9. Distolingual triangular groove
10. Distofacial triangular groove

As a point of clarification, it should be mentioned that triangular grooves are primary grooves that separate a marginal ridge from the triangular ridge of a cusp. These triangular grooves terminate in a triangular fossa. In studying the central groove, notice that the triangular groove is a continuation of the central groove. As the central groove goes toward the marginal ridge, it separates into two or three branches. The two outer Y-shaped branches curve between the marginal ridge and the triangular ridges of the buccal and lingual cusps. The part of the groove that lies between the cusp ridge and the marginal ridge is the triangular groove. The two triangular grooves are bisected by a third groove, which lies between them. This groove connects with the marginal ridge and is called the marginal groove.

SECOND MOLARS

Evidence of calcification	3 years
Enamel completed	7-8 years
Eruption	11-13 years
Root completed	14-16 years

A maxillary second molar supplements a first molar's function. Generally speaking, the differences that occur between the first and second molars are even more accentuated between the first and third molars. In other words, certain characteristics in form and development occur in a first molar that occur to a lesser degree in a second molar and possibly not at all in a third molar. What are these characteristics? Following is a list of several traits that may occur, but, in general, they have a tendency to be more accentuated in a second molar and most accentuated in a third molar.

1. The maxillary molar crowns are shorter occlusocervically and narrower mesiodistally in the second molars than in the first molars. The third molars continue to be smaller in all crown proportions, including buccolingually.

2. The molar crowns show more **supplemental (secondary) grooves** and pits on the second molars than on the first. The third molars show even more supplemental grooves, as well as **accidental (tertiary) grooves** and pits.

3. The oblique ridge is less prominent on the second molars and in some instances disappears almost entirely on the third molars.

4. The fifth lobe, or cusp of Carabelli, usually disappears on the second molars and occurs infrequently on the third molars.

5. The distolingual cusp is less developed on the maxillary second molars and disappears almost entirely on most maxillary third molars.

6. The occlusal outline of the second molars is less rhombiodal and more heart shaped. A third molar is even more heart shaped in occlusal outline.

7. The roots of the second molars have a tendency to lie closer together and may even be fused.

8. The mesiobuccal roots of the second and third molars have a greater tendency to curve toward the distal side in their apical third. The distobuccal root of a maxillary second molar is straighter than that of a maxillary first molar, with little or no mesial curvature. The third molar's distobuccal root has a tendency to curve toward the distal side in its apical third.

9. The roots of the second molars are almost as long as, sometimes even longer than, those of the first molars. The roots of the third molars are almost always smaller than those of either the first or second molars.

10. The second molars show more variety of form than the first molars, not only in the crown but also in root development. The third molars show unlimited variety in crown and root formations and are often congenitally missing.

Facial (Buccal) Aspect (Figs. 33-9 and 33-14, *A*)

The crown is shorter cervicoocclusally and narrower mesiodistally than that of a maxillary first molar. The distobuccal cusp is smaller.

The buccal roots are about the same length and are closer together. The distobuccal root is straighter up and down with no mesial curvature. The mesiobuccal root has a greater curvature toward the distal side at its apical third.

Lingual Aspect (Figs. 33-10 and 33-14, *B*)

There is no fifth cusp (cusp of Carabelli) on a maxillary second molar. The distolingual cusp is smaller than that of the first molars.

Mesial Aspect (Figs. 33-11 and 33-14, *D*)

Although the crown is shorter, its buccolingual measurement is about the same as that of a maxillary first molar. The roots are closer together.

Distal Aspect (Figs. 33-12 and 33-14, *E*)

The distobuccal cusp is smaller, thus more of the mesiobuccal cusp can be seen from this angle.

Occlusal Aspect (Figs. 33-13 and 33-14, *C*)

The occlusal outline of the crown of a maxillary second molar is less rhomboidal. The increase in size of the mesiolingual cusp and the absence of the cusp of Carabelli makes this possible. Also the distolingual cusp gets smaller.

The mesiodistal diameter of the crown is smaller, but the buccolingual diameter is about the same as that of a maxillary first molar.

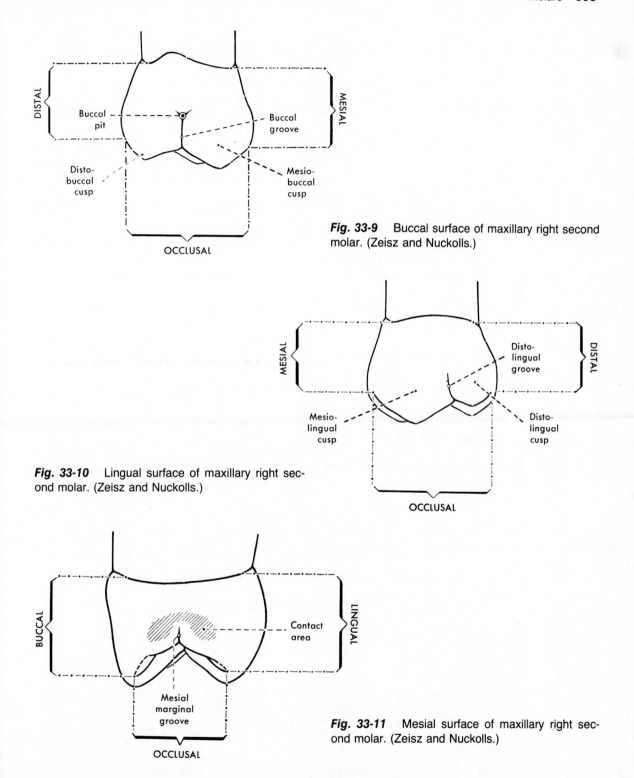

Fig. 33-9 Buccal surface of maxillary right second molar. (Zeisz and Nuckolls.)

Fig. 33-10 Lingual surface of maxillary right second molar. (Zeisz and Nuckolls.)

Fig. 33-11 Mesial surface of maxillary right second molar. (Zeisz and Nuckolls.)

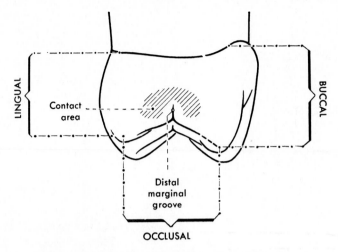

Fig. 33-12 Distal surface of maxillary right second molar. (Zeisz and Nuckolls.)

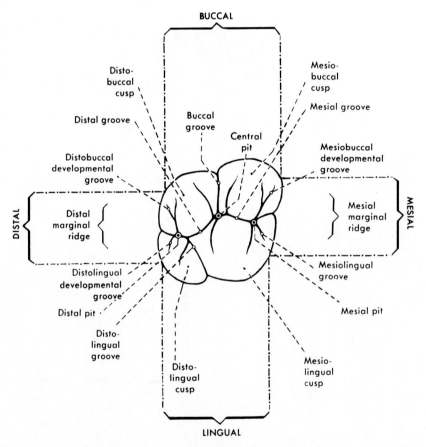

Fig. 33-13 Occlusal surface of maxillary right second molar. (Zeisz and Nuckolls.)

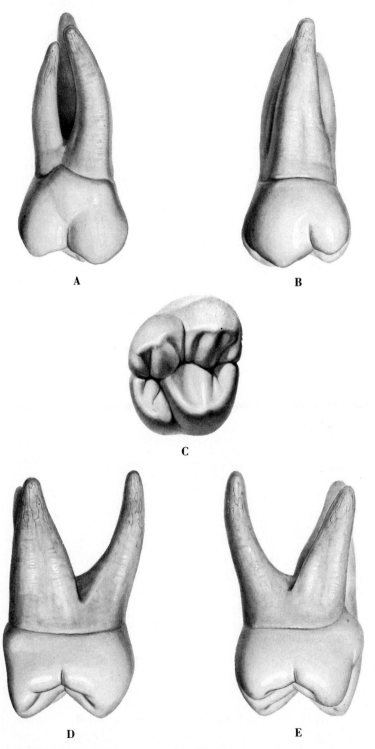

Fig. 33-14   Maxillary right second molar. **A,** Buccal view. **B,** Lingual view. **C,** Occlusal view. **D,** Mesial view. **E,** Distal view. (Zeisz and Nuckolls.)

The mesiobuccal and mesiolingual cusps are just as developed as in a first molar. The distobuccal cusp is just barely smaller, and the distolingual cusp noticeably smaller.

More supplemental grooves and pits are present on a maxillary second molar than on a maxillary first molar.

THIRD MOLARS

Evidence of calcification	7 years
Enamel completed	12-16 years
Eruption	17-22 years
Root completed	18-25 years

A maxillary third molar varies more than any other maxillary tooth in size, shape, and relative position to the other teeth. Rarely is it as well developed as a maxillary second molar. It often appears as a developmental anomaly or does not form at all. What term is descriptive of the latter situation?

The crown of a third molar is shorter than that of a second molar. The roots tend to fuse, resulting in one fused root.

The occlusal outline of a maxillary third molar is heart shaped. The distolingual cusp is poorly developed or even absent (Figs. 33-15).

Mention should be made at this point of the tendency of third molars to become impacted. If a tooth does not erupt because it is obstructed by bone or another tooth, or if it is prevented from eruption because of the angle at which it is situated within the bone, it is said to be impacted. Third molars, maxillary or mandibular, have a greater tendency to be impacted than any other teeth.

The impaction of third molars is to a large extent caused by an underdeveloped jaw and hence insufficient space to accommodate them. Thus they are blocked out and prevented from erupting.

Our ancestors' need for third molars was critical. The eruption of the third molars helped to push together the remaining teeth, especially necessary if a portion of or a whole tooth was lost through attrition or accident.

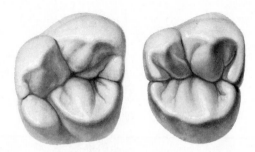

Fig. 33-15 Occlusal view of maxillary third molars. (Zeisz and Nuckolls.)

As civilization advanced, survival became less dependent on keeping one's teeth. More and more persons survived without third molars. Today congenital absence of third molars presents no problem whatsoever. A modern genetic trend in humans, which is becoming more dominant, is congenitally missing third molars. More and more persons will never have one or more third molars formed, and they will suffer no consequences because of it.

ROOTS (Figs. 33-16 to 33-19)

Maxillary molars are **trifurcated** and have three roots—mesiobuccal, distobuccal, and lingual—connected to a single **root trunk.** These trifurcated roots give maxillary molars sturdy anchorage against forces that would tend to displace them. The lingual root is the longest, and the distobuccal is the shortest.

All three roots are usually visible from the buccal view. The two buccal roots incline distally, with the mesiobuccal root starting to curve at its middle third. The distal root is usually straighter and tends to curve mesially at its middle third.

A deep developmental groove runs buccally between the bifurcation and the cervical line. The point of bifurcation of the two buccal roots is located about 4 mm above the cervical line. The point of bifurcation of deciduous molars is much less. Deciduous molars have a shorter root trunk than permanent molars. The buccal roots

Comparison chart of maxillary molars

Aspect	First molar	Second molar	Third molar
Buccal	Widest of the three mesio-distally	Intermediate in width mesiodistally	Smallest in width
	Buccal cusps equal in height	Distobuccal cusps slightly shorter than mesiobuccal	Distobuccal cusps much shorter than mesiobuccal
	Distobuccal root apex curves toward mesial	Distobuccal root straight	All roots show pronounced distal inclination
Lingual	Distolingual cusp well formed	Distolingual cusps smaller in width and height	Distolingual cusp usually missing
Mesial	Mesial marginal ridge tubercles numerous and pronounced	Mesial marginal ridge tubercles less numerous and less pronounced	Mesial marginal ridge tubercles absent
Occlusal	Crown outline square to rhomboidal	Rhombiodal form more pronounced in crown outline	Triangular or heart-shaped crown outline
	Oblique ridge smaller	Oblique ridge often absent	
Roots	Wide apart	Closer together	Usually fused

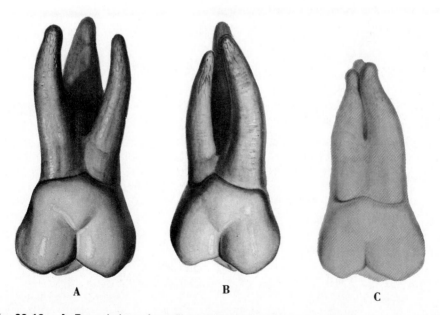

A   B   C

Fig. 33-16 **A,** Buccal view of maxillary right molars. **A,** First molar. **B,** Second molar. **C,** Third molar. Notice how roots tend to be closer together when molars are further distally. Third molar roots are often fused. (Zeisz and Nuckolls.)

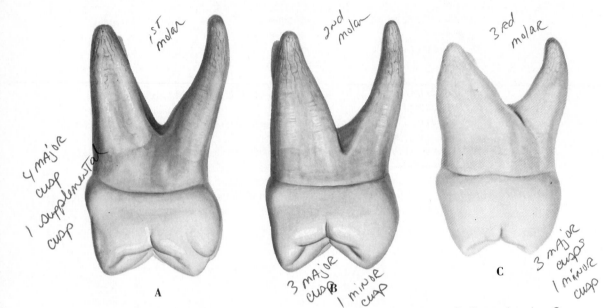

1st molar

2nd molar

3rd molar

4 major cusp 1 supplemental cusp

3 major cusp 1 minor cusp

3 major cusps 1 minor cusp

A   B   C

Fig. 33-17 Mesial view of maxillary right molars. **A,** First molar. **B,** Second molar. **C,** Third molar. Notice first molar has longest roots and third molar has shortest. (Zeisz and Nuckolls.)

of deciduous molars flare apart rather than curve toward each other.

The following are several characteristics of maxillary molar roots.

1. The roots become shorter the further posterior the maxillary molar. The maxillary first molar has the longest roots, and the third molar the shortest.

2. The roots become less divided the further posterior the maxillary molar. The roots of the maxillary first molar are much more divided than those of the second or third molar. The third molar often tends to have fused roots.

3. The roots become more varied in shape, size, and direction of curvature the more posterior the maxillary molar.

PULP CAVITY (Figs. 33-18 and 33-19)

The pulp cavity of maxillary molars consists of a pulp chamber and three main pulp canals, one for each root. The lingual root canal is by far the largest. The distobuccal is the smallest. The mesiobuccal is slightly larger than the distobuccal.

There is a tendency for the maxillary first molar to have four root canals, with two canals in the mesiobuccal root. In the fused-root form there may be only one large root with one root canal. If there are four roots, as in some maxillary third molars, there may be four root canals, one for each root.

There usually is one pulp horn for each cusp. The maxillary molars would then have four pulp horns—mesiobuccal, distobuccal, mesiolingual, and distolingual.

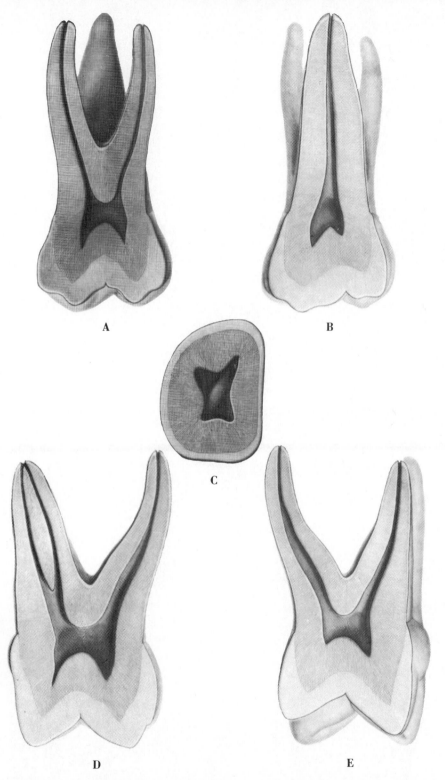

Fig. 33-18 Pulp cavity of maxillary right first molar. **A,** Mesiodistal section, buccal view. **B,** Distomesial section, lingual view. **C,** Cross section, occlusal view. **D,** Linguobuccal section, mesial view. **E,** Buccolingual section, distal view. Notice that mesiobuccal root has two root canals within one root. (Zeisz and Nuckolls.)

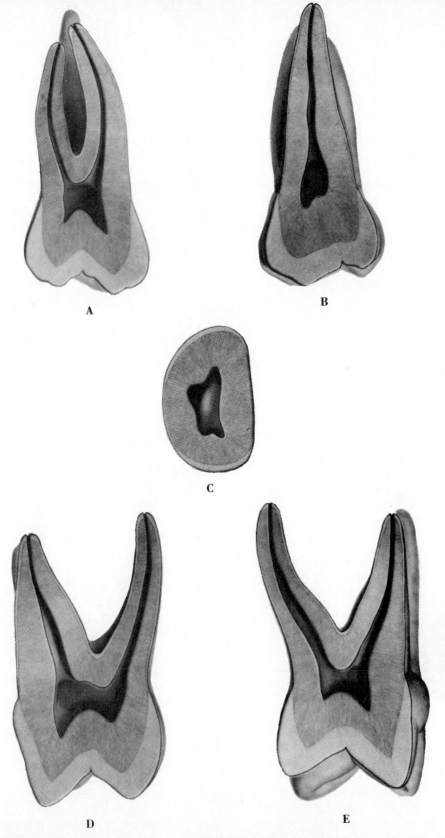

A

B

C

D

E

Fig. 33-19 For legend see opposite page.

PERTINENT DATA
Maxillary First Molars

	Right	Left
Universal Code	3	14
International Code	16	26
Palmer notation	6⌋	⌊6
Number of roots		3
Number of pulp horns		4
Number of cusps		4
		5 (including cusp of Carabelli)
Number of developmental lobes		5

Location of proximal contact areas
MESIAL: Middle third
DISTAL: Middle third
Height of contour
FACIAL: Cervical third, 0.5 mm
LINGUAL: Middle third, 0.5 mm
Identifying characteristics
A cusp of Carabelli may be present. The occlusal outline is square or rhomboidal rather than triangular. The distolingual cusp is well developed. There is a prominent oblique ridge and distal facial and lingual grooves. The crown is nearly as wide mesiodistally as buccolingually. The three roots are widely separated.

Maxillary Second Molars

	Right	Left
Universal Code	2	15
International Code	17	27
Palmer notation	7⌋	⌊7
Number of roots		3
Number of pulp horns		4
Number of cusps		4
Number of developmental lobes		4

Location of proximal contact areas
MESIAL: Middle third
DISTAL: Middle third

Height of contour
FACIAL: Cervical third, 0.5 mm
LINGUAL: Middle third, 0.5 mm
Identifting characteristics
These teeth are similar to maxillary first molars except that the fifth cusp is usually absent and the distolingual cusp is less well developed. The oblique ridge is less prominent. The crown is shorter occlusocervically and narrower mesiodistally. It is just as wide buccolingually. The occlusal outline of the crown is rhomboidal to heart shaped. The three roots are less separated.

Maxillary Third Molars

	Right	Left
Universal Code	1	16
International Code	18	28
Palmer notation	8⌋	⌊8
Number or roots		1 to 4
Number of pulp horns		1 to 4
Number of cusps		3 to 5
Number of developmental lobes		4

Location of proximal contact areas
MESIAL: Middle third
DISTAL: None
Height of contour
FACIAL: Cervical third, 0.5 mm
LINGUAL: Middle third, 0.5 mm
Identifying characteristics
These teeth vary more in form than any others. They usually do not have a distolingual cusp. The occlusal outline is heart shaped, with three cusps. The roots, usually three, have a tendency to be very close together or to fuse with an extreme distal inclination.

REVIEW QUESTIONS
1. Which cusp of a maxillary first molar has the widest mesiodistal measurement?

Fig. 33-19 Pulp cavity of maxillary right second molar. **A,** Mesiodistal section, buccal view. **B,** Distomesial section, lingual view. **C,** Cross section, occlusal view. **D,** Linguobuccal section, mesial view. **E,** Buccolingual section, distal view. (Zeisz and Nuckolls.)

2. Which two cusps join to form the oblique ridge?

3. Which of the five cusps is the least developed? *carabelli*

4. Which of the four functional cusps is least developed? DL

5. On which cusp is the tubercle of Carabelli located? DL

6. Which cusps surround the central fossa? Distal fossa?

7. Are the terms "mesiolingual groove" and "developmental groove of the cusp of Carabelli" synonymous? SAME thing

8. Are the terms "distolingual groove" and "distal oblique groove" synonymous? SAME thing

9. Are the terms "mesiolingual triangular groove" and "mesiolingual groove" synonymous?

10. If a mesial pit is present on a maxillary first molar, in which fossa will it occur? Where is the distal pit found?
    a. central fossa
    b. distal fossa
    c. mesial triangular fossa
    d. distal triangular fossa

11. Which of the following is more likely to be present only on maxillary first molars?
    a. oblique ridge
    b. distolingual cusp
    c. cusp of Carabelli
    d. distobuccal root with its apex curved slightly toward the mesial side

12. Of the three roots of a maxillary molar, which is most likely to help differentiate the maxillary first, second, and third molars from each other? MB root curve more D.

13. Which cusp is more likely to be smaller on a maxillary second molar than on a maxillary first molar?
    a. distobuccal cusp
    b. distolingual cusp

14. The roots of a maxillary second molar lie closer together than the roots of which tooth?
    a. maxillary first molar
    b. maxillary third molar

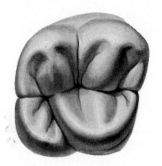

Fig. 33-20

15. Which two cusp ridges make up the transverse oblique ridge? ML → DB

16. Identify the tooth and label the developmental grooves in Fig. 33-20.

Mandibular molars

The permanent mandibular molars are larger than any other mandibular teeth. There are three on each side—the first, second, and third mandibular molars. They occupy the posterior segment of each mandibular quadrant. Like their maxillary antagonists, they show a progressive decrease in size the more posterior the tooth. Which molars will therefore be the smallest? 3rd molar

The crowns of the mandibular molars are shorter cervicoocclusally than those of the teeth anterior to them, but in all other dimensions the molars are larger. The roots are not as long as some of the mandibular roots, but their bifurcation results in excellent anchorage.

The crowns of the mandibular molars are wider mesiodistally than buccolingually. Is this also true of the maxillary molars? If not, how is it different? opposite

Certain traits distinguish mandibular molars from maxillary molars.

1. Mandibular molars, as a rule, have only two roots, one mesial and one distal. How many do the maxillary molars have? 3

2. Generally there are four major cusps on

mandibular molars; if a fifth cusp is present, it is a minor cusp.

3. The crowns are always broader mesiodistally than buccolingually.

4. Mandibular molars have two buccal cusps that are nearly equal in size. They also have two lingual cusps that are almost equal in size.

A first mandibular molar is often considered the anchor tooth in the mandibular dentition because it is the first permanent mandibular tooth to erupt. Eruption occurs around 6 years of age.

The mandibular molars function as chewing or grinding tools.

FIRST MOLARS

Evidence of calcification	Birth
Enamel completed	3 years
Eruption	6 years
Root completed	9-10 years

The mandibular first molars are usually the first permanent teeth to erupt. They are the only mandibular molars that usually have five cusps—two buccal and two lingual, which are major, and one distal, which is minor.

Mandibular molars generally have two roots, one mesial and one distal. What other teeth have two roots? Are the roots mesial and distal or buccal and lingual?

The mandibular first molars are normally the largest teeth in the mandibular arch, with a crown usually about 1 mm longer mesiodistally than buccolingually. *mesial ROOT broader*

Facial (Buccal) Aspect (Figs. 33-21 and 33-26, *A*)

From the buccal view, the one distal and two buccal cusps can be seen. The mesiobuccal cusp is the widest of the three; the distal cusp is the smallest. The mesiobuccal and distobuccal cusps are approximately equal in height and are separated by the mesiobuccal groove. This mesiobuccal groove often ends in a buccal pit. The distal cusp is much more conical in shape and is smaller in height and width than the other two. It is separated from a distobuccal cusp by a distobuccal groove. The cervical line on a mandibular first molar dips apically toward the root bifurcation. Whereas the entire distal profile of the

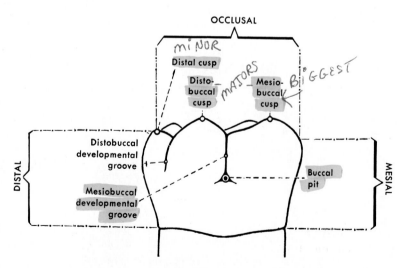

Fig. 33-21 Buccal surface of mandibular right first molar. (Zeisz and Nuckolls.)

crown is convex, only the mesial profile of the crown is convex at the middle and occlusal thirds; the cervical third is concave. Both the mesial and distal crown profiles converge toward the cervical side so that the cervical third of the crown is narrower than the occlusal third.

The roots of this tooth are well formed. The mesial root is almost perpendicular to the middle third of the root. From this point it curves distally toward its apex, which is located directly below its apex, which is located directly below and in line with the mesiobuccal cusp. The distal root shows little curvature and projects distally from the root base. The two roots are widely separated at their apices but share a common root base.

Lingual Aspect (Figs. 33-22 and 33-26, *B*)

Two cusps of almost equal size, mesiolingual and distolingual, make up the lingual profile. The lingual developmental groove separates these two cusps. The lingual cusps are higher and more pointed than the two buccal cusps.

A portion of the distal cusp can be seen from the mesial aspect. The tooth is wider on the buc-

cal than on the lingual side. From the lingual view notice the convergence from the distal to the distolingual cusp.

The mesial and distal profiles of the lingual aspect are both convex. The crest of contour, which represents the contact area, is somewhat higher on the mesial than on the distal side; however, both are in the middle third of the tooth.

The bifurcation of the two roots begins with the bifurcation groove on the root trunk located directly in line with the lingual developmental groove.

The lingual surface is rather flat in comparison with the convex buccal surface. The cervical line is rather straight mesiodistally.

Mesial Aspect (Figs. 33-23 and 33-26, *D*)

From the mesial aspect, two cusps can be seen, the mesiolingual and the mesiobuccal. The mesiolingual is the higher and more conical of the two.

Only one root, the mesial, can be seen from the mesial view.

The mesial marginal ridge has a prominent

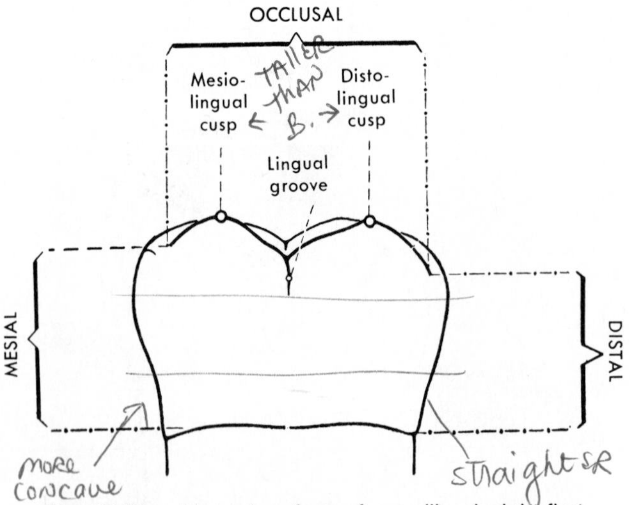

higher than D.

Fig. 33-22 Lingual surface of mandibualr right first molar. (Zeisz and Nuckolls.)

crest, which is divided by the mesial marginal groove, located lingual to the center of the crown.

The buccal profile is marked by the buccocervical ridge—a slight bulge in the cervical third of the buccal surface.

The lingual height of contour is located at the center of the middle third of the tooth on the lingual surface.

The cervical line tends to curve occlusally about 1 mm in the center of the mesial surface. It is located higher on the lingual than on the buccal side by almost 1 mm.

The buccolingual measurements of the crown, root, and cusps are all greater on the mesial than on the distal surface. The mesial cusp is also higher than the distal cusp.

Distal Aspect (Figs. 33-24 and 33-26, *E*)

The distolingual cusp is the largest of the three cusps visible from the distal aspect. The distobuccal cusp is next in size, and the distal cusp is the smallest. The distobuccal groove can be seen separating the latter two cusps. The distal marginal ridge, not so wide as the mesial marginal ridge, is bisected by the distal marginal groove. This groove is lingual to the center of the tooth.

The crown of a first molar tapers and converges distally, so that if a specimen of the tooth is held with the distal surface of the crown at a right angle to the line of vision, a greater portion of the occlusal surface is visible than from the mesial aspect. The distal contact area is located on the distal cusp and is centered over the distal root.

Occlusal Aspect (Figs. 33-25 and 33-26, *C*)

The occlusal view of a mandibular first molar shows five cusps, four major and one minor. All five are functional. What is the minor cusp? What differentiates a major cusp from a minor cusp?

The occlusal outline of the tooth is pentagonal and shows a tapering convergence toward the distal and lingual sides. Not only are the mesial cusps wider buccolingually than the distal cusps, but the mesiodistal measurement of the three buccal cusps together is much larger than the same measurement for two lingual cusps combined.

The mesiobuccal cusp is wider than either of

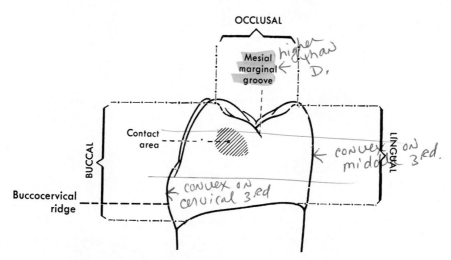

Fig. 33-23 Mesial surface of mandibular right first molar. (Zeisz and Nuckolls.)

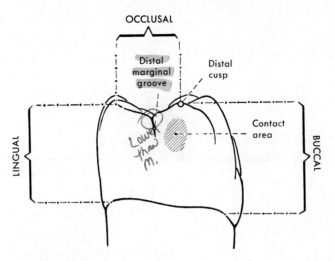

OCCLUSAL

Distal marginal groove

Distal cusp

Lower than M.

Contact area

LINGUAL

BUCCAL

Fig. 33-24 Distal surface of mandibular right first molar. (Zeisz and Nuckolls.)

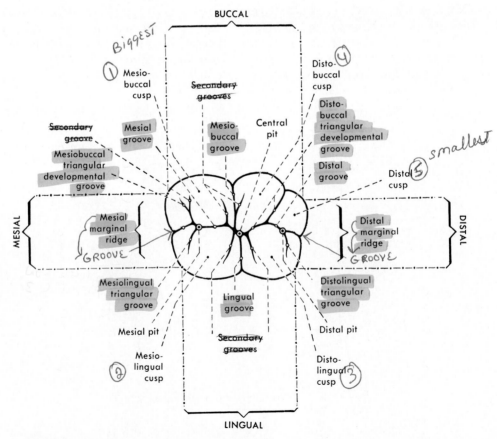

BUCCAL

BIGGEST ①

Mesio-buccal cusp

Secondary grooves

Disto-buccal cusp ④

Secondary groove

Mesial groove

Mesio-buccal groove

Central pit

Disto-buccal triangular developmental groove

smallest ⑤

Mesiobuccal triangular developmental groove

Distal groove

Distal cusp

Mesial marginal ridge

GROOVE

Distal marginal ridge

GROOVE

MESIAL

DISTAL

Mesiolingual triangular groove

Lingual groove

Distolingual triangular groove

Mesial pit

Secondary grooves

Distal pit

Mesio-lingual cusp ②

Disto-lingual cusp ③

LINGUAL

Fig. 33-25 Occlusal surface of mandibular right first molar. (Zeisz and Nuckolls.)

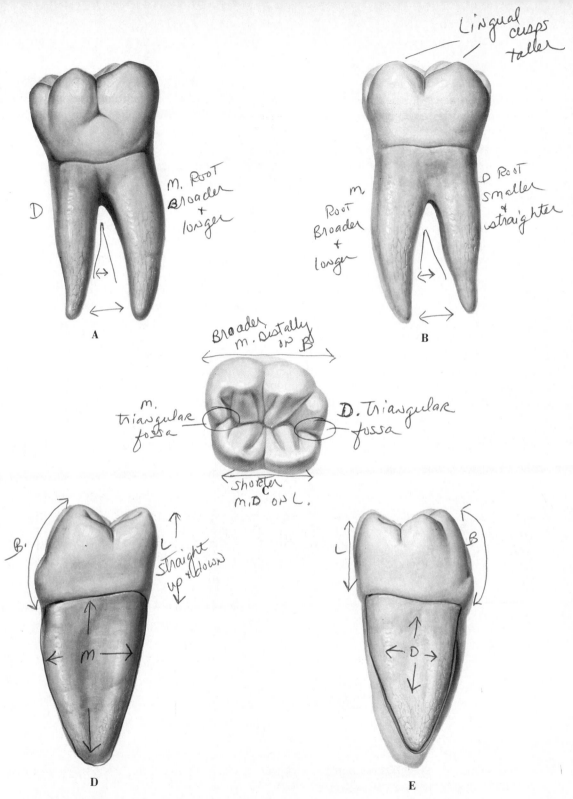

Fig. 33-26 Mandibular right first molar. **A,** Buccal view. **B,** Lingual view. **C,** Occlusal view. **D,** Mesial view. **E,** Distal view. (Zeisz and Nuckolls.)

the lingual cusps, which are about the same size. The distobuccal cusp is smaller than any of these three, and the distal is the smallest of all five.

The developmental grooves that separate these cusps are the **central developmental groove,** the **mesiobuccal developmental groove,** the **distobuccal developmental groove,** and the **lingual developmental groove.** All the developmental grooves converge at the cental pit in the center of the central fossa. The central fossa of the occlusal surface is a concave area bordered by the distal slope of the mesiofacial cusp, the mesial and distal slopes of the distofacial cusp, the mesial slope of the distal cusp, the distal slope of the mesiolingual cusps, and the mesial slope of the distolingual cusp. Two other fossae are present, the mesial triangular fossa (just inside the mesiodistal marginal ridge) and the distal triangular fossa (a slight depression that is just mesial to the central portion of the distal marginal ridge).

The mesiobuccal groove separates the mesiofacial and distofacial cusps and extends onto the buccal surface. The distobuccal groove separates the distofacial and distal cusps. The lingual groove separates the two lingual cusps and continues onto the lingual surface. The two buccal grooves and the lingual groove form a Y-shaped pattern on the occlusal surface of the crown.

Mesial and distal marginal ridge grooves may also be present. Several supplemental grooves radiate from the mesial and distal pits (mesial and distal pits are usually found in the mesial and distal triangular fossa, respectively).

SECOND MOLARS

Evidence of calcification	2-3 years
Enamel completed	7-8 years
Eruption	11-13 years
Root completed	14-15 years

The mandibular second molars resemble the mandibular first molars, buccally and lingually, except that there usually is not a fifth, or distal, cusp. The roots of the second molar are shorter, closer together, and more distally inclined.

All four cusps of the mandibular second molars are nearly equal in size. Occlusally the second molars have a more rectangular shape than the first molars have.

Facial (Buccal) Aspect (Figs. 33-27 and 33-32, A)

Facially the first and second molars are similar, except that a second molar crown is not so long mesiodistally and is slightly shorter cervicoocclusally. A second molar has only two buccal cusps separated by a single buccal groove. These two cusps, the mesiobuccal and the distobuccal, are equal in their mesiodistal measurements.

The roots of a second molar may be somewhat shorter and are usually located closer together than the roots of a first molar. They are also more distally inclined in relation to the occlusal plane of the crown. The roots of a third molar are angled even more distally in relation to the occlusal plane.

Lingual Aspect (Figs. 33-28 and 33-32, B)

The crown converges far less lingually than that of a first molar because there is no distal cusp. The two lingual cusps, mesiolingual and distolingual, are nearly the same size and are separated by a lingual groove. This groove sometimes terminates in a lingual pit. The contact areas are at a lower level mesially and especially distally.

Mesial Aspect (Figs. 33-29 and 33-32, D)

The cervical line shows less curvature than a first molar does, and the mesial root is less broad. Otherwise the mesial view is the same for both molars.

Distal Aspect (Figs. 33-30 and 33-32, E)

On the distal view, the most noticeable difference between the first and second molars is the absence of a distal cusp. The contact area is therefore centered both buccolingually and cervicoocclusally.

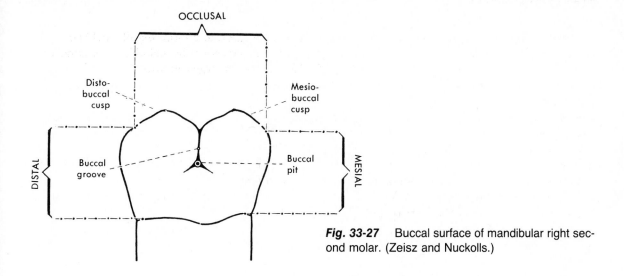

OCCLUSAL

Disto-
buccal
cusp

Mesio-
buccal
cusp

DISTAL

Buccal
groove

Buccal
pit

MESIAL

Fig. 33-27 Buccal surface of mandibular right second molar. (Zeisz and Nuckolls.)

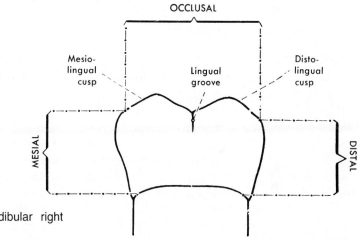

OCCLUSAL

Mesio-
lingual
cusp

Lingual
groove

Disto-
lingual
cusp

MESIAL

DISTAL

Fig. 33-28 Lingual surface of mandibular right second molar. (Zeisz and Nuckolls.)

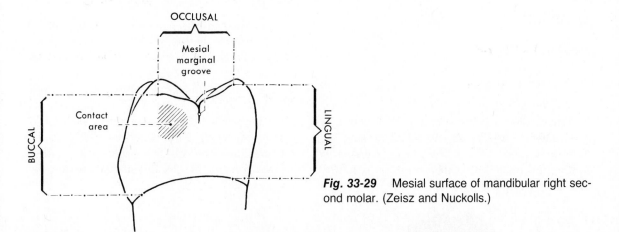

OCCLUSAL

Mesial
marginal
groove

Contact
area

BUCCAL

LINGUAL

Fig. 33-29 Mesial surface of mandibular right second molar. (Zeisz and Nuckolls.)

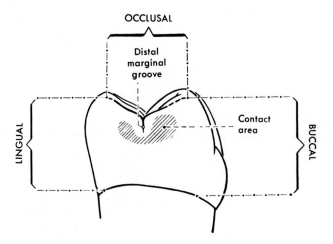

Fig. 33-30 Distal surface of mandibular right second molar. (Zeisz and Nuckolls.)

Occlusal Aspect (Figs. 33-31 and 33-32, *C*)

The occlusal outline of a second molar is rectangular. All four cusps are equal in size.

The developmental grooves are the buccal groove, the lingual groove, and the central developmental groove. They traverse the occlusal surface in a cross (+) pattern. There are more secondary grooves than on a first molar. The four triangular grooves include a distofacial, a distolingual, a mesiofacial and a mesiolingual. Three pits may be present—a mesial, a distal, and a central.

THIRD MOLARS

Evidence of calcification	8-10 years
Enamel completed	12-16 years
Eruption	17-21 years
Root completed	18-15 years

Like the maxillary third molars, the mandibular third molars are irregular and unpredictable. The crown is usually shorter in all dimensions than on second molars, though it is possible to find a third molar larger than even a first molar. This is an exception and not the rule.

The occlusal outline of the crown is more oval than rectangular, though the crown usually resembles those of the mandibular second molars. The two mesial cusps are larger than the two distal cusps. The occlusal surface has a very wrinkled appearance, with an irregular groove pattern and numerous pits. (Fig. 33-33).

The roots of the third molars are usually shorter than those of the second molars and are inclined acutely to the distal side. They are also very close together and often fused.

ROOTS

Mandibular molars have two roots, one mesial and one distal, with a single root trunk (bifurcated root). The mesial root is the longer and the stronger of the two. The mesial root curves mesially and then turns distally in the apical portion. The distal root is usually quite straight and may curve mesially or distally at its apical third.

The root trunk is bifurcated very close to the cervical line. The trunk is very short and is grooved on the buccal and lingual surfaces toward the bifurcation.

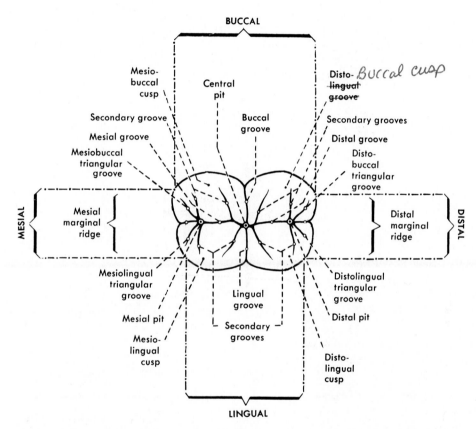

BUCCAL

Mesio-
buccal
cusp

Central
pit

Disto- *Buccal cusp*
~~lingual~~
~~groove~~

Buccal
groove

Secondary groove

Secondary grooves

Mesial groove

Distal groove

Mesiobuccal
triangular
groove

Disto-
buccal
triangular
groove

MESIAL

Mesial
marginal
ridge

Distal
marginal
ridge

DISTAL

Mesiolingual
triangular
groove

Distolingual
triangular
groove

Mesial pit

Lingual
groove

Distal pit

Mesio-
lingual
cusp

Secondary
grooves

Disto-
lingual
cusp

LINGUAL

Fig. 33-31 Occlusal surface of mandibular right second molar. (Zeisz and Nuckolls.)

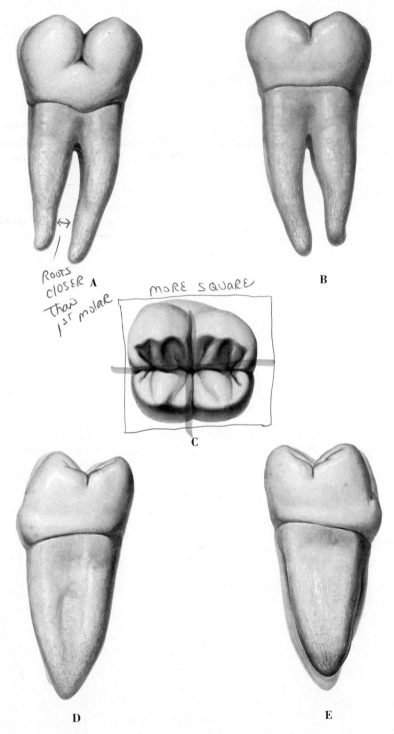

Fig. 33-32 Mandibular right second molar. **A,** Buccal view. **B,** Lingual view. **B,** Lingual view. **C,** Occlusal view. **D,** Mesial view. **E,** Distal view. (Zeisz and Nuckolls.)

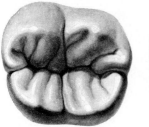

Fig. 33-33 Occlusal view of two mandibular right third molars. (Zeisz and Nuckolls.)

The following are characteristics of mandibular molar roots:

1. The roots become shorter the further posterior the molar. The mandibular first molar is therefore the longest.
2. The roots are less divided the further posterior the molar.

3. The roots become more varied in shape, size, and direction the more posterior the tooth (Figs. 33-34 and 33-35).

PULP CAVITY

The pulp cavity of the mandibular molars consists of a pulp chamber and three pulp canals, the distal, the mesiobuccal, and the mesiolingual.

The distal root canal is much larger than the other two canals and is the only canal in the distal root. The mesial root houses two root canals, the mesiobuccal and the mesiolingual. Often these two canals join into one single apical foramen; sometimes there is only one canal in the mesial root. On rare occasions there are two canals in the distal root, just as in the mesial root.

There are five pulp horns, one for each cusp. In the four-cusp form there are only four pulp horns. Which pulp horn is missing? (*Hint:* In the four-cusp form, which cusp is missing?)

 # pulp horns = # cusps

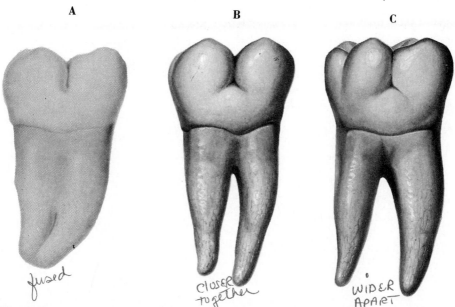

A   B   C

fused   *closer together*   *WIDER APART*

Fig. 33-34 Buccal view of mandibular right molars. **A,** Third molar. **B,** Second molar. **C,** First molar. Notice how roots get closer together and become shorter from first molar to third molar. Third molar roots are often fused.

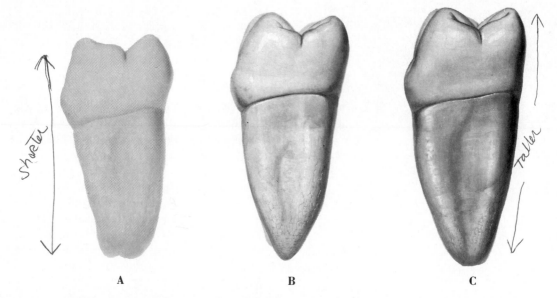

Shorter

Taller

A   B   C

Fig. 33-35 Mesial view of mandibular right molars. **A,** Third molar. **B,** Second molar. **C,** First molar. (Zeisz and Nuckolls.)

The first molar is more likely to have three root canals (distal, mesiobuccal, and mesiolingual) and five pulp horns. Although the second molar may have two canals (the mesial and the distal, one in each root), it is more likely to have three root canals. The second molar has only four pulp horns. Third molars resemble second molars in pulpal anatomy (Figs. 33-36 and 33-37).

PERTINENT DATA
Mandibular First Molars

	Right	Left
Universal Code	30	19
International Code	46	36
Palmer notation	6⌐	⌐6
Number of roots		2
Number of pulp horns		5
Number of cusps		5
Number of developmental lobes		5

Location of proximal contact areas
MESIAL: Middle third
DISTAL: Middle third

Height of contour
FACIAL: Cervical third, 0.5 mm
LINGUAL: Middle third, 1 mm
Identifying characteristics

The five cusps make these the largest mandibular teeth. They are wider mesiodistally than buccolingually. The crown converges lingually and slightly distally. The three buccal cusps are separated by two buccal grooves. The two lingual cusps are separated by one lingual groove. These three grooves converge to form a Y pattern. There are two roots, a mesial and a distal, and three root canals (the mesial root has two root canals).

Mandibular Second Molars

	Right	Left
Universal Code	31	18
International Code	47	37
Palmer notation	7⌐	⌐7
Number of roots		2
Number of pulp horns		4
Number of cusps		4
Number of developmental lobes		4

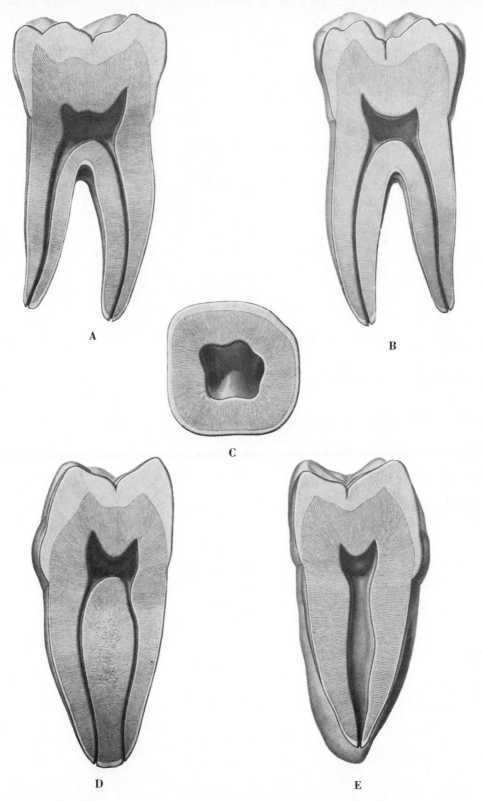

Fig. 33-36 Pulp cavity of mandibular right first molar. **A,** Mesiodistal section, buccal view. **B,** Distomesial section, lingual view. **C,** Cross section, occlusal view. **D,** Linguobuccal section, mesial view. **E,** Buccolingual section, distal view.

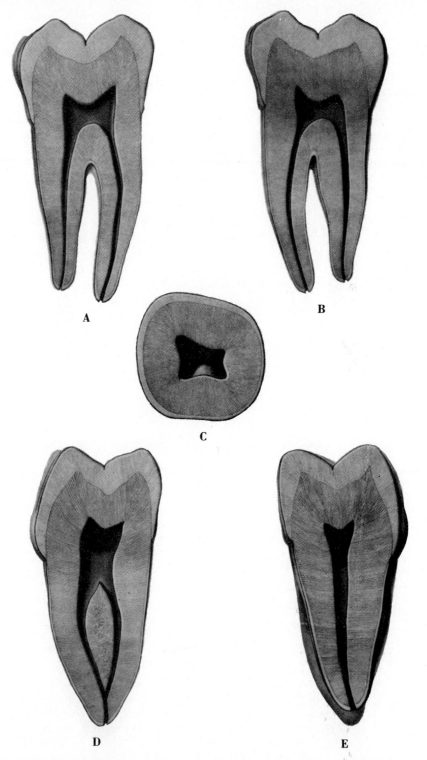

Fig. 33-37 Pulp cavity of mandibular right second molar. **A,** Distomesial section, buccal view. **B,** Mesiodistal section, lingual view. **C,** Cross section, occlusal view. **D,** Buccolingual section, mesial view. **E,** Linguobuccal section, distal view. (Zeisz and Nuckolls.)

Comparison chart of mandibular molars

Aspect	First molar	Second molar	Third molar
Buccal	Crown has widest mesiodistal diameter	Smaller crown than first molar	Smallest crown
	Three buccal cusps—mesiobuccal, distobuccal, and distal	Two buccal cusps, mesiobuccal and distobuccal	Two buccal cusps, mesiobuccal and distobuccal
	Two buccal grooves	One buccal groove	One buccal groove
	Roots widely separated and relatively vertical	Roots closer together and inclined distally	Roots short, fused, with pronounced distal inclination
Mesial	Mesial root broad	Mesial root not as broad	Same as second molar
Occlusal	Pentagonal outline	Rectangular outline	Ovoid outline
	Mesial and distal profiles straight, converging lingually	Mesial and distal profiles curved; no lingual convergence	Mesial and distal profiles highly curved; no lingual convergence
	Main grooves form Y pattern	Main grooves form a cross (+)	Grooves show no set pattern
	Large occlusal surface relative to total crown area seen from occlusal side	Occlusal table same as in first molar	More supplementary and accessory grooves
Roots	Wide apart and longest	Closer together	Usually fused, curved, shorter

Location of proximal contact areas
MESIAL: Middle third
DISTAL: Middle third
Height of contour
FACIAL: Cervical third, 0.5 mm
LINGUAL: Middle third, 1 mm
Identifying characteristics
These molars have four cusps of nearly equal size. The crown is smaller in all dimensions and has less lingual convergence. There is only one buccal groove and one lingual groove, which join together on the occlusal surface as they bisect the central developmental groove. The groove pattern is therefore a cross (+). The two roots are closer together and incline slightly distally. There is one root canal in the distal root. The mesial root can have one or two root canals.

Mandibular Third Molars

	Right	Left
Universal Code	32	17
International Code	48	38
Palmer notation	8⌋	⌊8
Number of roots	2 (fused into 1)	
Number of pulp horns	4 or 5	
Number of cusps	4 or 5	
Number of developmental lobes	4 or 5	

Location of proximal contact areas
MESIAL: Middle third
DISTAL: Middle third
Height of contour
FACIAL: Cervical third, 0.5 mm
LINGUAL: Middle third, 1 mm

Identifying characteristics

These are the most variable mandibular teeth in form. They usually resemble the mandibular second molars, with four cusps and a shallower, smaller central fossa, with more secondary and tertiary grooves. A five-cusp form is not unusual. The two roots (mesial and distal) are often fused and inclined toward the distal side.

REVIEW QUESTIONS

1. When the first and second molars of the mandibular arch are compared, which of the following is *not* true?
   a. There is only one groove visible from the facial surface on a second molar.
   b. The crown is larger both mesiodistally and faciolingually on a second molar.
   c. There is less lingual convergence on a second molar.
   d. Both have two roots.

2. When the mandibular first and second molars are compared, in what way are the two different?
   a. The first has more roots and root canals. NO
   b. The second has more pulp horns. NO
   c. The second does not have a distal cusp.
   d. The first has a different height of contour. NO

3. The lingual height of contour on all mandibular molars
   a. measures 0.5 mm.
   b. measure more than 0.5 mm. → 1 mm
   c. measures less than 0.5 mm.
   d. varies considerably from the first to the third molar.

4. An important factor concerning personal oral hygiene is that the mandibular molars
   a. do not have an oblique ridge, which helps deflect the food onto the gums. False
   b. have a greater amount of lingual contour and are therefore hard to clean. False

5. Which of the following is *not* true of a mandibular second molar?
   a. It has four cusps of nearly equal size.
   b. It has three root canals, with two in the mesial root.
   c. It has five cusps. False
   d. It has four developmental lobes.

6. Which of the following is a list of correct names for the cusps of a mandibular first molar?
   a. mesiolingual, mesiofacial, distolingual, distofacial, cusp of Carabelli
   b. central, mesial, distal, facial, lingual NO
   c. mesiolingual, mesiofacial, distolingual, distofacial, distal
   d. distolingual, distofacial, mesiolingual, mesiofacial

7. The roots of a mandibular first molar are
   a. facial and lingual.
   b. mesial, distal, and central.
   c. facial, lingual, and middle.
   d. mesial and distal.

8. When comparing all maxillary and mandibular molars, fused roots would most likely be found on which of the following?
   a. first molars
   b. second molars
   c. third molars
   d. all of the above

9. What is a major difference between first and second molars, whether maxillary or mandibular?
   a. First molars usually have four cusps, and second molars have three.
   b. First molars usually have five cusps, and second molars have four.
   c. First molars have more supplemental grooves.
   d. Second molars are wider mesiodistally.

10. Which of the following is true concerning maxillary and mandibular molars?
    a. Both have oblique ridges.
    b. Only maxillary molars have oblique ridges.
    c. Neither have oblique ridges.
    d. Only mandibular molars have oblique ridges.

11. Two root canals are commonly found in
    a. the lingual root of maxillary first molars.
    b. the distal root of mandibular first molars.
    c. the mesial root of mandibular first molars.
    d. none of the above.
12. "Furcation" refers to
    a. the absence of a particular characteristic of the root anatomy.
    b. the splitting of a root trunk into terminal roots.
    c. the division of root canals from the root trunk.
    d. none of the above.

34

Deciduous Dentition

OBJECTIVES

- To identify the various deciduous teeth
- To recognize whether a tooth is primary or secondary
- To know the eruption dates of the primary and secondary teeth
- To understand the essential differences between deciduous and permanent teeth
- To understand the importance and functions of deciduous teeth
- To compare the dental anatomical feature of deciduous teeth, not only with the other deciduous teeth but also with their permanent counterparts

The deciduous dentition is made up of primary teeth in humans. These teeth are shed and then replaced by their permanent successors. This process of shedding the deciduous teeth and replacement by the permanent teeth is called exfoliation. Exfoliation begins 2 or 3 years after the deciduous root is completely formed. At this time the root begins to resorb at its apical end, and resorption continues in the direction of the crown until the entire root is resorbed and the tooth finally falls out.

The primary, or deciduous, dentition consists of 20 teeth, each quadrant containing two incisors, one canine, and two molars (Fig. 34-1).

The first deciduous teeth to erupt, about 8 months after birth, are the mandibular central incisors. The maxillary central incisors usually erupt about a month later. As in the permanent teeth, the primary mandibular teeth usually erupt

before the maxillary. Following is an approximate eruption schedule of the deciduous teeth. (See Fig. 24-6.)

Central incisors	8-12 months
Lateral incisors	9-13 months
First molars	13-19 months
Canines	16-22 months
Second molars	25-33 months

ESSENTIAL DIFFERENCES BETWEEN DECIDUOUS AND PERMANENT TEETH

1. The deciduous anteriors are smaller than their permanent successors in both their crown and root proportions. Deciduous molars are wider mesiodistally than the permanent premolars, which will take their places.
2. The roots of deciduous anterior teeth are narrower and longer in comparison with crown length, as well as tooth length and width, than are the permanent teeth roots.
3. The roots of deciduous posterior teeth are very narrow at their cervical enamel junctions where the crowns join the roots. In addition the root trunks of deciduous molars are very short.
4. The cervical ridge of enamel at the cervical third of the anterior crown labially and lingually is much more prominent in the deciduous dentition. These bulky ridges extend out from the very narrow cervical necks of the teeth.
5. The buccocervical ridges on the deciduous molars are much more pronounced, especially on first molars. These cervical prominences give deciduous crowns a bulbous ap-

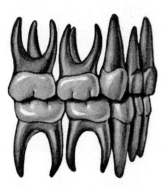

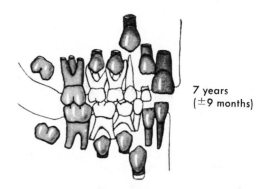

7 years
(±9 months)

Fig. 34-1   Deciduous teeth. (Massler and Schour.)

Fig. 34-2   Premolars rest between deciduous molar roots. Gray teeth are permanent; white teeth are primary. (Massler and Schour.)

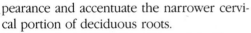

pearance and accentuate the narrower cervical portion of deciduous roots.

6. The buccal and lingual surfaces of deciduous molars taper occlusally above the cervical curvatures much more than the permanent molar surfaces. This results in a much narrower **occlusal table** of the occlusal surface buccolingually.

7. The roots of the deciduous molars are more slender and longer than the roots of the permanent teeth. These roots also flare apically to allow room between the roots for the developing permanent tooth crowns (Fig. 34-2).

8. The deciduous teeth are usually lighter in color than the permanent teeth. The deciduous teeth have a whiter color with a bluish cast. Permanent teeth have more yellow, grey, or brown tones.

9. The pulp chambers are relatively large in comparison with the deciduous crowns that envelop them.

10. The pulp horns extend rather high occlusally, placing them much closer to the enamel than in the permanent teeth.

11. The dentin thickness between the pulp chambers and the enamel is much less than in the permanent teeth.

12. The enamel is relatively thin and has a consistent depth (Fig. 34-3).

IMPORTANCE OF DECIDUOUS TEETH

The importance of the deciduous teeth cannot be stressed enough. These teeth are extremely important for the proper development of the muscles of mastication, the formation of the bones of the jaws, and the eventual location, alignment, and occlusion of the permanent teeth. Indeed, the succedaneous teeth develop as buds from the deciduous tooth buds.

The deciduous teeth maintain a place for the permanent teeth. It is the function of the deciduous teeth to allow for bone growth of the dental arches by their eruption.

As the bone continues to grow, the deciduous teeth develop spaces between them called "primate spaces."

The spaces between the deciduous canines and first molars and those between the first and second molars are called "leeway spaces." They allow an extra margin of space for the eruption of the permanent canine, first premolar, and second premolar. Leeway space is necessary because several offsetting factors are present. First, the mesiodistal measurement of the two permanent premolars combined is less than the sum of the mesiodistal measurement of the deciduous molars. Although this allows extra room for the premolars, the permanent canine requires more room than the deciduous canine, which is

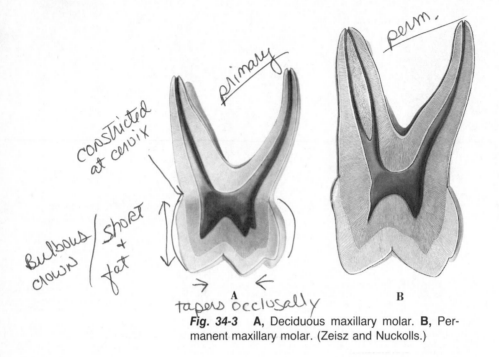

primary

perm.

constricted at cervix

Bulbous crown / short + fat

tapers occlusally

Fig. 34-3 **A,** Deciduous maxillary molar. **B,** Permanent maxillary molar. (Zeisz and Nuckolls.)

smaller. Second, growth allows the possibility of leeway space, but this is offset by the phenomenon of mesial drift. The first permanent molar tends to move mesially; thus the amount of space reserved for the permanent premolars is shortened. If a deciduous molar is prematurely lost or a decayed interproximal space is not restored, a permanent molar will push into this space and block out the premolar. There is very little extra space, if any. (See Fig. 25-3).

In addition, the resorption of the deciduous roots helps to guide their erupting permanent replacements into the proper location. The succedaneous teeth follow the resorbing root through the bone until the deciduous tooth exfoliates from a lack of root anchorage. When a deciduous tooth exfoliates, its permanent replacement can often be seen directly underneath it. Sometimes a thin layer of gum may be covering it; usually it is not completely impacted with bone.

MAXILLARY CENTRAL INCISORS
Labial Aspect (Figs. 34-4 and 34-7, *A*)

A deciduous central incisor's mesiodistal diameter is greater than its cervicoincisal length, whereas a permanent central incisor's cervicoincisal length is greater than its mesiodistal diameter. No mamelons are visible.

Lingual Aspect (Figs. 34-5 and 34-7, *B*)

From the lingual aspect, the crown shows well-developed marginal ridges and a highly developed cingulum.

Mesial and Distal Aspects (Figs. 34-6 and 34-7, *D* and *E*)

From the proximal aspects, the crown appears wide in relation to its total length. Because of its short length, the labiolingual measurements make the crown appear thick, even at the incisal third. The mesiocervical curvature is greater than the distal curvature.

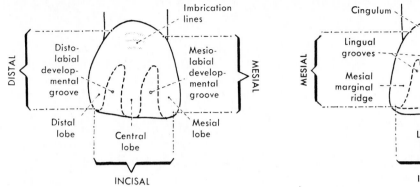

Fig. 34-4 Labial surface of maxillary right central incisor. (Zeisz and Nuckolls.)

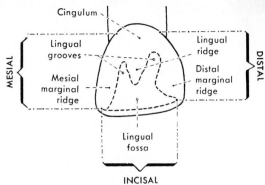

Fig. 34-5 Lingual surface of maxillary right central incisor. (Zeisz and Nuckolls.)

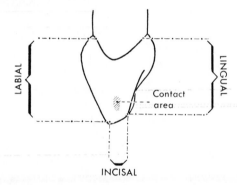

Fig. 34-6 Mesial surface of maxillary right central incisor. (Zeisz and Nuckolls.)

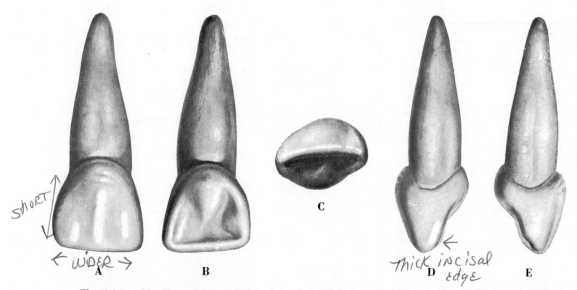

Fig. 34-7 Maxillary right central incisor. A, Labial view. B, Lingual view. C, Incisal view. D, Mesial view. E, Distal view. (Zeisz and Nuckolls.)

Incisal Aspect (Fig. 34-7, *C*)

From the incisal surface, the crown appears much wider mesiodistally than labiolingually. The incisal edge appears nearly straight.

MAXILLARY LATERAL INCISORS

A lateral incisor's crown is smaller in all dimensions, except that the cervicoincisal length is greater than its mesiodistal width. In all other ways it appears similar to a central incisor. The root appears much longer in proportion to the crown when compared with the central (Fig. 34-8).

Roots of Maxillary Incisors

The root appears constricted at the cervical third. It is twice as long as the crown and tapers evenly toward a blunt apex. There is a mesial concavity on the root surface, but the distal surface is generally convex. The lateral surface is longer and more tapered than the central.

MANDIBULAR CENTRAL INCISORS
Labial Aspect (Figs. 34-9 and 34-13, *A*)

Mamelons, or grooves, may be visible. The crown appears wide in comparison with its permanent successor. The mesial and distal sides of the crown taper evenly from the contact areas. The root may be two to three times the height of the crown. It is very narrow and is also conical in shape.

Lingual Aspect (Figs. 34-10 and 34-13, *B*)

The lingual surface appears smoothly contoured and tapers toward the cingulum. The marginal ridges are less pronounced than those of the primary maxillary incisors.

Mesial and Distal Aspects (Figs. 34-11 and 34-13, *D* and *E*)

From the mesial aspect, the incisal ridge is centered over the root. The labial and lingual cervical contours are quite convex, much more

so than those of the permanent mandibular incisors. Cervical curvature is greater on the mesial than on the distal side.

Incisal Aspect (Figs. 34-12 and 34-13, *C*)

The incisal ridge is centered over the crown of the tooth. The labial surface appears flat with a slight convexity, whereas the lingual surface appears concave.

MANDIBULAR LATERAL INCISORS

The mandibular lateral incisors are wider and longer than the central incisors, and their cingulums more developed. Labiolingually the lateral incisors are also wider. There is a tendency for the incisal ridge to slope distally, and its distal margin is more rounded (Fig. 34-14).

Roots of Mandibular Incisors

The root of the deciduous mandibular lateral is longer than the central, narrower, and more tapered. It is less blunt at the apex. The lateral has a distal longitudinal groove and a mesial depression running lengthwise.

The central is just a little shorter and does not have any grooves or depressions on its root surfaces.

MAXILLARY CANINES
Labial Aspect (Figs. 34-15 and 34-23, *A*)

A canine is bulkier than the primary incisors in every aspect. The crown is more constricted at the cervix in relation to its mesiodistal width and more convex on its mesial and distal surfaces. The facial lobes are well developed, and a sharp cusp is evident. The root is about twice as long as the crown and more slender than that of its permanent successor.

Lingual Aspect (Figs. 34-16 and 34-23, *B*)

The mesial and distal marginal ridges, incisal ridges, and cingulum are all very pronounced. A tubercle may extend from the cusp tip to the lin-

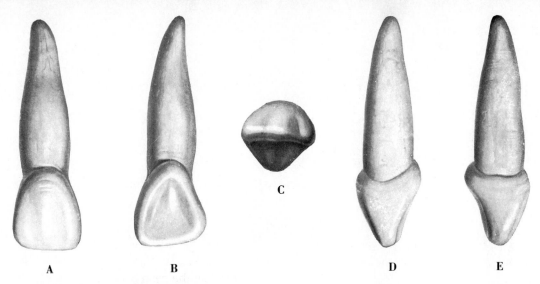

A   B   D   E

Fig. 34-8   Maxillary right lateral incisor. **A,** Labial view. **B,** Lingual view. **C,** Incisal view. **D,** Mesial view. **E,** Distal view. (Zeisz and Nuckolls.)

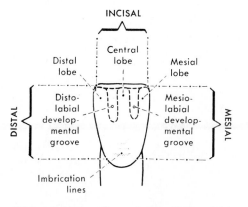

Fig. 34-9   Labial surface of mandibular right central incisor. (Zeisz and Nuckolls.)

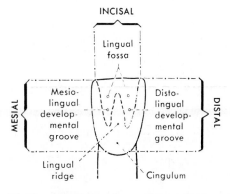

Fig. 34-10   Lingual surface of mandibular right central incisor. (Zeisz and Nuckolls.)

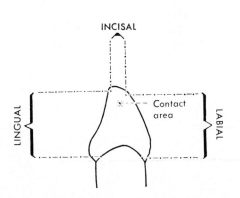

Fig. 34-11   Distal surface of mandibular right central incisor. (Zeisz and Nuckolls.)

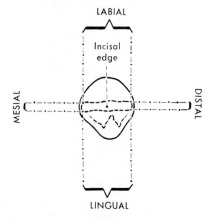

Fig. 34-12   Incisal edge of mandibular right central incisor. (Zeisz and Nuckolls.)

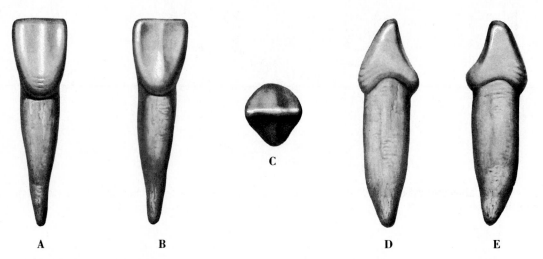

Fig. 34-13 Mandibular right central incisor. **A,** Labial view. **B,** Lingual view. **C,** Incisal view. **D,** Mesial view. **E,** Distal view. (Zeisz and Nuckolls.)

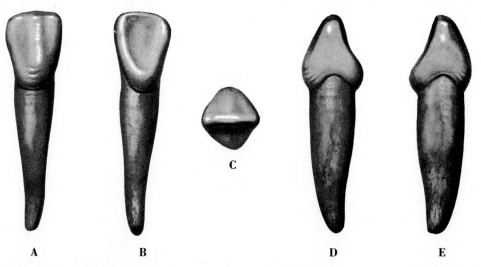

Fig. 34-14 Mandibular right lateral incisor. **A,** Labial view. **B,** Lingual view. **C,** Incisal view. **D,** Mesial view. **E,** Distal view. (Zeisz and Nuckolls.)

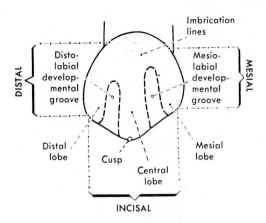

Fig. 34-15   Labial surface of maxillary right canine. (Zeisz and Nuckolls.)

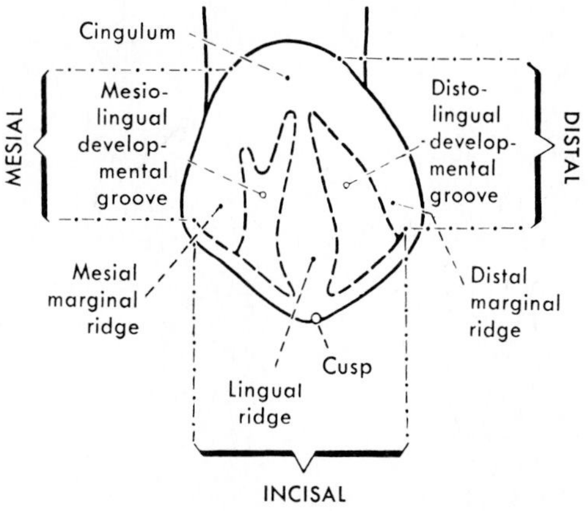

Fig. 34-16   Lingual surface of maxillary right canine. (Zeisz and Nuckolls.)

gual ridge. The lingual ridge extends from the cusp tip to the cingulum and divides the lingual surface into mesiolingual and distolingual fossae.

Mesial and Distal Aspects (Figs. 34-17 and 34-23, *D* and *E*)

The outline form is similar to that of a lateral or central incisor, except that a canine is much

wider at the cervical third of the crown. Both the crown and the root at the cervical third are wider labiolingually.

Incisal Aspect (Figs. 34-18 and 34-23, *C*)

From the incisal view, the crown is rhomboidal—like a square that has been slightly shifted. The labial ridge is relatively pronounced, and the

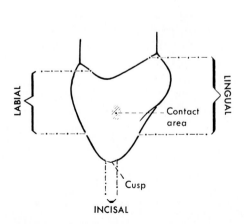

Fig. 34-17   Mesial surface of maxillary right canine. (Zeisz and Nuckolls.)

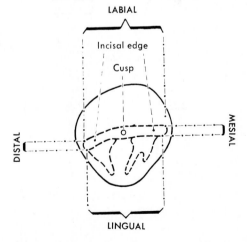

Fig. 34-18   Incisal edge of maxillary right canine. (Zeisz and Nuckolls.)

cingulum is obvious. The tip of the cusp is slightly distal to the center of the tooth.

MANDIBULAR CANINES
Labial Aspect (Figs. 34-19 and 34-24, A)

Compared with a maxillary canine, the labial surface is much flatter, with shallow developmental grooves. The distal cusp ridge is longer than that on a maxillary canine. The root is long, narrow, and almost twice the length of the crown, though shorter and more tapered than that of a maxillary canine.

Lingual Aspect (Figs. 34-20 and 34-24, B)

The most obvious difference between the maxillary and mandibular canines is the presence of a slight concavity called the lingual fossa. Instead of two lingual fossae, there is one. The lingual surface is less prominent than that on a maxillary canine, and the crown converges lingually so that it is narrower on the lingual than on the labial side.

Mesial and Distal Aspects (Figs. 34-21 and 34-24, D and E)

The outline form resembles an incisor, with the incisal ridge centered over the crown labiolingually. The labiolingual measurements are smaller than those of a maxillary canine.

Incisal Aspect (Figs. 34-22 and 34-24, C)

The incisal ridge is straight and centers over the crown labiolingually. The lingual surface shows a definite tapering toward the cingulum. The labial surface from this aspect presents a flat surface with a slight convexity, whereas the lingual surface presents a flattened surface that is slightly concave.

Roots of Canines

The roots of the deciduous canines are almost twice as long as their crowns. They are thicker than the roots of the incisors, and their apices are more blunt. The mandibular root is slightly shorter than the maxillary and more tapered. Both have roots that taper to the lingual side, as well as toward the apical. They are triangular in cross section.

MAXILLARY FIRST MOLARS
Buccal Aspect (Figs. 34-25 and 34-35, A)

The deciduous maxillary first molar is a blend of premolar and molar. It does not resemble any other tooth, deciduous or permanent. It is wider buccolingually than mesiodistally.

It has two major cusps, a mesiobuccal and a mesiolingual. There is a distobuccal cusp, but it is only about half as large as the mesiobuccal cusp.

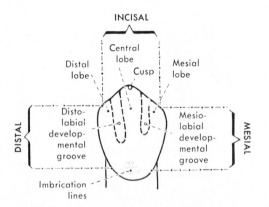

Fig. 34-19 Labial surface of mandibular right canine. (Zeisz and Nuckolls.)

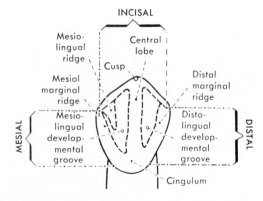

Fig. 34-20 Lingual surface of mandibular right canine. (Zeisz and Nuckolls.)

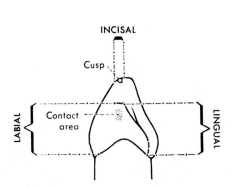

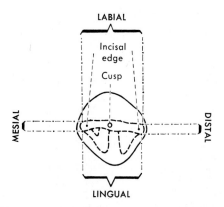

Fig. 34-21   Mesial surface of mandibular right canine. (Zeisz and Nuckolls.)

Fig. 34-22   Incisal edge of mandibular right canine. (Zeisz and Nuckolls.)

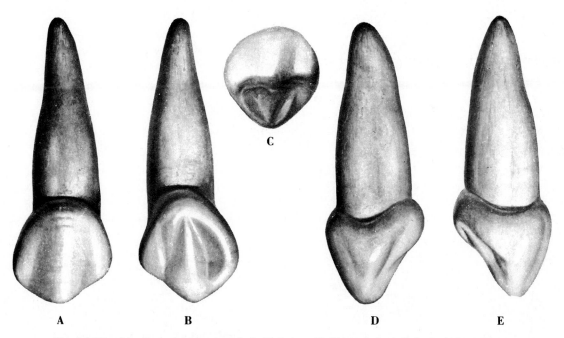

A   B   C   D   E

Fig. 34-23   Maxillary right canine. **A,** Labial view. **B,** Lingual view. **C,** Incisal view. **D,** Mesial view. **E,** Distal view. (Zeisz and Nuckolls.)

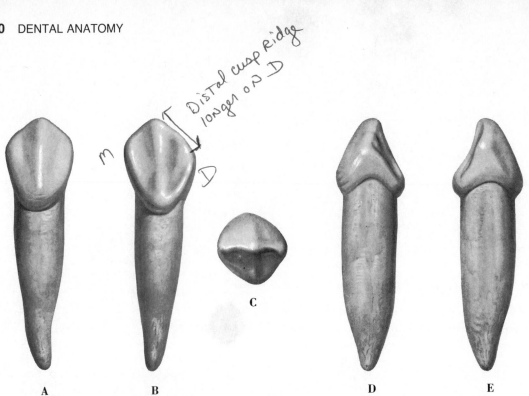

Distal cusp ridge longer on D

Fig. 34-24 Mandibular right canine. **A,** Labial view. **B,** Lingual view. **C,** Incisal view. **D,** Mesial view. **E,** Distal view. (Zeisz and Nuckolls.)

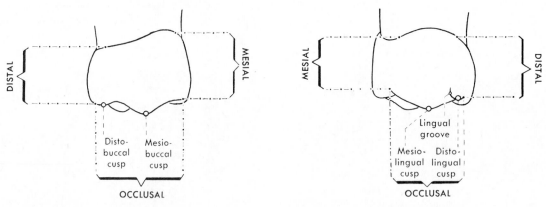

Fig. 34-25 Buccal surface of maxillary right first molar. (Zeisz and Nuckolls.)

Fig. 34-26 Lingual surface of maxillary right first molar. (Zeisz and Nuckolls.)

Lingual Aspect (Figs. 34-26 and 34-35, *B*)

The crown converges toward the lingual surface.

The mesiolingual cusp is the longest and sharpest cusp on this tooth. The distolingual cusp is small and rounded, if present at all. There is also a type of deciduous maxillary first molar that has only three cusps—one lingual and two buccal.

The lingual root is larger than the other two roots. A tiny tubercle can sometimes be seen on the mesiolingual cusps, but it cannot be called a cusp of Carabelli.

Mesial Aspect (Figs. 34-27 and 34-35, *D*)

The buccolingual measurement at the cervical third is greater than the same measurement at the occlusal third. This is true of all molar teeth, but it is more evident on the deciduous teeth. The mesiolingual cusp is more pronounced and longer in size than the mesiobuccal cusp. The most obvious difference between the deciduous and permanent molars is that the deciduous first molars have an extreme convexity in the cervical third of the buccal surface (buccocervical ridge). This convexity appears to be overdeveloped when compared with that of the permanent and deciduous teeth. It is a major characteristic of the deciduous maxillary first molars. The cervical line curves slightly toward the occlusal side.

Distal Aspect (Figs. 34-28 and 34-35, *E*)

The crown appears to be narrower distally than mesially. The distobuccal cusp is more developed than the distolingual, which is not always present. The cervical convexity (buccocervical ridge) on the buccal surface does not continue onto the distal surface.

Occlusal Aspect (Figs. 34-29 and 34-35, *C*)

The crown converges in a lingual direction so that the occlusal table appears triangular. The crown may have three or four cusps. If four are present, two will be on the buccal and two on the lingual. If three cusps develop, only one will be lingual.

The occlusal surface is similar to that of the permanent molars except that the occlusal table is smaller in comparison. On the three-cusp form there is only a central and a mesial pit (no distal pit), and an oblique ridge often unites the mesiolingual with the distofacial cusps. The central groove connects the two fossae—the central fossa and the mesial triangular fossa. The buccal developmental groove is well developed and divides the two buccal cusps occlusally. The mesial, mesiofacial triangular, mesial marginal, and mesiolingual triangular grooves originate in the mesial pit. The distal, facial, and mesial developmental grooves radiate from the central pit.

On the four-cusp form, there are three fossae,

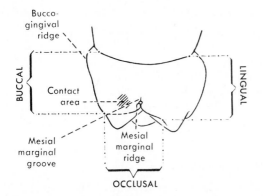

Fig. 34-27 Mesial surface of maxillary right first molar. (Zeisz and Nuckolls.)

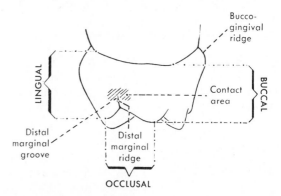

Fig. 34-28 Distal surface of maxillary right first molar. (Zeisz and Nuckolls.)

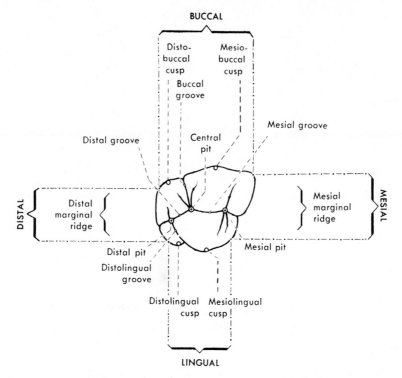

BUCCAL

Disto-buccal cusp

Mesio-buccal cusp

Buccal groove

Mesial groove

Distal groove

Central pit

DISTAL

Distal marginal ridge

Mesial marginal ridge

MESIAL

Distal pit

Mesial pit

Distolingual groove

Distolingual cusp

Mesiolingual cusp

LINGUAL

Fig. 34-29 Occlusal surface of maxillary right first molar. (Zeisz and Nuckolls.)

mesial, central, and distal. A small pit is usually present in each fossa. Grooves originating at the distal pit are the distofacial triangular, the distolingual, and the distal marginal. An oblique ridge runs from the distobuccal cusp to the mesiolingual cusp.

Roots of Maxillary First Molars

There are three roots, two buccal and one lingual. They are long, slender, and very flared. The lingual root is longer and more curved and tips back toward the buccal at the apex. The mesiobuccal root is the next longest; the distobuccal is the shortest and the straightest.

The root trunk becomes trifurcated immediately above the cervical line. The root trunk is proportionately small when compared to the length of the roots. Each root has a single root canal.

MAXILLARY SECOND MOLARS
Buccal Aspect (Figs. 34-30 and 34-36, A)

A deciduous maxillary second molar resembles a permanent maxillary first molar, though it is much smaller. From the buccal view two equal-sized buccal cusps, with a buccal groove between them, are visible. As on a deciduous first molar, the crown is narrow at its cervix, compared with its mesiodistal measurement at the contact area. A deciduous second molar is much larger than a deciduous first molar both in crown and root formation. The two buccal cusps are about equal in size. How is this different from the cusps of a deciduous first molar?

Lingual Aspect (Figs. 34-31 and 34-36, B)

From the lingual view the crown shows three cusps—a mesiolingual, a distolingual, and a supplemental cusp. The mesiolingual cusp is large

1). Maxillary first molar - Left (#14)   Wandat
Szzy

2). Mandibular right 2cnd premolar (#29)

3). Mandibular right central incisor (#26)

4). Maxillary #≠ Left 3rd molar (#16)

5). Mandibular left lateral incisor (#23)

(1)

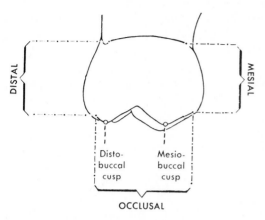

Fig. 34-30   Buccal surface of maxillary right second molar. (Zeisz and Nuckolls.)

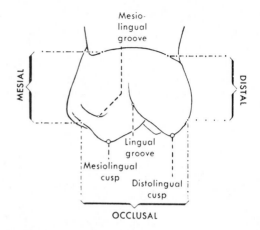

Fig. 34-31   Lingual surface of maxillary right second molar. (Zeisz and Nuckolls.)

and well developed. The distolingual cusp is more developed than that of a deciduous first molar but still small in comparison with the two buccal and the mesiolingual cusps. The supplemental cusp, which resembles a cusp of Carabelli, is a fifth cusp on this tooth. It is poorly developed and is located on the lingual surface of the mesiolingual cusp. It is separated from the mesiolingual cusp by a developmental groove. A lingual developmental groove separates the mesiolingual and distolingual cusps.

Mesial Aspect (Figs. 34-32 and 34-36, *D*)

From the mesial view this tooth resembles a permanent molar, though it is smaller. In comparison with a deciduous first molar, the crown is 0.5 mm longer and about 2 mm wider buccolingually, and the roots are up to 2 mm longer. The lingual root curves much the same way as those of the first molars. The supplemental fifth cusp is visible lingual and apical to the mesiolingual cusp, which is large in comparison with the mesiobuccal cusp.

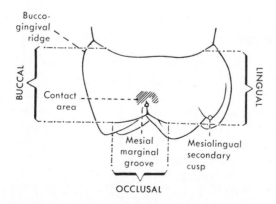

Fig. 34-32   Mesial surface of maxillary right second molar. (Zeisz and Nuckolls.)

Distal Aspect (Figs. 34-33 and 34-36, *E*)

From the distal view the crown appears smaller than from a mesial aspect, but not to the same degree as found on a deciduous maxillary first molar. The distobuccal and distolingual cusps are about the same length. A rather straight cervical line is evident both distally and mesially.

Occlusal Aspect (Figs. 34-34 and 34-36, *C*)

From the occlusal view this tooth resembles a permanent first molar. It has four well-developed cusps and one supplemental cusp—mesiobuccal, distobuccal, mesiolingual, distolingual, and the fifth cusp. The developmental grooves (pits, oblique ridge, and so forth),

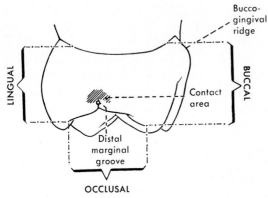

Fig. 34-33   Distal surface of maxillary right second molar. (Zeisz and Nuckolls.)

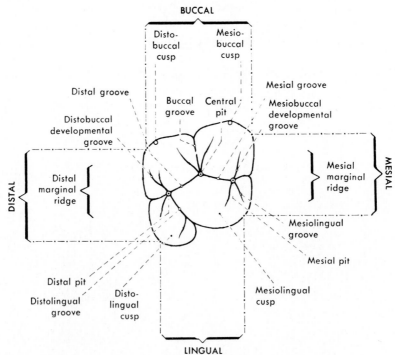

Fig. 34-34   Occlusal surface of maxillary right second molar. (Zeisz and Nuckolls.)

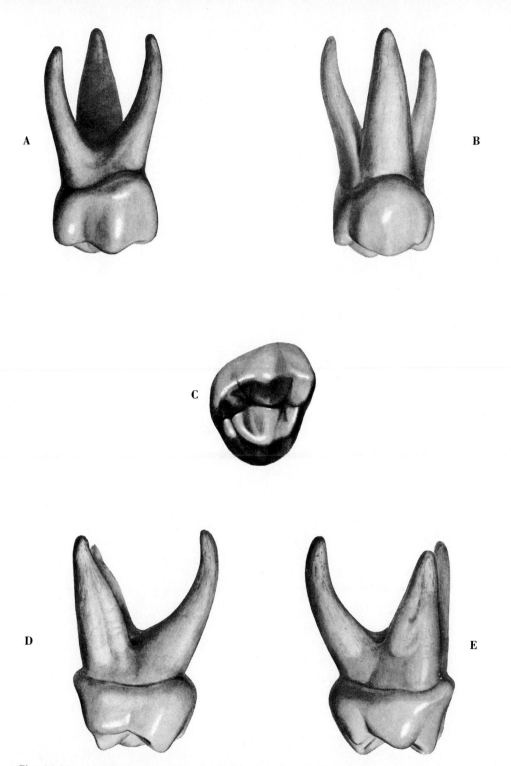

Fig. 34-35 Maxillary right first molar. **A,** Buccal view. **B,** Lingual view. **C,** Occlusal view. **D,** Mesial view. **E,** Distal view. (Zeisz and Nuckolls.)

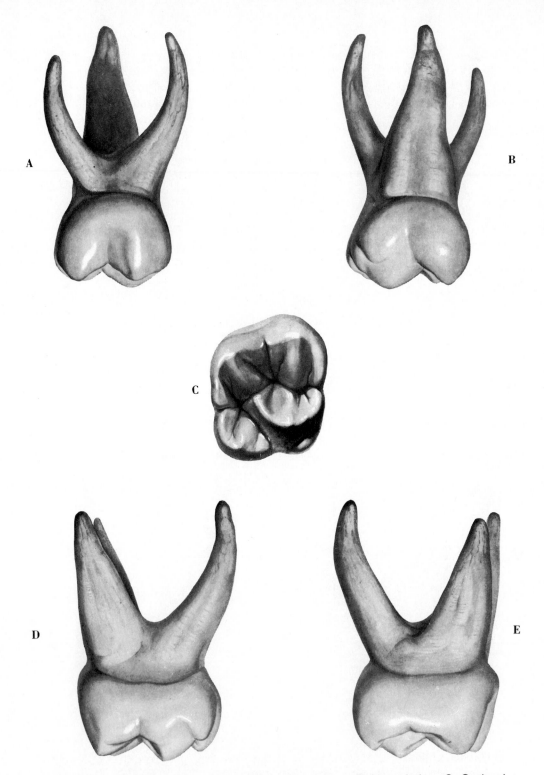

Fig. 34-36   Maxillary right second molar. **A,** Buccal view. **B,** Lingual view. **C,** Occlusal view. **D,** Mesial view. **E,** Distal view. (Zeisz and Nuckolls.)

though less defined, are almost identical to those found on a permanent first molar. The mesiolingual cusp is the largest and the distolingual the smallest, except for the fifth cusp.

Roots of Maxillary Second Molars

There are three roots, two buccal and one lingual. Like the deciduous first molar, the deciduous maxillary second molar's longest root is the lingual and its shortest is the distobuccal. Unlike the first molar the mesiobuccal root may be as long as the lingual. The root trunk is short, and each of the roots has only one root canal.

MANDIBULAR FIRST MOLARS
Buccal Aspect (Figs. 34-37 and 34-47, A)

A primary mandibular first molar does not resemble any of the other teeth, deciduous or permanent. Its mesial outline is rather flat straight up and down, whereas the distal outline is rather convex, converging sharply toward the cervical line. This makes the distal contact area fairly convex. The distal portion of the crown is shorter than the mesial portion.

Two rather distinct buccal cusps are present, but the developmental groove between them is not always evident. The mesial cusp is larger than the distal cusp. The crown is wider mesiodistally than buccolingually.

The roots are long, slender, and flared, with the mesial root curving slightly distally in its apical third. The point of bifurcation is very close to the cervical line of the crown, a characteristic of all deciduous molars. Observe the curvature of the cervical line.

Lingual Aspect (Figs. 34-38 and 34-47, B)

The crown and root converge lingually on the mesial half of the crown; distally they do not converge. The mesiolingual cusp is long and sharp, whereas the distolingual cusp is more rounded and not so long. The mesial marginal ridge is so well developed that it almost appears to be another cusp.

The cervical line is almost straight across, being quite different from the cervical line on the buccal aspect. Buccally the cervical line curves apically on the mesial half of the tooth.

Mesial Aspect (Figs. 34-39 and 34-47, D)

The most characteristic feature of this tooth is an extremely bulbous curvature on its buccal surface at the cervical third. This extreme buccocervical convexity can easily be seen on the mesial view and causes the occlusal table to appear rather narrow from cusp tip to cusp tip.

The mesiobuccal cusp is longer than the mesiolingual cusp, since the cervical line curves up-

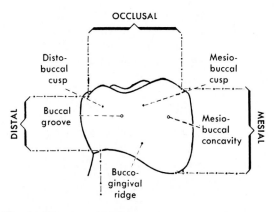

Fig. 34-37   Buccal surface of mandibular right first molar. (Zeisz and Nuckolls.)

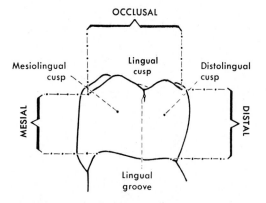

Fig. 34-38   Lingual surface of mandibular right first molar. (Zeisz and Nuckolls.)

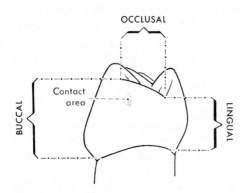

Fig. 34-39 Mesial surface of mandibular right first molar. (Zeisz and Nuckolls.)

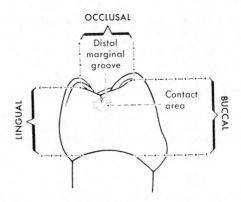

Fig. 34-40 Distal surface of mandibular right first molar. (Zeisz and Nuckolls.)

ward from the buccal to the lingual side. The buccal surface is flat from the tip of the mesiobuccal cusp to the crest of the buccocervical curvature. Although this buccocervical curvature is quite pronounced, the remainder of the buccal surface above the curvature is rather flat and tipped at a sharp angle toward the buccal cusp.

Distal Aspect (Figs. 34-40 and 34-47, *E*)

The distal aspect of the crown does not display such an extreme buccocervical curvature. The height of the cusps, buccal and lingual, appears more uniform, and the cervical line is almost straight across buccolingually. The distobuccal and distolingual cusps are not so developed as the two mesial cusps. Furthermore, the distal marginal ridge is not as well defined as the mesial marginal ridge. The distal root is rounder and shorter, tapers apically, and houses only one root canal.

The distal surface is more convex than the mesial; therefore the distal contact area is more rounded and convex than the mesial.

Occlusal Aspect (Figs. 34-41 and 34-47, *C*)

The occlusal outline of the crown is rhomboidal. From this view the prominence of the me-

siobuccal surface is apparent. The mesiobuccal cervical ridge is quite evident and gives the tooth a rhomboidal shape that tapers distally. The mesiolingual cusp appears to be the widest cusp. The mesial marginal ridge is well developed. A buccal developmental groove may be present. A distinct transverse ridge runs between the mesiofacial and the mesiolingual cusps. This ridge divides the occlusal surface into two fossae: one contains the mesial pit and the other the central and distal pits, and all are joined by a central developmental groove. A lingual groove radiates from the central pit between the two lingual cusps. A facial groove runs from the central pit to the buccal surface between the two buccal cusps. Mesial and distal triangular fossae, as well as mesial and distal marginal and triangular grooves, can be seen in Fig. 34-47, *C*.

Roots of Mandibular First Molars

The deciduous mandibular first molar has two roots, a mesial and a distal. They are rather flat, broad, and flared widely apart. The mesial has a longitudinal developmental groove running the length of its root. This root has two root canals. The distal root is the shorter and thinner of the two; it has only one canal.

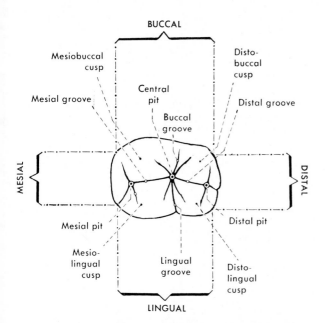

Fig. 34-41 Occlusal surface of mandibular right first molar. (Zeisz and Nuckolls.)

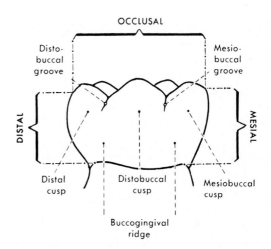

Fig. 34-42 Buccal surface of mandibular right second molar. (Zeisz and Nuckolls.)

MANDIBULAR SECOND MOLARS
Buccal Aspect (Figs. 34-42 and 34-48, *A*)

A primary mandibular second molar resembles a permanent mandibular first molar except that it is smaller and has the typical deciduous molar constriction at the cervix of the crown.

Mesiobuccal and distobuccal developmental grooves divide the buccal surface occlusally into three cusps. The three buccal cusps are the mesiofacial, the distofacial, and the distal. The term "buccal" can be substituted for "facial." What would the names of the three cusps then be? These cusps are about the same length and width; the distobuccal (distofacial) cusp is a little longer than the other two.

Characteristically the roots of a second molar are long and slender, flaring mesiodistally at their middle and apical thirds. These roots are often twice as long as or longer than the crown. The point of bifurcation of the roots starts imme-

diately below the cervical line of the crown. How is this different from a permanent first molar's roots?

Lingual Aspect (Figs. 34-43 and 34-48, *B*)

From the lingual view a short lingual groove can be seen dividing two cusps of about equal dimensions. The two lingual cusps, the mesiolingual and the distolingual, are not so wide as the three buccal cusps. The tooth therefore converges lingually. The cervical line is straight.

Mesial Aspect (Figs. 34-44 and 34-48, *D*)

The mesial view of the crown resembles that of a permanent mandibular first molar. However, its buccal surface shows a cervical bulge typical of deciduous molars. This crest of contour on the buccal side is notably less than on a deciduous first molar. Like a deciduous first molar, a flattened buccal surface angles occlusally from this

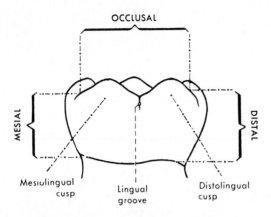

Fig. 34-43 Lingual surface of mandibular right second molar. (Zeisz and Nuckolls.)

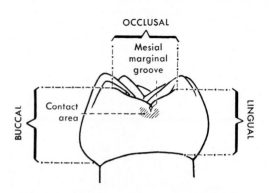

Fig. 34-44 Mesial surface of mandibular right second molar. (Zeisz and Nuckolls.)

crest of contour. This presents a proportionately smaller occlusal table than on the permanent mandibular molars.

The mesial marginal ridge is rather high, giving the cusp the appearance of being shorter. The lingual cusp is longer than the buccal cusp, since the cervical line extends upward from the buccal to the lingual side.

The mesial root is broad, flat, and blunted at the apex and houses two canals.

Distal Aspect (Figs. 34-45 and 34-48, *E*)

The crown is not so wide distally as it is mesially, nor is the distal marginal ridge as high or as long as the mesial marginal ridge. The cervical line has the same upper inclination buccolingually as the mesiocervical line.

Three cusps can be seen from the distal view: the distofacial, the distal, and the distolingual. Because the tooth converges distally, portions of the mesiofacial and mesiolingual cusps are also visible.

Although the distal root is more tapered at its apical end, it does resemble the mesial root with its broad and flattened surface. The distal root has one canal. Does this differ from the distal root of a deciduous mandibular first molar?

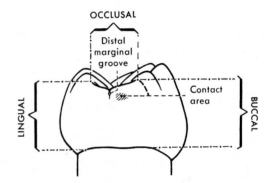

Fig. 34-45 Distal surface of mandibular right second molar. (Zeisz and Nuckolls.)

Occlusal Aspect (Figs. 34-46 and 34-48, *C*)

The three buccal cusps are similar in size, as are the two lingual cusps. However, the total mesiodistal width of the three buccal cusps is much more than the total mesiodistal width of the two lingual cusps. This allows the tooth to converge lingually.

The mesiofacial, distofacial, and lingual grooves radiate from the central pit in a Y shape. A central developmental groove joins the mesial triangular fossa and pit. Scattered over the oc-

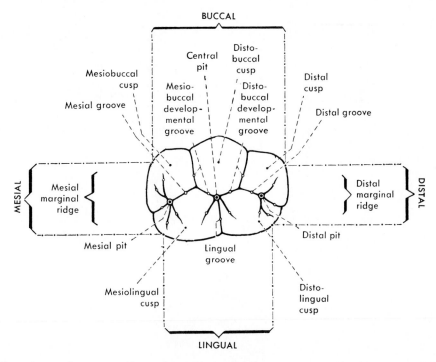

BUCCAL

Central
pit

Disto-
buccal
cusp

Mesiobuccal
cusp

Mesio-
buccal
develop-
mental
groove

Disto-
buccal
develop-
mental
groove

Distal
cusp

Mesial groove

Distal groove

MESIAL

Mesial
marginal
ridge

Distal
marginal
ridge

DISTAL

Distal pit

Mesial pit

Lingual
groove

Mesiolingual
cusp

Disto-
lingual
cusp

LINGUAL

Fig. 34-46 Occlusal surface of mandibular right second molar. (Zeisz and Nuckolls.)

clusal surface are supplemental grooves located on the triangular ridges and fossae. The mesial marginal ridge is more pronounced than the distal marginal ridge.

The crown converges both distally and lingually. This convergence is similar to that seen in a permanent first molar, but the distal cusp in a permanent molar is much smaller than the two other buccal cusps. On a deciduous molar the three buccal cusps are almost equal in size and development. All three buccal cusps of the deciduous molars are small in comparison with those of the permanent molars. This gives the deciduous tooth crown a narrower buccolingual dimension in comparison with its mesiodistal dimensions.

Roots of Mandibular Second Molars

The roots of the deciduous mandibular second molar are twice as long as the crown. They are long, slender, and very flared. The root trunk, like all deciduous molars, is very short, bifurcating immediately below the cervix of the tooth.

The two roots are the mesial and the distal. The mesial has two root canals. The mesial root may have a longitudinal groove dividing it buccolingually. The distal root has only one root canal, and no grooves divide the root surface itself.

Pulp Cavities of Deciduous Teeth

The pulp cavities of deciduous teeth mirror the outer form of the teeth except that the pulp horns are longer and more pointed (Figs. 34-49 and 34-50). Compared with the permanent teeth, the pulp chambers are large in proportion to the tooth size and the pulp horns are more extreme. The mandibular deciduous molars are like miniature permanent teeth with larger-sized pulp chambers, root canals, and pulp horns (Fig. 34-51.) *Text continued on p. 447.*

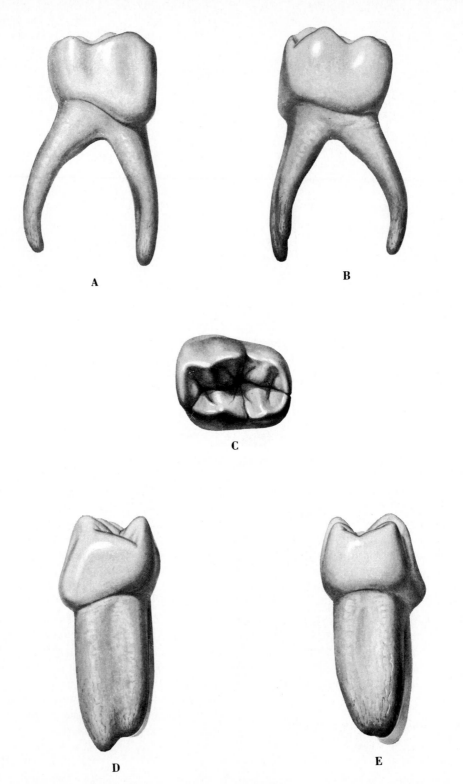

Fig. 34-47 Mandibular right first molar. **A,** Buccal view. **B,** Lingual view. **C,** Occlusal view. **D,** Mesial view. **E,** Distal view. (Zeisz and Nuckolls.)

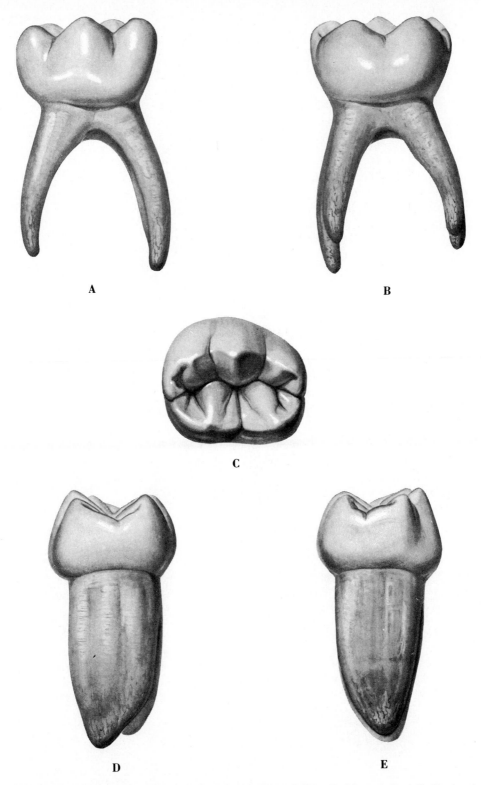

Fig. 34-48 Mandibular right second molar. **A,** Buccal view. **B,** Lingual view. **C,** Occlusal view. **D,** Mesial view. **E,** Distal view. (Zeisz and Nuckolls.)

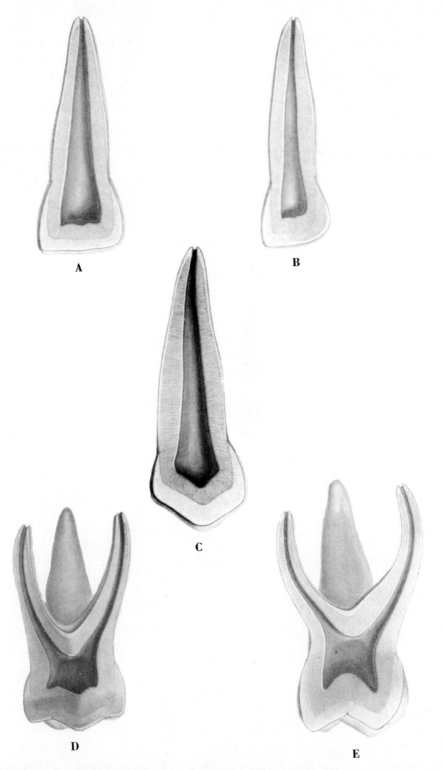

Fig. 34-49 Maxillary right deciduous teeth, facial views. **A,** Central incisor. **B,** Lateral incisor. **C,** Canine. **D,** First molar. **E,** Second molar. (Zeisz and Nuckolls.)

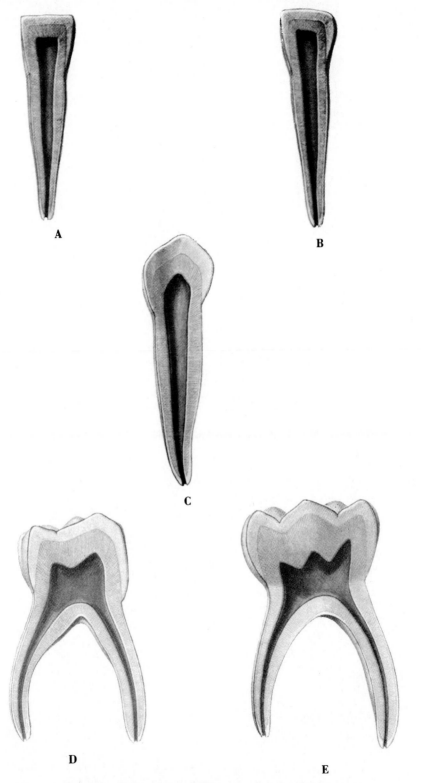

Fig. 34-50 Mandibular right deciduous teeth, facial views. **A,** Central incisor. **B,** Lateral incisor. **C,** Canine, **D,** First molar. **E,** Second molar. (Zeisz and Nuckolls.)

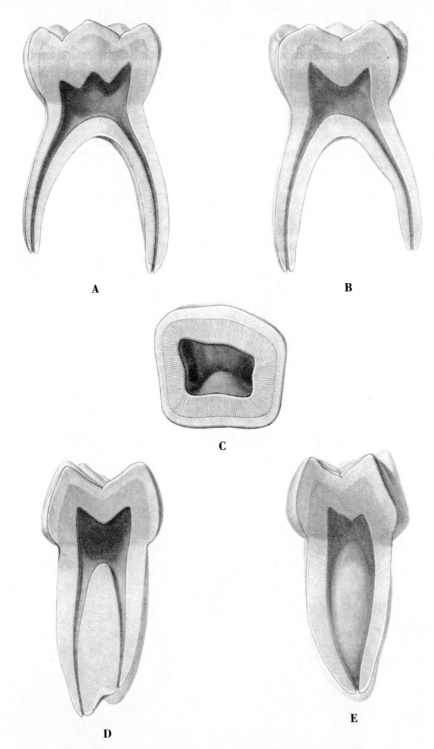

Fig. 34-51 Mandibular right deciduous second molar. **A,** Buccal view. **B,** Lingual view. **C,** Occlusal view. **D,** Mesial view. **E,** Distal view. (Zeisz and Nuckolls.)

REVIEW QUESTIONS

1. Give two terms that are synonymous with what are commonly called "baby teeth."
2. What is meant by the term exfoliation, and how does it occur?
3. How many deciduous teeth are there? How many are molars? How many are incisors? How many are premolars?
4. What are the eruption dates of the following?
   a. deciduous maxillary incisors
   b. deciduous mandibular incisors
   c. deciduous canines
   d. deciduous first molars
5. Which teeth usually erupt first, maxillary or mandibular?
6. Name twelve essential differences between deciduous and permanent teeth.
7. What cervical bulge of enamel is more pronounced on the deciduous teeth than on the permanent teeth?
8. Which deciduous tooth is least like any in the permanent dentition?
   a. primary maxillary second molar
   b. primary mandibular first molar
   c. primary mandibular second molar
9. Give one special characteristic that is unique to each type of deciduous molar.
10. Rewrite the twelve essential differences between deciduous and permanent teeth in summary form.

TEST

1. A small elevation of enamel that may be found on the surface of a tooth is a
   a. cusp.
   b. tubercle.
   c. sulcus.
   d. fossa.

2. Of the permanent premolars, the one that is most likely to have two root canals is the
   a. maxillary first premolar.
   b. maxillary second premolar.
   c. mandibular first premolar.
   d. mandibular second premolar.

3. Which of the following is *least* typical for the maxillary second premolar?
   a. The lingual cusp is slightly shorter than the facial cusp.
   b. The facial cusp is slightly smaller than the lingual cusp.
   c. The two cusps are approximately the same length.
   d. The facial cusp is shorter and more blunt compared to the lingual cusp.

4. When the two cusps of the maxillary first premolars are compared,
   a. the facial cusp is longer but not wider.
   b. the lingual cusp is both shorter and narrower.
   c. the facial cusp is shorter but wider.
   d. the lingual cusp is both longer and wider.

5. Which of the following is *not* true of maxillary first premolars?
   a. commonly bifurcated root
   b. single root trunk
   c. facial cusp tip displaced to the distal from midline
   d. the roots are the mesial and distal

6. The last of these teeth to erupt are
   a. the mandibular first premolars.
   b. the maxillary canines.
   c. the maxillary first premolars.
   d. the mandibular canines.

7. Of the following, the least likely to bifurcate is the
   a. maxillary second premolar.
   b. mandibular canine.
   c. mandibular first premolar.
   d. mandibular second premolar.

8. The least likely to have two root canals is
   a. the mesiobuccal root of a maxillary molar.
   b. the mesial root of the mandibular molar.
   c. an upper premolar.
   d. a mandibular canine.

9. Which of the following are the first permanent teeth to erupt?
   a. maxillary first molars
   b. mandibular first molars
   c. mandibular centrals
   d. maxillary centrals

10. Which of the following have the least cervical contact areas?
    a. central incisors
    b. third molars
    c. canines
    d. premolars

11. Which of the following are class traits of all molars?
    a. Molars have the largest occlusal surfaces of any teeth in the dentition.
    b. Molars have three to five major cusps.
    c. Molars have two functional cusps and two afunctional cusps.
    d. Molars have two or three roots.
    e. a, b, d

f. a, c, d

g. a, b, c

h. a, d

i. a, b

12. The distobuccal and mesiolingual cusps on the occlusal table of a maxillary molar are usually connected by a ridge. This ridge is termed
   a. the transverse ridge. ✓
   b. the triangular ridge.
   c. the Carabellian ridge.
   d. the oblique ridge. ✓
   e. a and d. ✓

13. The maxillary incisors in a class II, division II malocclusion are
   a. retruded. ✓
   b. protruded.
   c. edge to edge.
   d. end to end.

14. Maxillary laterals exhibit
   a. the same number of lobes as first molars.
   b. the same number of lobes as first premolars. ✓
   c. two labial and two lingual lobes.
   d. three lobes only.

A 9-year-old boy presents himself with a large gingival abscess at the gingival crest of his deciduous maxillary first right molar. The tooth is loose and painful upon percussion.

15. We could expect this 9-year-old patient to exhibit
   a. no permanent teeth at all other than first molars.
   b. a mixed dentition. ✓
   c. evidence of facial trauma.
   d. evidence of severe periodontal disease.

16. We would consider the following types of treatment appropriate:
   a. root canal
   b. periodontal surgery
   c. removal of the affected tooth ✓
   d. splinting the deciduous molars together

17. If this molar was removed, which of the following is *not* true?
   a. A space maintainer is probably not needed.
   b. The permanent replacement could be expected soon.
   c. His eruption pattern is earlier than most children his age. ✓
   d. Not much evidence of the deciduous root would be present.

18. From the occlusal view, which tooth is wider on the lingual than on the buccal?
   a. maxillary central incisor
   b. mandibular first molar
   c. maxillary first molar ✓
   d. mandibular first premolar
   e. mandibular second premolar

19. The cusp of Carabelli of the maxillary first molar may be
   a. absent. ✓
   b. located lingual to the distolingual cusp.
   c. the third largest cusp.
   d. all of the above.

20. The longest and shortest cusps of the maxillary first molar are the
   a. mesiofacial and distofacial.
   b. mesiolingual and distofacial.
   c. mesiolingual and distolingual. ✓
   d. distofacial and distolingual.

21. In class I occlusion, the mandibular lateral incisor
   a. opposes the maxillary lateral incisor and canine.
   b. opposes only the maxillary lateral incisor.
   c. opposes maxillary central and lateral incisors. ✓
   d. is free of contact with opposing teeth.

22. As compared with the permanent mandibular central incisor, the root of the mandibular lateral incisor is
   a. larger in all dimensions. ✓
   b. longer but not wider.
   c. wider but not longer.
   d. the same size.

23. Morphologically, the mandibular lateral incisor is almost identical to the mandibular central incisor, with which difference?
   a. The mandibular lateral incisor is usually

slightly larger.

b. The mandibular lateral incisor has an elongation of the distoincisal angle distolingually.

c. When the mandibular lateral incisor is viewed incisally, the crown appears to be slightly rotated on its base.

d. All of the above are true.

24. In comparison with the permanent maxillary canine, the permanent mandibular canine has a mesiodistal crown width that is

a. somewhat wider.

b. somewhat narrower.

c. identical.

d. a great deal wider.

25. In comparison with the mandibular canine, the maxillary canine

a. has a relatively longer crown.

b. is less likely to be bifurcated.

c. has a less pronounced cingulum.

d. has less prominent lingual features.

26. Which of the following anterior teeth exhibits the most deviation in tooth morphology?

a. mandibular central incisor

b. maxillary canine

c. maxillary lateral incisor

d. mandibular lateral incisor

27. The smallest permanent tooth in the mouth is the

a. maxillary central incisor.

b. mandibular central incisor.

c. maxillary lateral incisor.

d. mandibular lateral incisor.

28. Which of the following anterior teeth is most likely to have two root canals?

a. mandibular lateral incisor

b. maxillary canine

c. maxillary central incisor

d. mandibular canine

29. Mesiodistal measurements of the crowns of anterior teeth as seen from an incisal view indicate that the crowns are

a. wider at the mesial than the distal.

b. wider at the distal than the mesial.

c. wider at the lingual than the facial.

d. wider at the facial than the lingual.

30. Which of the following is the largest, longest, and strongest root of the maxillary molar?

a. facial

b. lingual

c. mesiofacial

d. distofacial

31. Which of the following cusps is frequently missing from the maxillary third molar?

a. mesiofacial

b. distofacial

c. distolingual

d. mesiolingual

32. The oblique ridge of maxillary molars crosses the occlusal surface obliquely from

a. mesiofacial to mesiolingual.

b. mesiolingual to distofacial.

c. distofacial to distolingual.

d. mesiofacial to distolingual.

33. Where is the lingual height of contour located on the mandibular molars?

a. middle third

b. occlusal third

c. cervical third

d. at the junction of occlusal and middle third

34. The mandibular molars are aligned in the alveolar bone in such a way that their crowns are

a. tilted to the distal and facial side.

b. tilted to the lingual but upright otherwise.

c. upright in all directions.

d. tilted to the mesial and lingual side.

35. The permanent mandibular first molar usually has

a. two root canals in the mesial root, one in the distal.

b. one root canal in the lingual root, one in the facial.

c. two root canals in both the mesial and distal roots.

d. one root canal in each root.

36. The four most frequently found congenitally missing teeth are

a. maxillary first premolar, maxillary lateral,

mandibular lateral, and third molar.
- b. maxillary third molar and lateral, and mandibular canine and third molar.
- c. maxillary third molar, mandibular third molar, maxillary lateral, and mandibular second bicuspid.
- d. maxillary third molar and first bicuspid, and mandibular third molar and canine.

37. The greatest convexity of the facial surface of anterior teeth is
- a. different from that of the posterior teeth.
- b. the cervical third.
- c. the middle third.
- d. the junction of middle and incisal thirds.

38. Which of the following is *not* a set trait of the deciduous dentition?
- a. Most primary teeth are smaller than the analogous permanent teeth.
- b. The crowns of primary teeth seem long relative to their total length when compared with the permanent teeth.
- c. In the anterior primary teeth, the labial and lingual surfaces bulge conspicuously in the cervical third.
- d. Primary crowns are milk white in color.
- e. The enamel is thinner in primary teeth and the pulp chamber is larger.

39. What is the most distinguishing feature of the maxillary first deciduous molar?
- a. cusp relationship
- b. buccal cervical ridge
- c. mesial profile
- d. occlusal outline

40. A child, 14 months of age, should normally have which deciduous teeth present in the mouth (all four quadrants)?
- a. centrals, laterals, canines, first molars, second molars
- b. centrals, laterals, canines, first molars
- c. centrals, laterals, first molars, second molars
- d. centrals, laterals, canines
- e. centrals, laterals, first molars

41. Which of the following deciduous teeth do not resemble any other deciduous teeth or permanent teeth?
- a. deciduous mandibular first molar
- b. deciduous mandibular second molar
- c. deciduous maxillary first molar
- d. deciduous maxillary second molar
- e. a and c

42. Which has three roots?
- a. mandibular molars
- b. maxillary premolars
- c. deciduous maxillary molars
- d. maxillary molars
- e. a, c, and d
- f. c and d

43. The cusp of Carabelli of the maxillary first molar is sometimes
- a. located on the distolingual cusp.
- b. missing entirely.
- c. located on the lingual surface.
- d. located on the mesiolingual cusp.
- e. a, c, and d.
- f. b, c, and d.

44. The smallest tooth in the human dentition is the
- a. deciduous mandibular central.
- b. deciduous mandibular lateral.
- c. permanent mandibular central.
- d. permanent lower lateral.

45. The permanent mandibular incisors differ from the permanent maxillary incisors in the following way.
- a. Maxillary incisors are smaller.
- b. Mandibular lateral is larger than the central.
- c. Maxillary have fewer pits and less developed marginal ridges.
- d. Mandibular have more developed cingulums.

46. What is the excess space called that is available for the permanent canine and premolars?
- a. freeway space
- b. primate space
- c. interdental space
- d. leeway space
- e. horizontal overjet

SECTION FOUR

REFERENCES

SUGGESTED READINGS

Andrews LF: The six keys to normal occlusion, Amer J Orthod 62(3):296, September 1972.

Angle EH: Treatment of malocclusion of the teeth and fractures of the maxillae: Angle's system, ed 6, Philadelphia, 1900 SS White Dental Manufacturing Co.

Ash MM: Wheeler's atlas of tooth form, ed 5, Philadelphia, 1984, WB Saunders Co.

Ash MM: Wheeler's dental anatomy, physiology, and occlusion, ed 6, Philadelphia, 1984, WB Saunders Co.

Ayer WA: Thumb-finger sucking and bruxing habits in children. In Bryant P, Gale E, and Rugh J, (editors): Oral motor behavior: impact on oral conditions and dental treatment, NIH Publications No. 79-1845, Washington, DC, 1979, US Government Printing Office.

Begg PR: Stone age man's dentition, Amer J Orthod 40:298, 1954.

Berry DC and Singh BP: Effect of electromyographic biofeedback therapy on occlusion contacts, J Prosthet Dent 51:397, 1984.

Dawson PE: Evaluation, diagnosis, and treatment of occlusal problems, ed 2, St Louis, 1989, The CV Mosby Co.

DuBrul EL: Sicher's oral anatomy, ed 8, St Louis, 1988, Ishiyaku EuroAmerica, Inc.

Farman AG and Escobar V: Duplication of oral and maxillofacial structures, Quintessence International, 17(11):731, 1986.

Grahnen H and Granath LE: Numerical variations in primary dentition and their correlation with permanent dentition, Odontol Rev 12:348, 1961.

Kessler HP and Kraut RA: Dentigerous cyst associated with an impacted mesiodens, Gen Dent 48:47, 1989.

King NM and Wei SH: Developmental defects of enamel: a study of 12 year olds in Hong Kong, JADA 112:835, 1986.

Kraus BS, Jordan E, and Abrams L: Dental anatomy and occlusion, Philadelphia, 1973, BC Decker, Inc.

Mangold WG et al.: New community residents' preferences for dental service information, JADA 112:840, 1986.

Massler M and Schour I: Atlas of the mouth in health and disease, ed 2, Chicago, 1975, American Dental Association.

Mohl ND: A textbook of occlusion, Lombard, IL, 1988, Quintessence.

Mourino AP and Camm JH: Multiple anomalies of a newborn: report of a case, JADA 114:335, 1987.

Proffit WR, Fields HW, and Nixon WL: Occlusal forces in normal and long-face adults, J Dent Res 62:566, 1983.

Ramfjord S and Ash MM: Significance of occlusion in the etiology and treatment of early, moderate, and advanced periodontitis, J Periodontal 52:511, 1981.

Ramfjord S and Ash MM: Occlusion, ed 3, Philadelphia, 1983, WB Saunders Co.

Renner RP: An introduction to dental anatomy and esthetics, Lombard, IL, 1985, Quintessence.

Woelfel JB: Dental anatomy: its correlation with dental health service, ed 3, Philadelphia, 1984, Lea & Febiger.

ILLUSTRATION SOURCES

Kraus BS, Jordon RE, and Abrams L: Dental anatomy and occlusion, Baltimore, 1969, The Williams & Wilkins Co.

Massler M and Schour I: Atlas of the mouth in health and disease, ed 2, Chicago, 1958 and 1973, American Dental Association.

Ross IF: Occlusion: a concept for the clinician, St Louis, 1970, The CV Mosby Co.

Wheeler RC: A textbook of dental anatomy and physiology, Philadelphia, 1965, WB Saunders Co.

Zeisz RC and Nuckolls J: Dental anatomy, St Louis, 1949, The CV Mosby Co.

TEST ANSWERS

SECTION TWO

1. b
2. d
3. f
4. b
5. b
6. c
7. b
8. g
9. b
10. b
11. c
12. b
13. d
14. d
15. b
16. b
17. b
18. c
19. c
20. a
21. b
22. c
23. e
24. d
25. d
26. d
27. e
28. c

29. a
30. d
31. b
32. d
33. a
34. c
35. b
36. d
37. e—None of the above. They develop posterior to the primary teeth.
38. c
39. c
40. c
41. a
42. d
43. b
44. d
45. c
46. d
47. d

SECTION THREE

1. e—None of the above. There are 22 bones.
2. f
3. f
4. e—None of the above. It is in body of mandible.
5. d
6. c
7. d
8. b
9. d
10. d
11. f
12. d
13. d
14. a
15. c
16. c
17. d
18. d
19. b
20. c

21. c
22. b
23. b
24. c
25. e—None of the above. The buccinator does it.
26. e
27. e
28. d
29. a
30. e
31. f—None of the above. The internal carotid artery has no branches in the neck.
32. d
33. b
34. a
35. d
36. b
37. d
38. e
39. d
40. d
41. d
42. e—None of the above. It is the anterior superior alveolar.
43. d
44. e
45. e
46. b
47. b
48. d

SECTION FOUR

1. b
2. a
3. b
4. b
5. d
6. b
7. d
8. d
9. b
10. a
11. a
12. e
13. a
14. b
15. b
16. c
17. c
18. c
19. a
20. c
21. c
22. a
23. d
24. b
25. b
26. c
27. b
28. d
29. d
30. b
31. c
32. b
33. a
34. d
35. a
36. c
37. b
38. b
39. b
40. e
41. e
42. f
43. f
44. a
45. b
46. d

GLOSSARY

A band Dark microscopic band in the middle of a muscle sarcomere. The A band contains the myosin and parts of the actin myofilaments.

abducens Sixth cranial nerve (VI); has to do with eye movement.

abrasion Mechanical wearing away of teeth by abnormal stresses. This could result from abnormal toothbrushing habits or other abnormal stresses on the teeth.

accessional Permanent teeth that do not replace deciduous teeth but rather become an accession (an addition) to the deciduous or succedaneous teeth, or both types.

accessory nerve Eleventh cranial nerve (XI); supplies motor control to trapezius and sternomastoid muscles in the neck, as well as muscles of pharynx, larynx, and soft palate.

accessory root canals Extra openings into the pulp; usually located on the sides of the roots or in the bifurcations.

accidental grooves Tertiary grooves that occur on third molars; smaller than primary or secondary grooves and occur with no uniformity.

acellular cementum Cementum that has no cells trapped in it.

acini Bulbous or tubular endpieces of a gland that produce secretions; pronounced as'i-nī.

acquired Pertaining to something obtained by oneself; not inherited.

acquired occlusion See *centric occlusion*

acromegaly Disease resulting from an excess of growth hormone, which causes some bones in the body to continue to grow after normal growth has been completed.

actin One of the myofilaments in muscle, which is thinner than myosin; located in the I band and part of the A band.

action Function of a muscle; the work accomplished when a muscle contracts or shortens.

afferent Refers to a nerve fiber carrying sensory messages *to* the brain.

afunctional Not performing a purpose or action.

agranulocytes White blood cells without granules in their cytoplasm; lymphocytes and monocytes.

ala Latin for 'wing,' referring to the sides of the nostrils of the nose; plural *alae.*

alignment Arrangement of teeth in a row.

allergenic Being hypersensitive to something.

allergic reaction Body's reaction to an allergen, as in hives.

alveolar bone Bone that forms the sockets for the teeth.

alveolar bone proper See *cribriform plate.*

alveolar crest Highest part of the alveolar bone closest to the cervical line of the tooth.

alveolar crest group Alveolodental fibers running from the cementum to the alveolar crest of bone.

alveolar eminences Bulges on the facial surface of alveolar bone that outline the position of the roots.

alveolar mucosa Mucosa between the mucobuccal fold and gingiva.

alveolar process Part of the bone in the maxillae and mandible that forms the sockets for the teeth. See *alveolar bone.*

alveolodental fibers Periodontal fibers that run between the tooth and alveolar bone.

alveolus (alveoli) Cavity, or socket, in the alveolar process in which the root of the tooth is held.

ameloblast Enamel-forming cell that arises from oral ectoderm.

amelogenesis imperfecta A hereditary form of enamel hypocalcification.

amylase Digestive enzyme that breaks starch down into simpler compounds.

anatomical crown That part of the tooth covered by enamel.

anemia Deficiency of red blood cells or hemoglobin to carry oxygen.

angle of the mandible Point at the lower border of

the body of the mandible where it turns up onto the ramus.

Angle's classification   System of dental classifications based primarily on the relationship of the permanent first molars to each other and to a lesser degree on the relationship of the permanent canines to each other.

ankyloglossia   See *tongue-tie.*

ankylosis   Fusion of the cementum of a tooth with alveolar bone.

anodontia   No teeth at all are present in the jaw.

anomaly   Any noticeable difference or deviation from that which is ordinary or normal.

antagonists   Having opposing, or opposite, action to something else.

anterior   Situated in front of; a term commonly used to denote the incisor and canine teeth or the area toward the front of the mouth.

anterior auricular muscle   Muscle of facial expression that extends from in front of the ear into the skin of the ear.

anterior coupling   The touching of the anterior teeth during centric occlusion.

anterior ethmoid sinus   Frontmost group of ethmoid air cells.

anterior nasal spine   Small projection of the maxillae at the bottom of the nasal aperture.

anterior pillar   Fold of tissue extending down in front of the tonsil.

anterior superior alveolar artery   Branch of the infraorbital artery to the maxillary incisors, canines, and premolars.

anterior superior alveolar nerve   Branch of the infraorbital nerve that serves maxillary incisors and canines.

antihistamine   Drug that controls the body's histamine reaction, which causes congestion of tissues.

aorta   Large vessel carrying oxygenated blood from the heart to the remainder of the body.

apatite crystals   Small crystals of mineral deposits.

apex (apices)   End point, or furthest tip, as of the tooth root.

apical end of cell   Narrow end of a pyramidal cell forming the lumen of a duct.

apical foramen   Aperture, or opening, at or near the apex of a tooth root through which the blood and nerve supply of the pulp enters the tooth.

apical group   Alveolodental fibers that attach from the base of the alveolus to the apex of the tooth.

apposition   Addition, as to the surface of bone or any hard substance. One of the processes that takes place in bone growth and remodeling.

arch, dental   See *dental arch.*

arthritis   Inflammation of body joints.

articular disc   Fibrous disc between the condyle and the mandibular fossa.

articular eminence   Slope of temporal bone in front of the mandibular fossa.

atrophic   Pertaining to the wasting away of a tissue, organ, or part from disease, defective nutrition, or lack of use.

atrophy   Wasting away of a tissue, organ, or part from disease, defective nutrition, or lack of use.

attached gingiva   Tightly adherent gingiva that extends from free gingiva to alveolar mucosa.

attachment apparatus   See *attachment unit.*

attachment epithelium   The cells that attach the gingiva to the tooth. These originally are cells of the reduced enamel epithelium.

attachment unit   Subdivision of the periodontium; cementum, periodontal ligament, and alveolar bone.

attrition   Process of normal wear on the crown.

auriculotemporal nerve   Branch of the third division of the trigeminal nerve that supplies the skin over the ear and the parotid gland.

autonomic nervous system   Automatic nervous system of the body that is not willfully controlled. It controls the functions of the glands and smooth and cardiac muscle.

axon   Process of the neuron that carries the message from the cell body to the next neuron.

balancing side   Term used in denture construction to denote the side of the denture that must be balanced to prevent the denture from tipping. In natural dentition it occurs when the buccal cusps of the mandibular teeth are located directly under the lingual cusps of the maxillary teeth. These cusps actually touch.

basal end of cell   Broad outer end of a pyramidal cell forming a duct; end of any tall cell resting on a basement membrane.

basal layer   Bottom layer in multiple-layered epithelium; layer that undergoes cell division.

basophils   White granulocyte blood cells that play a role in phagocytosis and possible allergic reactions.

bell stage   Third stage of enamel organ formation in which the crown form is established.

biconcave discs   Discs that have a depression in the middle on both sides.

bicuspid   See *premolars*.

bifurcation   Division into two parts or branches, as any two roots of a tooth.

bisecting angle   Technique of taking radiographs that slightly compromises accuracy of the image.

body of the mandible   Horizontal portion of the mandible, excluding the alveolar process.

bolus of food   A ball of food that has been chewed and mixed with saliva and is ready to be swallowed.

bone   Hard connective tissue that forms the framework of the body. The hardness is attributable to the hydroxyapatite crystal.

brachiocephalic artery   Branch of the aorta that carries blood to the right arm and right side of the head.

brachiocephalic veins   Paired veins that drain the right and left arms and sides of the head. These two veins unite to form the superior vena cava.

branchial arches   See *pharyngeal arches*.

bruxism   Abnormal grinding of the teeth.

bucca   Latin word for cheek.

buccal   Pertaining to the cheek; toward the cheek or next to the cheek. Also called facial.

buccal branch   Branch of the maxillary artery that goes to the cheek and buccal gingiva.

buccal contour   Posterior teeth; see *facial contours*.

buccal developmental groove   Groove that separates the buccal cusps on a buccal surface.

buccal embrasure   See *embrasure*.

buccal glands   Small minor salivary glands in the cheek.

buccal nerve   Branch of the third division of the trigeminal nerve that supplies the skin and mucosa of the cheek and buccal gingiva.

buccinator   Muscle of facial expression that extends from the back buccal portion of the maxillae and mandible and pterygomandibular raphe, forward in the cheek to the corner of the mouth.

buccopharyngeal membrane   Membrane that separates the stomodeum from the foregut.

bud stage   First stage of development of the enamel organ. It develops from the dental lamina.

bundle bone   Extra thickness of bone added to the cribriform plate.

calcification   Process by which organic tissue becomes hardened by a deposit of calcium salts within its substance. The term, in a liberal sense, connotes the deposition of any mineral salts that contribute to the hardening and maturation of hard tissue.

canal   Long tubular opening through a bone.

cancellous bone   See *spongy bone*.

canine eminence   Extra bulk of bone on the labial aspect of the maxillae, overlying the roots of the canine teeth.

canine fossa   Depression in the maxillae below the infraorbital foramen.

canine rise   During lateral excursion, the only teeth to touch are the maxillary and mandibular canines on the side toward which the jaw is moving.

canines   Third teeth from the midline, at corner of mouth; used for grasping; also called cuspids.

cap stage   Second stage of enamel organ development.

capsule   Fibrous band of tissue surrounding a joint.

cardiac muscle   Striped, involuntarily controlled muscle of the heart.

carotid canal   Canal in the base of the skull for the passage of the internal carotid artery.

cartilage   Type of firm connective tissue that gives form to different parts of the body, such as ears, trachea, and larynx.

cell   Basic functioning component of the body; capable of reproducing itself in most instances. Tissues are made up of groups of cells.

cell body   Central part of a neuron containing the nucleus.

cell membrane   Wall surrounding the cell.

cellular cementum   Cementum that has cells trapped in it.

cellular inclusions   Storage products in a cell not actually used to maintain the cell under normal circumstances.

cementoblasts   Cells that form cementum.

cementocytes   Cementoblasts that have become entrapped in cementum.

cementoenamel junction (CEJ)   Junction of enamel of the crown and cementum of the root. This junction forms the cervical line around the tooth.

cementoma   Cementum tumor at root tip that destroys surrounding bone.

cementum   Layer of bonelike tissue covering the root of the tooth.

central developmental groove   Developmental groove that crosses the occlusal surface of a tooth from the mesial to the distal side; divides the tooth into buccal and lingual parts.

central developmental pit   Pit that occurs in the central fossa.

central fossa   Fossa that occurs in the center of the central groove.

central groove   See *central developmental groove*.

central nervous system   Brain and spinal cord.

centric occlusion (central occlusion)   Relationship of the occlusal surfaces of one arch to those of the other when the jaws are closed and the teeth are in maximum intercuspation.

centric relation   Arch-to-arch relationship of the maxilla to the mandible when the condyles are in their most upward position and the mandible is in its most posterior position and the jaw is most braced by its musculature.

cervical   That portion of a tooth near the junction of the crown and root. Pertaining to the neck region, for example, nerves of the neck.

cervical crest   Gingival tissue located near the cervical line of the tooth.

cervical embrasure   Embrasure or spillway located cervical to the contact area of the teeth.

cervical line   Line formed by the junction of the enamel and cementum on a tooth.

cervical third   That portion of the crown or root of a tooth at or near the cervical line.

cervicoenamel ridge   Any prominent ridge of enamel immediately near the cervical line on the crown of a tooth.

cervix   Constricted structure; the narrow region at the junction of the crown and root of the tooth.

choana   Region at the posterior end of the nasal septum where it opens into the nasal pharynx; means 'funnel.'

chondroblasts   Cells that form cartilage.

chondrocytes   Cartilage-forming cells that have surrounded themselves with their secretory product.

chorda tympani   Branch of the facial nerve (VII) that joins with the lingual nerve to carry taste sensations from the anterior two thirds of the tongue and secretomotor fibers to the submandibular and sublingual glands.

cilia   A movable, hairlike process on the apical end of a columnar cell that helps to move substances over the surface of the cells.

cingulum   Lingual lobe of anterior teeth.

circumferential lamellae   Growth layers in bone around the outermost portion of the bone.

circumvallate papillae   Large V-shaped row of papillae lying on the posterior dorsum of the tongue.

class I occlusal relationship   Normal relationship between maxillary and mandibular molars.

class II occlusal relationship   When a mandibular molar is posterior to its normal position.

class III occlusal relationship   When a mandibular molar is anterior to its normal position.

cleft lip   Gap in the upper lip occurring during development.

cleft palate   Lack of joining together of the hard or soft palates.

clinical crown   That part of the tooth protruding out of the gingiva.

clinical root   That part of the tooth embedded in the gingiva and socket.

coalescence   Joining of two lobes of a tooth.

coccygeal   Relating to the tailbone area; single pair of nerves in the tailbone region.

col   Area of an interdental papilla that lies cervical to the interproximal contact of the tooth.

collagen   Nonelastic, primary fiber of connective tissue.

common carotid artery   Main blood vessel on either side of the neck that supplies most of the head.

compound tubuloalveolar   Glandular arrangement that has a branching duct system with secreting cells at the ends of the ducts arranged like tubes with a bulbous endpiece.

compressor naris   Muscle in flared part of nostrils that closes them.

concavity   Depression in a surface.

concha   See *superior nasal concha*.

concrescence   Two adjacent teeth that fuse by their cementum.

condylar neck   Constricted part of ramus of mandible, just below the condyle.

congenital   Occurring at or before birth; may or may not be hereditary.

congenitally missing   Condition of having never been developed.

conical tooth   A supernumerary tooth that is cone shaped.

connective tissue   One of the four basic tissues made up of cells, fibers, ground substance (glue), and sometimes crystal. Bone, cartilage, and blood are special types of connective tissue.

contact area   Area of contact of one tooth with another in the same arch.

contact point   Specific point at which a tooth from one arch occludes with another tooth from the opposing arch.

contour   Shape of the tooth.

convenience occlusion   See *centric occlusion*.

convexity   Bulge in a surface.

copula   Pharyngeal-arch structure that forms posterior third of tongue.

coronal suture   Suture between the frontal bone and the two parietal bones; also called the frontoparietal suture.

coronoid notch   Notch in the upper surface of the mandibular ramus, just anterior to the condyle.

coronoid process   Bony projection at upper anterior ramus of mandible; point of attachment for temporal muscle.

corrugator   Muscle from the bridge of the nose to the lateral part of the eyebrow.

cortical plate   Dense bone on the buccal and lingual surfaces of the alveolar bone.

cortisone   An anti-inflammatory drug.

cranial nerves   Twelve pairs of nerves originating from the brain.

craniosacral outflow   Another name for the parasympathetic nervous system.

cribriform plate   Bone that forms the actual wall of the tooth socket.

cribriform plate of ethmoid   Small perforations of ethmoid bone beside the crista galli that provide passages for olfactory nerves from the nasal to the cranial cavity.

crista galli   Small bony projection of ethmoid bone in the anterior cranial fossa; helps attach the dura mater covering of the brain.

cross-bite   Condition in which the cusps of a tooth in one arch exceed the cusps of a tooth in the opposing arch, buccally or lingually.

cross section   Cutting through a tooth perpendicular to the long axis.

crown   That part of the tooth covered with enamel.

crypt   Term used to describe the early tooth socket.

curve of Spee   Anatomical line beginning at the tip of the canines and following the buccal cusps of premolars and molars when viewed from the buccal aspect of the first molars.

curve of Wilson   Curve that follows the cusp tips, as seen from a frontal view.

cusp   Major pointed or rounded eminence on or near the occlusal surface of a tooth.

cusp of Carabelli   Fifth lobe of a maxillary first molar.

cyst   Sac of fluid lined by epithelium that may grow to varying sizes.

cytoplasm   Fluid substance of cells.

dead tracts   Empty dentinal tubules resulting from death of odontoblasts and their processes in that area.

debrided   Having already accomplished the removal (debridement) of nerve tissue and other debris from the pulp cavity to leave a surgically cleaned area.

deciduous   That which will be shed; specifically, the first dentition of human or animal.

deglutition   Action of swallowing.

dendrite   Single process or multiple processes of a neuron that pick up impulses from other neurons and carry them to the cell body of its neuron.

dens in dente   An invagination of the outer surface of the tooth crown turning inward upon itself.

dental arch   All the teeth in either the maxillary or mandibular jaw that form an arch.

dental lamina   Embryonic downgrowth of oral epithelium that is the forerunner of the tooth germ.

dental papilla   Mesodermal structure partially surrounded by the inner enamel epithelial cells. The dental papilla forms the dentin and pulp.

dental sac   Several layers of flat mesodermal cells partially surrounding the dental papilla and enamel organ; forms the cementum, periodontal ligament, and some alveolar bone.

dentin (formerly **dentine)**   Hard calcified tissue forming the inside body of a tooth, underlying the cementum and enamel and surrounding the pulpal tissue.

dentinal tubule   Space in the dentin occupied by odontoblastic process.

dentinocemental junction   Location in root where the dentin joins the cementum.

dentinoenamel junction   Line marking the junction of the dentin and the enamel.

dentinogenesis imperfecta   Hereditary imperfect dentin formation.

dentition   General character and arrangement of the teeth, taken as a whole, as in carnivorous, herbivorous, and omnivorous dentitions. Primary dentition refers to the deciduous teeth, secondary dentition to the permanent teeth. Mixed dentition refers to a combination of permanent and deciduous teeth in the same dentition.

depression   Lowering of the mandible or opening of the mouth.

depressor anguli oris   Muscle of facial expression that extends from the lower border of the mandible at the canine area up to the corner of the lower lip.

depressor labii inferioris   Muscle that goes from the chin area up into the middle part of the lower lip.

descending palatine artery   Branch of the maxillary artery that supplies the hard and soft palates.

descending palatine nerve   Branch of the second division of the trigeminal nerve to the hard and soft palates.

developmental depression   Noticeable concavity on the formed crown or root of a tooth; occurs at the junction of two lobes, as on the mesial surface of maxillary first premolars, or at the furcation of roots.

developmental grooves   Fine depressed lines in the enamel of a tooth that mark the union of the lobes of the crown.

developmental lines   See *developmental grooves.*

developmental pit   Small hole formed by the junction of two or more developmental lines.

diastema   Any spacing between teeth in the same arch.

digastric fossae   Two small depressions on inferior surface of the mandible at the midline.

digastric muscle   Suprahyoid muscle extending from the mastoid process area to the midline of the mandible; retracts and lowers the mandible.

dilacerated   Said of developing tooth roots that become bent and crooked because of developmental problems.

dilacerated tooth   Tooth with sharply bent roots.

dilaceration   A sharp bend in the root or crown of the tooth.

dilator naris   Muscle going over the tip of nose that opens the nostrils.

disc derangement   When there is damage and displacement to the articular disc of the temporomandibular joint.

distal   Distant; farthest from the median line of the face, or from the origin of a structure.

distal contact area   See *contact area.*

distal marginal groove   Groove that crosses the distal marginal ridge.

distal oblique groove   Groove that separates the distolingual cusp from the remainder of the occlusal surface of an upper molar.

distal pit   Pit found in the distal fossa.

distal proximal surface   Proximal surface on the posterior side of a tooth.

distal step   The mandibular molars are more posterior than the maxillary molars.

distal third   Viewed from the facial or lingual surface, third of a surface farther from the midline.

distobuccal developmental groove   Developmental groove that extends on the buccal surface of a lower first or third molar between the distobuccal and distal cusps.

distoclusion   See *class II occlusal relationship.*

distolingual cusp   Most distal of the lingual cusps.

distolingual groove, distolingual developmental groove   See *distal oblique groove.*

DNA   Deoxyribonucleic acid; the substance in a cell nucleus that builds the genetic information to enable the cell to build a duplicate of itself or control products produced by the cell.

dorsum of the tongue   Top surface of the tongue.

dwarfed roots   Tooth with very short roots in comparison to the crown.

ectoderm   Outer embryonic germ layer that forms skin, salivary glands, hair, sweat glands, sebaceous glands, nerves, and so on.

edema   Swelling of tissue.

edge, incisal   See *incisal edge.*

efferent   Refers to a nerve fiber carrying motor messages *from* the brain.

elastic cartilage   Type of cartilage that has a large number of elastic fibers in it, for example, the ear.

elastic fiber   Fiber of connective tissue that has elastic properties. Many of these are found in the walls of large arteries.

elastin   Major component of elastic fibers of connective tissue.

elevation   Raising the mandible, or closing the mouth.

embrasure   Open space between the proximal surfaces of two teeth where they diverge buccally, labially, or lingually and occlusally from the contact area.

enamel   Hard calcified tissue that covers the dentin of the crown portion of a tooth.

enamel cuticle   Nasmyth's membrane; a thin membrane that covers the crown of a tooth at eruption.

enamel dysplasia   Abnormalities of enamel growth.

enamel hypocalcification   Enamel that is not as dense as regular enamel.

enamel hypoplasia   Enamel that is thin or pitted.

enamel lamellae   Imperfections or cracks in enamel formed by trauma or imperfect enamel formation.

enamel organ   Ectodermal epithelial structure that leads to the formation of tooth enamel.

enamel pearls   Small rounded elevations of enamel

that develop usually in the bifurcations or trifurcations of teeth; considered abnormal structures.

enamel rod Individual pillars of enamel formed by ameloblasts.

enamel spindle Odontoblastic process trapped in enamel at the dentinoenamel junction.

enamel tuft Area of hypocalcified enamel at the dentinoenamel junction.

endochondral bone formation Bone that forms by replacing a hyaline cartilage model.

endocrine Gland or type of secretion that is carried away from the producing cells by blood vessels; the secretion is used in other parts of the body to control certain functions; has no duct system.

endoplasmic reticulum Tubular system in a cell related to the cell's production of secretions such as protein.

endosteal Inside bone; in the center marrow area.

entoderm Inner germ layer of an embryo that forms the epithelial lining of organs such as the digestive tract, liver, lungs, and pancreas.

enzyme Agent capable of producing chemical changes in processes such as the digestion of foods.

eosinophils White granulocyte cells that have some phagocytosing properties and allergic properties.

epicranius See *occipitofrontalis.*

epiglottis Cartilage that helps cover laryngeal opening.

epinephrine Substance produced by the body or synthetically produced that causes many reactions; in dentistry, used to constrict blood flow in tissues.

epithelial Pertaining to epithelium.

epithelial attachment The substance produced by the reduced enamel epithelium that helps secure the attachment epithelium at the base of the gingival sulcus to the tooth.

epithelial diaphragm Deep part of the epithelial root sheath that is turned horizontally.

epithelial rests Cells from the epithelial root sheath that remain in the periodontal space and cells that remain at areas of embryonic fusion.

epithelial rests of Malassez See *epithelial rests.*

epithelial root sheath Downgrowth of the inner and outer enamel epithelium that outlines the shape and number of the roots.

epithelium Layer or layers of cells that cover the surface of the body or line the tubes or cavities inside the body; one of the four basic tissues.

equilibrium Sense of balance.

eruption Movement of the tooth as it emerges through surrounding tissue so that the clinical crown gradually appears longer.

eruptive stage Period of eruption from the completion of crown formation until the teeth come into occlusion.

ethmoid air cells Small, interconnecting bony compartments in the lateral nasal wall that form the ethmoid sinuses.

ethmoid bone Bone that forms a very small part of the anterior neurocranium, a part of the medial wall of the orbit, and a large part of the nasal cavity.

ethmoid bulla Oblong bulge in the middle meatus above the hiatus semilunaris, onto which opens the middle ethmoid air cells.

ethmoid sinus Group of small air cavities in the bone of the lateral wall of the nasal cavity.

excretory duct Duct that is surrounded by connective tissue between lobules of a gland, or is outside the gland and carrying the salivary fluid to the surface without changing it.

exfoliation Shedding or loss of a primary tooth.

exocrine Gland or type of secretion that is carried away from the producing cells by a duct system.

exostoses Small extra growths of bone on its surface; usually seen on the buccal cortical plate.

external auditory meatus Opening of the ear on the side of the skull.

external carotid artery Branch of the common carotid artery that supplies most of the head except the inside of the skull.

external jugular vein Vein that drains the superficial structures of the neck and flows eventually into the subclavian vein in the neck.

external oblique line The bony ridge running downward from the anterior border of the ramus of the mandible and out onto the lateral alveolar process and body.

extrinsic Originating outside a structure.

extrinsic factors External factors.

facial Term used to designate the outer surfaces of the teeth collectively (buccal or labial).

facial artery Branch of the external carotid artery that supplies the superficial face area.

facial contours Curvature of the facial surface of a tooth.

facial embrasure   See *embrasure.*

facial nerve   Seventh cranial nerve (VII), which serves the muscles of facial expression as well as most taste and gland control.

facial surface   See *facial.*

facial third   From a proximal view, the third of that surface closest to the facial side.

familial tendency   When an anomaly occurs more frequently than usual in one family.

fascia   Connective tissue covering muscles and separating muscle layers.

fascial spaces   Potential spaces between layers of muscles or layers of connective tissue.

fauces   Space between the left and right palatine tonsils.

FDI system   The Fédération Dentaire Internationale (International Dental Federation); system for tooth identification.

fibroblast   Basic cell of connective tissue that produces the collagen fiber.

fibrocartilage   Type of cartilage containing large quantities of collagen fibers.

fifth-cusp developmental groove   Groove that separates the cusp of Carabelli from the lingual surface on an upper molar.

filiform papillae   Small pointed projections that heavily cover most of the dorsum of the anterior two thirds of the tongue.

fissure   Deep cleft; developmental line fault usually found in the occlusal or buccal surface of a tooth; commonly the result of the imperfect fusion of the enamel of the adjoining dental lobes.

flange   Projecting edge; the edge of the denture.

fluorosis   Discolored enamel resulting from excessive fluoride intake while crown is developing.

flush terminal plane   The mandibular and maxillary second molars are even, with neither being anterior or posterior.

foliate papillae   Poorly developed papillae that appear as small vertical folds in the posterior part of the sides of the tongue.

foramen   Short circular opening through a bone.

foramen cecum   Depression in tongue two thirds of the way back that marks beginning point of development of thyroid gland; means 'blind aperture.'

foramen magnum   Large foramen in the base of the occipital bone.

foramen ovale   Oval-shaped foramen in the sphenoid bone at the base of the skull.

foramen rotundum   Foramen in the front part of the middle cranial fossa that opens into the pterygopalatine fossa behind and below the eye.

foregut   Front end of the gastrointestinal tube in the early developing embryo.

fossa   Round, wide, relatively shallow depression in the surface of a tooth as seen commonly in the lingual surfaces of the maxillary incisors or between the cusps of molars; also a shallow depression in bone.

free gingiva   Gingiva that forms the gingival sulcus.

frenulum   Little frenum or fold of tissue.

frontal bone   Bone that forms the forehead.

frontal prominence   Bulge in the forehead region that forms the upper facial area in the embryo.

frontal sinus   Air sinus in frontal bone above the eye that opens into the hiatus semilunaris in the middle meatus.

fronto-occipitalis   See *occipitofrontalis.*

frontoparietal suture   See *coronal suture.*

functional eruptive stage   See *posteruptive stage.*

fungiform papillae   Small circular papillae scattered throughout the anterior two thirds of the dorsum of the tongue.

fusion   Two teeth that fuse at their dentin while developing.

gemination   A tooth that partially or fully divides into two teeth while developing.

genial tubercles   Small projections for muscle attachment on the lingual surface of the mandible at the midline.

genioglossus   Extrinsic tongue muscle running from center of mandible up into tongue.

geniohyoid muscle   Suprahyoid muscle that extends from the genial tubercles to the hyoid bone.

germinative layer   See *basal layer.*

gingiva   Part of the gum tissue that immediately surrounds the teeth and alveolar bone.

gingival crest   Most occlusal or incisal extent of gingiva.

gingival crevice   Subgingival space that, under normal conditions, lies between the gingival crest and the epithelial attachment.

gingival embrasure   See *cervical embrasure.*

gingival fibers   Periodontal fibers in the gingiva.

gingival papillae   That portion of the gingiva found between the teeth in the interproximal spaces gingival to the contact area; also called interdental papillae.

gingival sulcus   Space between the free gingiva and the tooth surface.

gingival tissue   See *gingiva.*

gingival unit Subdivision of the periodontium.

gingivitis Inflammation involving the gingival tissues only.

glands of von Ebner Small, minor, serous salivary glands (lingual glands) that open into the crypts of the vallate papillae.

glossopharyngeal glands Small minor salivary glands in the tonsillar pillars.

glossopharyngeal nerve Ninth cranial nerve (IX), serving the muscles of the pharynx, taste, general sensation, and salivary glands.

glycogen Form of starch that by enzymes makes glucose (body sugar) or is made from glucose depending on body needs; stored as a cellular inclusion and readily available as instant energy.

goblet cells Single-celled glands that secrete mucus; found in epithelium of respiratory and digestive tracts from the stomach through the gastrointestinal tract.

Golgi apparatus Flat saclike layers in a cell that "package" the cell products for transportation outside the cell.

granular layer of Tomes Interglobular dentin in the root.

granulocytes White blood cells that have small or large granules in their cytoplasm; neutrophils, basophils, and eosinophils.

greater palatine artery Branch of the descending palatine artery to the hard palate.

greater palatine foramen Foramen on either side of the hard palate between the maxillae and palatine bones.

greater palatine nerve Branch of the descending palatine nerve that serves the hard palate.

greater wing of the sphenoid Part of the sphenoid bone projecting onto the side of the skull behind the zygomatic bone, as well as posterior part of orbit.

ground substance Gluelike substance that serves as the background for connective tissue, including cartilage and bone; composed of a substance known as a mucopolysaccharide.

group function During lateral excursion several teeth, not just a solitary canine, touch simultaneously. Usually the maxillary canine and the first and second premolars touch at the same time.

habitual occlusion See *centric occlusion*.

hamular process See *pterygoid hamulus*.

hard tissue Calcified or mineralized tooth tissues or bone.

haversian system System of blood vessels located within the bones to provide them with nourishment.

hematoma Escape of blood from injured blood vessel into tissue spaces.

hemoglobin Component in red blood cells that carries oxygen.

hereditary Inherited through the genes of parents.

Hertwig's epithelial root sheath See *epithelial root sheath*.

hiatus An opening.

hiatus semilunaris Curving depression beneath the middle nasal concha in the middle meatus. It has openings in it for the frontal, anterior ethmoid, and maxillary sinuses.

histamine Substance produced by some cells that causes swelling, or edema, of the tissues.

holocrine Method of secretion wherein the cell dies and releases its products.

horizontal group Group of alveolodental fibers.

hormones Chemical substances produced by the body that have certain effects on other organs or glands of the body.

Hutchinson's incisors Notched central incisors that develop as a result of congenital syphilis.

hyaline cartilage Type of cartilage that is very firm; sometimes replaced by bone. The larynx and trachea are examples of hyaline cartilage.

hydroxyapatite (sometimes spelled **hydroxylapatite**) The crystal that is found in hard substances of the body such as bone, cementum, dentin, and enamel.

hyoglossus Extrinsic tongue muscle running from hyoid bone up into lateral border of tongue.

hyoid Horseshoe-shaped bone in neck between mandible and larynx.

hyoid arch Second pharyngeal arch, which forms some of the structures in the neck.

hyoid muscles Muscles that attach to the free-floating hyoid bone in the neck.

hypercementosis Increased thickness of cementum, usually seen at the apex of the root.

hyperdontia More than the usual number of teeth.

hyperemia Congestion of blood seen in pulp.

hypocalcified enamel Condition in which there is either an insufficient number of enamel crystals or insufficient growth of the crystals.

hypoglosssal nerve Twelfth cranial nerve (XII); supplies motor control to the tongue muscles.

hypophyseal fossa Saddle-shaped depression on the body of the sphenoid bone located in the middle cranial fossa containing the pituitary gland.

hypoplastic enamel Thin enamel; may be hypocalcified as well.

I band   Light microscopic band at either end of the sarcomere. The I band contains only actin myofilaments.

imbrication lines   Horizontal lines best seen on the labial surfaces of anterior teeth. These are surface manifestations of the striae of Retzius.

immunity   Body's resistance to certain organisms or diseases.

impacted   Teeth not completely erupted that are fully or partially covered by bone or soft tissue.

incisal edge   Edge formed at the labioincisal line angle of an anterior tooth after an incisal ridge has worn down.

incisal embrasure   See *embrasure*.

incisal ridge   Rounded ridge form of the incisal portion of an anterior tooth.

incisal third   From a proximal, lingual, or labial view of an anterior tooth, third of the surface closest to the incisal edge.

incisive foramen   Foramen at the midline of the anterior palate region.

incisive papilla   Small, rounded, oblong mound of tissue directly behind or lingual to the maxillary central incisors and lying over incisive foramen.

incisors   Four center teeth in either arch; essential for cutting.

inferior alveolar branch or artery   Branch of the maxillary artery that supplies the lower teeth.

inferior alveolar nerve   Branch of the third division of the trigeminal nerve to the lower teeth.

inferior border of mandible   Lower edge of the lower jaw.

inferior meatus   Area sheltered over by the inferior nasal concha.

inferior nasal conchae   Small bones that project from the lower lateral walls of the nasal cavity.

inferior orbital fissure   Groovelike opening in the inferior lateral part of the orbit.

inferior pharyngeal constrictor muscle   Lowest of three muscles that form the throat wall and help to move food downward into the esophagus.

inflammatory reaction   Body's mechanism to combat harmful organisms by bringing more plasma and blood cells to injured area.

infrahyoid muscles   Muscles below the hyoid bone that attach to it.

infraorbital artery   Termination of the maxillary artery that passes out of the floor of the orbit through the infraorbital foramen; supplies the skin of the lower eyelid, upper lip, and side of the nose.

infraorbital foramen   Foramen just below the lower rim of the orbit in the maxillary bone.

infraorbital nerve   Termination of the second division of the trigeminal nerve that supplies the skin of the lower eyelid, nose, and upper lip.

infratemporal fossa   Area on side of skull immediately below the temporal fossa; pterygoid muscles and the maxillary artery are located there.

inherited   Passed on from parents or grandparents.

inner enamel epithelium (IEE)   Group of epithelial cells in the enamel organ that eventually form the enamel of the crown.

inorganic matrix   Hydroxyapatite crystals in the early matrix.

inorganic matter   Mineral deposits such as calcium or phosphorus.

insertion   End of muscle attached to more movable structure.

intercalated ducts   Short, small ducts that carry saliva from acini to striated ducts.

intercellular fluid   Fluid between cells; primarily consists of blood plasma.

intercuspal position (ICP)   See *centric occlusion*.

intercuspation   Relationship of the cusps of the premolars and molars of one jaw with those of the opposing jaw during any of the occlusal relationships.

interdental   Located between the teeth.

interdental papilla   Projection of gingiva between the teeth.

interglobular dentin   Areas of hypocalcified dentin between normal areas of dentin; found in both crown and root dentin.

interlobular ducts   Ducts between lobules of glands.

intermaxillary suture   Suture between the maxillae. It is seen below the nasal cavity and in the front portion of the hard palate.

internal acoustic meatus   Opening in the lateral part of the posterior cranial fossa for the facial and statoacoustic cranial nerves.

internal carotid artery   Branch of the common carotid artery that supplies the brain and inside of the skull.

internal jugular vein   Main vein that drains the brain and deep structures of the head and neck; flows into the brachiocephalic vein.

interparietal suture   See *sagittal suture*.

interproximal   Between the proximal surfaces of adjoining teeth in the same arch.

interproximal space   Triangular space between adjoining teeth; the proximal surfaces of the teeth form sides of the triangle; the alveolar bone, the base, and the contact area of the teeth form the apex.

interstitial lamellae Parts of old bone layers found between newly formed layers of bone.

intertubular dentin All dentin that is not tubular or peritubular.

intralobular ducts Ducts surrounded by acini in a gland. Some of them help change the saliva before it leaves the gland.

intramembranous bone formation Bone formed directly from mesenchymal cells that become osteoblasts.

intrinsic Lying entirely inside a structure.

intrinsic factors Internal factors.

involuntary muscle Not voluntary; unable to be willfully controlled.

jugular foramen See *jugular fossa.*

jugular fossa Depression in the base of the skull with an opening for the passage of the internal jugular vein and the IX, X, and XI cranial nerves from the skull.

junctional epithelium Epithelium that functions to hold mucosa, in the base of the gingival sulcus, to the tooth.

keratin Substance that makes up the surface cells of skin, hair, and nails.

keratinized cells Dead cells of the stratum corneum.

keratinized stratified squamous epithelium Multilayered epithelium, like skin; upper layers are dead cells; makeup is similar to the composition of hair.

keratohyalin granules Granules in the stratum granulosum, which finally help produce the dead layer of cells on the skin surface.

labia Latin word for lips; singular *labium.*

labial Of or pertaining to the lips; toward the lips.

labial frenum Fold of tissue that attaches the lip to the labial mucosa at the midline of the lips.

labial glands Small minor salivary glands in the lips.

lacrimal bone Small bone at the inner front of the orbit, forming part of the canal from the eye to the nose.

lacrimal groove Groove in the lacrimal bone for the lacrimal duct.

lambdoid suture Inverted V-shaped suture between the occipital and parietal bones; also known as the parieto-occipital suture.

lamina dura Radiographic term denoting cribriform plate and bundle bone.

larynx Voice box; trachea begins just below it.

lateral excursion Movement of the jaws sideways.

lateral lingual swellings Paired structures that arise from the internal pharyngeal arches that forms the anterior two thirds of the tongue.

lateral nasal process Embryological structure that forms the side of the nose and the area beneath the medial corner of the eye.

lateral pharyngeal Area or fascial space beside the throat wall.

lateral pharyngeal space See *lateral pharyngeal.*

lateral pterygoid muscle Muscle that extends from the pterygoid plate to the condyle and protrudes the mandible.

lateral pterygoid plate Thin wall of bone projecting backward from the pterygoid process on the lateral side.

leeway space The difference between the sum of the mesiodistal measurements of the deciduous canines plus the deciduous molars compared with mesiodistal measurements of the permanent canine and premolars in any one quadrant.

lesser palatine artery Branch of the descending palatine artery that goes to the soft palate.

lesser palatine nerve Branch of the descending palatine nerve that supplies the soft palate.

lesser petrosal nerve Branch of the glossopharyngeal nerve (IX) that carries secretomotor function to the parotid gland via the auriculotemporal nerve.

lesser wing of sphenoid Projection of the sphenoid bone that forms the posterior border of the anterior cranial fossa.

leukemia Cancer of white blood cells that chokes out red blood cell production.

levator anguli oris Muscle that goes from beneath the eye to the corner of the upper lip.

levator labii superioris Muscle that extends from below the eye to the middle part of the upper lip.

levator veli palatini Muscle of the soft palate that helps pull it back against the throat wall.

ligament Regularly arranged group of collagen fibers that attach bone to bone.

line angle Angle formed by two surfaces, for example, mesial and lingual; the junction is called the mesiolingual line angle.

lingual Pertaining to or affecting the tongue; next to or toward the tongue.

lingual artery Branch of the external carotid artery that supplies the tongue and floor of the mouth.

lingual contours Curvature of the lingual surface of a tooth.

lingual crest of curvature   Most convex or widest portion of the lingual surface of a tooth.

lingual developmental groove   Groove on the lingual surface that separates two lingual cusps; see *lingual groove.*

lingual embrasure   See *embrasure.*

lingual frenum   Fold of tissue that attaches the undersurface of the tongue to the floor of the mouth.

lingual glands   Minor salivary glands of the tongue.

lingual groove   Developmental groove that occurs on the lingual side of the tooth.

lingual nerve   Branch of the third division of the trigeminal nerve that supplies the general sensation to the tongue and floor of the mouth.

lingual surface   See *lingual.*

lingual third   From a proximal view, third of a surface closest to the lingual side.

lingual tonsils   Tonsil tissue on the dorsum of the posterior part of the tongue.

lingula   Small projection of bone just in front of the mandibular foramen.

lining mucosa   Mucosa of the soft palate, lips, cheeks, vestibule, and floor of the mouth.

lipid   Fatty substance found in cells as an inclusion; used as a reserve source of energy.

lobe   Part of a tooth formed by any one of the major developing centers that begin the calcification of the tooth.

lobe of Carabelli   See *cusp of Carabelli.*

long buccal nerve   Lower branch of the buccal nerve that supplies the mandibular buccal gingiva.

lower deep cervical   Group of lymph nodes in the lower lateral neck beneath the sternomastoid muscle.

Ludwig's angina   Infection in the fascial spaces beneath the chin.

lumbar   Relating to the lower back, for example, vertebrae or nerves of the lower back.

lumen   Inside of a tube or duct; inside diameter of the opening.

lymph nodes   Small bean-shaped structures connected to one another by very small tubules. They combat infections in the body.

lymphadenopathy   Enlarged lymph glands, or nodes; may be seen or felt when one has a sore throat, infected ears, and so on.

lymphatic vessels   Small tubes throughout the body that carry fluid from between the cells back into the vascular system.

lymphocytes   Kind of agranulocyte; active in the inflammatory process.

lymphoid tissue   Tissues made up of lymphocytes, which fight infections.

lysosomes   Small membrane-bound structures in a cell that act as a "garbage can" for the nonusable or harmful substances that find their way inside the cell.

macrodontia   Teeth are too large for the jaw.

macrophage   Cell of connective tissue that destroys other cells, usually from outside the body.

malocclusion   Abnormal occlusion of the teeth.

mamelon   One of the three rounded protuberances of the incisal surface of a newly erupted incisor tooth.

mandible   Lower jaw.

mandibular   Pertaining to the lower jaw.

mandibular arch   First pharyngeal arch that forms the area of the mandible and maxillae; the lower dental arch.

mandibular condyle   Rounded top of the mandible that articulates with the mandibular fossa.

mandibular division   Third part of the trigeminal nerve (V); frequently represented as V_3.

mandibular foramen   Opening on the medial surface of the ramus of the mandible for entrance of nerves and blood vessels to the lower teeth.

mandibular fossa   Depression on the inferior surface of the skull in the temporal bone that articulates with the condyle of the mandible.

mandibular notch   See *coronoid notch.*

mandibular process   That portion of the mandibular pharyngeal arch that goes to form the mandible.

mandibular tori   Bony growths on the lingual cortical plate of bone opposite the mandibular canines; also called torus mandibularis.

marginal developmental groove   See *marginal groove.*

marginal gingiva   See *free gingiva.*

marginal groove   Groove that crosses a marginal ridge.

marginal ridge   Ridge or elevation of enamel forming the margin of the surface of a tooth; specifically, at the mesial and distal margins of the occlusal surfaces of premolars and molars, and the mesial and distal margins of the lingual surfaces of incisors and canines.

marrow cavity   Hollow center of bone responsible for blood cell production and, later in life, for fat storage.

masseter muscle   Muscle on the lateral surface of the mandible that elevates it.

masseteric branch   Branch of the maxillary artery to the masseter muscle.

mast cells   Cells in connective tissue that release histamines.

mastication   Act of chewing or grinding.

masticatory mucosa   Mucosa of the hard palate and gingiva.

mastoid process   Large projection of temporal bone behind the ear.

matrix   Framework for a material; the framework for hard-tissue formation.

matrix band   Metal or plastic band fitted around a tooth when interproximal fillings are placed to prevent the filling material from squeezing out.

maxillae   Paired main bone of the upper jaw.

maxillary   Pertaining to the upper arch.

maxillary arch   Upper dental arch.

maxillary artery   Major branch of the external carotid artery that supplies the teeth, gingiva, cheeks, palate, and several other areas.

maxillary division   Second part of the trigeminal nerve (V); usually represented as V_2.

maxillary process   Upper portion of the mandibular pharyngeal arch that forms the maxillae.

maxillary sinus   Largest of the paired paranasal sinuses, located in the maxillae.

maxillary tuberosity   Bulging posterior surface of the maxillae behind the third molar region.

meatus   Space beneath the shelter of each of the nasal conchae.

medial nasal process   Embryological structures that form the bridge of the nose, the middle part of the upper lip, part of the nasal septum, and part of the anterior hard palate.

medial pterygoid muscle   Muscle running between the mandible and pterygoid plate that elevates the mandible.

medial pterygoid plate   Thin wall of bone projecting backward from the pterygoid process on the medial side.

median line   Vertical (central) line that divides the body into right and left; the median line of the face.

median palatine suture   Suture that goes down the middle of the hard palate. The anterior part of the suture may also be called part of the intermaxillary suture.

median raphe   A midline joining of the left and right pharyngeal constrictor muscles in the posterior throat wall; runs from the base of the skull above to the esophagus below.

megakaryocyte   Large cell in marrow that is forerunner of white blood cells.

melanin   Brown pigment in the skin. An increase in the amount of pigment is seen after sunburn and is produced by the melanocytes.

melanocytes   Pigment-producing cells located below the basal layer of epithelium. The pigment granules are incorporated into the basal cells and move up through the layers to the surface.

mental artery   Branch of the inferior alveolar artery that supplies the lower lip and gingiva adjacent to the lip.

mental branch   See *mental artery.*

mental foramen   Foramen on the lateral side of the mandible, below the premolars.

mental nerve   Branch of the inferior alveolar nerve that supplies the skin and mucosa of the lower lip and labial gingiva.

mental protuberance   Point of the chin on the anterior inferior surface of the midline of the mandible.

mental spines   See *genial tubercles.*

mentalis   Muscle that extends from the bone on the chin into the skin of the chin.

merocrine   Method of secretion wherein the droplets pass out of the cell by fusing with the cell membrane, eliminating the possibility of damage to the cell.

mesenchymal cell   Primitive cell of the mesodermal embryonic layer. This cell has the ability to form a number of different tissues. Some of these cells are available throughout life.

mesial   Toward or situated in the middle, for example, toward the midline of the dental arch.

mesial contact area   See *contact area.*

mesial developmental depression   Indented area on the mesial surface of a tooth.

mesial drift   Phenomenon of permanent molars continuing to move mesially after eruption.

mesial marginal developmental groove   See *mesial marginal groove.*

mesial marginal groove   Developmental groove that crosses the mesial marginal ridge.

mesial pit   Pit found in the mesial fossa.

mesial proximal surface   Proximal surface closest to the midline.

mesial step   The mandibular molars are more anterior than the maxillary molars.

mesial third   From a facial or a lingual view, third of the surface closest to the midline.

mesiobuccal developmental groove   Developmental groove that runs on the buccal surface of a lower first or third molar between the mesiobuccal and distobuccal cusps.

mesioclusion   See *class III occlusal relationship*.

mesiodens   Supernumerary teeth arising in the midline of the maxilla.

mesiolingual cusp   Most mesial of the lingual cusps.

mesiolingual developmental groove   Lingual developmental groove that separates the mesiolingual and distolingual cusps.

mesiolingual groove   See *mesiolingual developmental groove*.

mesoderm   Middle germ layer of the embryo that forms connective tissue, muscle, bone, cartilage, blood, and so on.

metabolism   Building up or breaking down of food accompanied by the production or use of energy.

microdontia   Teeth are too small for the jaw.

middle ethmoid sinus   Middlemost group of ethmoid air cells.

middle meatus   Area sheltered by the middle nasal concha.

middle nasal concha   Small projection of thin bone from the middle of the lateral nasal wall.

middle pharyngeal constrictor muscle   The middle of three muscles that form the throat wall and help to move food downward into the esophagus.

middle superior alveolar nerve   Branch of the infraorbital nerve that supplies the maxillary premolars and usually the mesiobuccal root of the maxillary first molar.

middle third   See *mesial third*.

midline   Imaginary line that divides the body into right and left halves.

midsagittal plane   Divides the body vertically into right and left halves.

migration (movement)   The flow of connective tissue in the upper lip that aids in the formation of the lip.

mitochondria   Small organelles in a cell that produce energy and control the metabolism of the cell; singular *mitochondrion*.

mitotic division   Process of cell division that leads to development of two cells from one.

mixed dentition   State of having primary and permanent teeth in the dental arches at the same time.

molars   Large posterior teeth used for grinding.

monocytes   White agranulocytes that have phagocytic properties.

mortality rate   Death rate; number of deaths in a certain population for a certain reason; usually measured in percentage, or may be the number of deaths per 1,000, 10,000, 100,000, and so on.

mucogingival junction   Point at which the alveolar mucosa becomes gingiva.

mucosa   Moist epithelial linings of oral cavity and respiratory and digestive systems.

mucous   Pertaining to mucus, the thick viscous secretion of a gland.

mucous acini   Salivary unit that produces viscous saliva.

mulberry molars   Molars with multiple cusps that are caused by congenital syphylis.

multiple root   Root with more than one branch.

muscle   One of the four basic tissues; has the property of contraction or shortening of the fibers, which accomplishes work. There are three types of muscle: skeletal, cardiac, and smooth.

muscle of uvula   The small muscular projection that extends downward from the posterior of the soft palate.

myelin sheath   Covering around axons or dendrites of some nerves.

myelinated   Covered with myelin; a nerve that has a myelin sheath.

mylohyoid line   Diagonal line on the medial surface of the mandible for attachment of the mylohoid muscle.

mylohyoid muscle   Suprahyoid muscle that forms the floor of the mouth.

mylohyoid nerve   Branch of the inferior alveolar nerve to the mylohyoid muscle and anterior belly of the digastric muscle.

myoepithelial cell   An epithelium-like cell that is found around glands and can contract like a muscle to help squeeze the secretions out of the ducts of the glands.

myofiber   Single muscle fiber or muscle cell.

myofibril   Small muscle fiber; when grouped together, they make up a myofiber.

myofilaments   Smallest thick and thin filaments in a myofibril which are responsible for contraction.

myosin   One of the myofilaments located in the A band; thicker than actin.

nasal aperture   Opening of nasal cavity in skull.

nasal bone   Bones that form the bridge of the nose.

nasal pits   Depressions in the developing facial area that deepen into the nasal passages.

nasal septum   Wall between the left and right sides of the nasal cavity, made up of the ethmoid and vomer bones.

nasalis   Nasal muscle of facial expression; divided into dilator naris and compressor naris.

Nasmyth's membrane   See *primary enamel cuticle.*

nasopalatine nerve   Continuation of pterygopalatine nerve that supplies lingual gingiva of maxillary incisors.

nervous tissue   One of the four basic tissues. Groups of cells (neurons) carry messages to and from the brain and perform many other tasks.

neurocranium   Part of the skull that surrounds the brain.

neuron   Nerve cell.

neutroclusion   See *class I occlusal relationship.*

neutrophils   Granulocytes whose granules do not stain brightly. This is one of the major cell groups involved in the inflammatory process.

nodular   Characterized by nodes or knot-like swellings.

nonsuccedaneous   Permanent teeth that do not succeed or replace deciduous teeth.

nonworking side   Opposite side from which the mandible is moved.

nucleus   Control center of the cell. DNA and RNA are found here to control cell division and production.

oblique groove   See *distolingual groove.*

oblique group   Group of alveolodental fibers.

oblique ridge   Ridge running obliquely across the occlusal surface of the upper molars. It is formed by the union of the triangular ridge of the distobuccal cusp with the distal portion of the triangular ridge of the mesiolingual cusp.

occipital bone   Bone of the base and back of the skull. The foramen magnum is found in the basal portion.

occipital condyles   Thick smooth surfaces on the basal part of the occipital bone just lateral to the foramen magnum. They articulate with the cervical vertebrae.

occipitofrontalis   Muscle of facial expression in the scalp region extending from front to back.

occluding   Contacting opposing teeth.

occlusal   Articulating or biting surface.

occlusal embrasure   See *embrasure.*

occlusal plane   Side view of the occlusal surfaces.

occlusal relationship   Way in which the maxillary and mandibular teeth touch each other.

occlusal stress   Pressures on the occlusal surfaces of teeth.

occlusal surface   See *occlusal.*

occlusal table   As seen from an occlusal view, area bordered by the cusp tips and marginal ridges.

occlusal third   From a proximal, lingual, or buccal view of a posterior tooth, the third of a surface closest to the occlusal surface.

occlusal trauma   Injury brought about by one tooth prematurely hitting another during closure of the jaws.

occlusion   Relationship of the mandibular and maxillary teeth when closed or during excursive movements of the mandible; when the teeth of the mandibular arch come into contact with the teeth of the maxillary arch in any functional relationship.

oculomotor nerve   Third cranial nerve (III); aids in the movement of the eye.

odontoblast   Dentin-forming cell that originates from the dental papilla.

odontoblastic process   Cellular extension of the odontoblast, which is located along the full width of the dentin.

odontoma   A tumor made up of enamel, dentin, cementum, and pulp.

olfactory epithelium   Modified respiratory epithelium found in the superior nasal cavity containing nerves that allow the sensation of smell.

olfactory nerve   First cranial nerve (I); transmits sensations of smell.

omohyoid muscle   Infrahyoid muscle that extends from the shoulder blade to the hyoid bone.

opaque   Not easily able to transmit light.

open bite   Space left between the teeth when the jaws close.

open contact   Space between adjacent teeth in the same arch; an interproximal opening instead of a contact area where the teeth touch.

ophthalmic division   First part of the trigeminal nerve (V); usually represented as V_1.

optic nerve   Second cranial nerve (II); conducts visual stimuli.

oral epithelium   Lining membrane of the oral cavity; stratified squamous epithelium.

oral pharynx   The area behind the oral cavity that runs from the palatine tonsils to the back wall of the throat.

orbicularis oculi   Muscle that goes around the eye and eyelid.

orbicularis oris   Muscle that encircles the mouth; has many muscles running into it and blending with it.

orbit   Bony opening for the eye in the skull.

organelles   Means 'little organs'; the functioning components in cells; they aid in the vital functions of the cells.

organic matrix   Noncalcified framework in which crystals grow.

origin   End of a muscle that is attached to the less movable structure.

ossicles   Small bones of the middle ear.

osteoblasts   Cells that form bone.

osteoclast   Multinucleated cell that is responsible for destroying bone, as well as cementum and dentin.

osteocyte   Osteoblast that has surrounded itself with bone.

ostium of the maxillary sinus   Opening of the maxillary sinus into the nasal cavity beneath the middle nasal concha.

outer enamel epithelium (OEE)   Outer epithelial layer of the enamel organ; serves as a protection for the developing enamel.

overbite   Relationship of the teeth in which the incisal ridges of the maxillary anterior teeth extend below the incisal edges of the mandibular anterior teeth when the teeth are placed in a centric occlusal relationship.

overhanging restoration   Excess of filling material extending past the confines of the tooth preparation; an overextension of filling material.

overjet   Relationship of teeth in which the incisal ridges or buccal cusp ridges of the maxillary teeth extend facially to the incisal ridges or buccal cusp ridges of the mandibular teeth when the teeth are in a centric occlusal relationship.

palatal   Pertaining to the palate or roof of the mouth.

palatal process of the maxillae   Part of the maxillae that forms the anterior part of the hard palate.

palatal shelves   Projections of the maxillary processes that form the hard and soft palates.

palatine bone   Bone that forms the posterior part of the hard palate and the lateral nasal cavity.

palatine glands   Minor salivary glands in the hard and soft palates.

palatine tonsils   Normally just called tonsils; found at the side of the throat opposite the back of the tongue.

palatoglossal arch   See *anterior pillar.*

palatoglossal fold   See *anterior pillar.*

palatoglossal muscle   Muscle that extends from the soft palate down into the sides of the tongue. The mucosa over this muscle forms the anterior pillar of the throat.

palatomaxillary suture   See *transverse palatine suture.*

palatopharyngeal arch   See *posterior pillars.*

palatopharyngeal fold   Posterior tonsillar pillar running from soft palate down to pharynx.

palatopharyngeal muscle   Muscle that extends from the soft palate down into the lateral pharyngeal wall. The mucosa over this muscle forms the posterior pillar of the throat.

Palmer notation system   System of coding the teeth using brackets, numbers, and letters.

pancreas   Organ in the abdominal cavity behind the stomach that produces many of the enzymes necessary for the digestion of food.

papillary gingiva   Gingiva that forms the interdental papillae.

parakeratinized layer   Stratum corneum where some cells are dead and some are still alive.

parakeratinized stratified squamous epithelium   Multilayered epithelium in which top layers of cells are not completely dead.

paralleling technique   Method of taking radiographs that supposedly gives the most accurate representation of proper tooth dimensions; requires the use of special film holders.

paramolar   Small supernumerary tooth located buccally or lingually to a molar.

paranasal sinuses   Four pairs of cavities in bones around the nasal cavity.

parapharyngeal   See *lateral pharyngeal.*

parasympathetic nervous system   Part of the autonomic (automatic) nervous system that originates from some of the cranial nerves and some of the sacral nerves. It controls a number of functions, including stimulation of the salivary glands.

parathyroid gland   Small gland embedded in the thyroid gland that helps control calcium metabolism in the body.

parietal bone   Pair of bones that form the upper lateral part of the skull.

parieto-occipital suture   See *lambdoid suture.*

parotid gland   Large salivary gland on the side of the face in front of the ear.

passive eruption   Condition in which the tooth does not move but the gingival attachment moves farther apically.

peg-shaped lateral   Poorly formed maxillary lateral incisor with a cone-shaped crown.

periapical   Around the tip of a tooth root.

periodontal   Surrounding a tooth.

periodontal membrane or ligament Collagen fibers attached to the teeth roots and alveolar bone, serving as an attachment of the tooth to the bone.

periodontium Supporting tissues surrounding the teeth.

periosteum Fibrous and cellular layer that covers bones and contains cells that become osteoblasts.

peripheral nervous system Made up of the nerves originating from the spinal cord and brain (spinal and cranial nerves).

periphery Circumferential boundary; outer border.

peristaltic contractions The rhythmic waves of contraction of the smooth muscle of the gut wall that moves the food through the digestive tract.

peritubular dentin Dentin immediately surrounding the tubule. It is slightly more calcified than the rest of the dentin.

phagocytes Cells that destroy various microorganisms.

pharyngeal Relating to the pharynx or throat.

pharyngeal arches Development tissue in upper throat areas from which develop a number of structures in that region.

pharyngeal plexus of nerves Fibers of the glossopharyngeal (IX) and vagal (X) cranial nerves that supply the pharyngeal, or throat, wall.

pharynx Throat area, from the nasal cavity to the larynx.

pheresis Process of removing platelets from a blood donor and then pumping the collected blood, minus the platelets, back into the donor.

philtrum Small depression at the midline of the upper lip.

pillars Folds of tissue appearing in front of and behind the palatine tonsils.

piriform aperture See *nasal aperture.*

pit Small pointed depression in dental enamel, usually at the junction of two or more developmental grooves; a small hole anywhere on the crown.

pituitary gland Master controlling endocrine gland located in the middle cranial fossa.

plasma Fluid part of the blood without the cells.

plasma cell One of the cells that helps produce antibodies.

platysma Broad muscle in the neck going from the mandible down into the upper chest region.

point angles Meeting of three surfaces at a point to form a corner; angles formed by the junction of three surfaces, for example, the mesiolingual occlusal point angle.

posterior Situated toward the back, as premolars and molars.

posterior auricular muscle Muscle extending from behind the ear into the back of the ear.

posterior ethmoid sinus Posteriormost group of ethmoid air cells.

posterior mediastinum Space in the chest behind the heart and between the lungs.

posterior nasal aperature See *choana.*

posterior nasal spine Pointed bony projection at posterior end of the hard palate.

posterior pillars Folds of tissue behind the tonsil that contain the palatopharyngeus muscle.

posterior superior alveolar artery Branch of the maxillary artery that enters the maxillary tuberosity and supplies the maxillary molars.

posterior superior alveolar nerve Part of the second division of the trigeminal nerve that enters the maxillary tuberosity and supplies the maxillary molars, generally excluding mesiobuccal root of first molar.

posterior teeth Teeth of either jaw to the rear of the incisors and canines.

posteruptive stage Period of eruption from the time the teeth occlude until they are lost and characterized by occlusal wear of teeth and compensating eruption.

potential spaces Areas between two layers of tissue that are normally closed but may be spread apart, as in a tissue space infection.

preameloblast Cell in the intermediate stage between an inner enamel epithelial cell and an ameloblast.

preeruptive stage Period of time when the crown of the tooth is developing.

prefunctional eruptive stage See *eruptive stage.*

premature contact area The area where an upper and a lower tooth touch and hit each other before the rest of the teeth occlude together.

premaxilla Bony area of the upper jaw that includes the alveolar ridge for the incisors and the area immediately behind it.

premolars Permanent teeth that replace the primary molars.

preventive considerations Ideas relating to the prevention of dental disease rather than the treatment of the disease after it occurs.

primary attachment epithelium Remains of reduced enamel epithelium that provides initial attachment of mucosa at base of gingival sulcus.

primary dentin Dentin formed from the beginning of calcification until tooth eruption.

primary dentition   First set of teeth; baby teeth; milk teeth; deciduous teeth.

primary enamel cuticle   Keratinlike covering on the surface of the enamel; the final product of the ameloblast.

primary nodes   First group of lymph nodes to be involved in the spread of infection.

primary palate   The early developing part of the hard palate that comes from the medial nasal process and forms a V-shaped wedge of tissue that runs from the incisive foramen forward and laterally between the lateral incisors and canines of the maxilla.

primary teeth   See *deciduous.*

primate spaces   The diastema present mesial to the maxillary canine and also present distal to the mandibular canine. A characteristic usually present in primates such as apes, monkeys, and man.

procerus   Muscle going from the bridge of the nose to the medial part of the eyebrow.

prosthetic appliance   Any constructed appliance that replaces a missing part.

protein   One of the basic components of many foodstuffs and much of the body. Proteins are made up of small units known as amino acids, strung together in long chains.

protrude   See *protrusion.*

protrusion   Condition of being thrust forward, as protrusion of the anterior teeth, referring to the teeth being too far labial; the forward movement of the mandible.

proximal   Nearest, next, immediately adjacent to; distal or mesial.

proximal contact areas   Proximal area on a tooth that touches an adjacent tooth on the mesial or distal side.

proximal surface   See *proximal.*

pseudostratified columnar epithelium   Single layer of cells appearing as many layers because the cells have various heights; found primarily in the respiratory tract.

pterygoid branches   Branches of the maxillary artery that supply the medial and lateral pterygoid muscles.

pterygoid fossa   Depression between the medial and lateral pterygoid plates.

pterygoid hamulus   Small curving process projecting downward from the medial pterygoid plate of the sphenoid bone.

pterygoid plexus of veins   Meshwork of veins behind the maxillary tuberosity that flows into the maxillary veins.

pterygoid processes   Large downward projections of the sphenoid bone behind the maxillae.

pterygomandibular raphe   Band of connective tissue of tendon that connects the posterior end of the buccinator muscle with the anterior end of the superior constrictor of the pharynx.

pterygopalatine artery   Branch of the maxillary artery for the nasal cavity that joins the greater palatine artery in the anterior hard palate.

pterygopalatine fossa   Space behind and below the orbit; location of maxillary nerve and last part of maxillary artery.

pterygopalatine nerve   Branch of the second division of the trigeminal nerve that goes to the mucosa of the nasal cavity and anterior hard palate.

pulmonary artery   Blood vessel that carries blood from the heart to the lungs to pick up oxygen.

pulmonary veins   Blood vessels that carry blood back to the heart from the lungs.

pulp canal   Canal in the root of a tooth that leads from the apex to the pulp chamber. Under normal conditions it contains dental pulp tissue.

pulp cavity   Entire cavity within the tooth, including the pulp canal and pulp chamber.

pulp chamber   Cavity or chamber in the center of the crown of a tooth that normally contains the major portion of the dental pulp. The pulp canals lead into the pulp chambers.

pulp, dental   Highly vascular and innervated connective tissue contained within the pulp cavity of the tooth. The dental pulp is composed of arteries, veins, nerves, connective tissues and cells, lymph tissue, and odontoblasts.

pulp horn (horn of pulp)   Extension of pulp tissue into a thin point of the pulp chamber in the tooth crown.

pulp stones   Small dentinlike calcifications in pulp.

Purkinje's fibers   Specialized heart muscle fibers that carry nerve impulses.

pyramidal cells   Cuboidal cells in smaller ducts that are pushed into a pyramid shape because of the smaller diameter of the inside (lumen) versus the outside.

quadrants   One fourth of the dentition. The four quadrants are divided into right and left, maxillary and mandibular.

radiopacities   Whitish region on an x-ray film.

ramus of the mandible   Vertical portion of mandible.

Rathke's pouch   Outpouching in the embryonic oral cavity that becomes part of the pituitary gland.

recession   Migration of the gingival crest in an apical direction, away from the crown of the tooth.

red blood cells   Most numerous of the blood cells, responsible for carrying oxygen to the rest of the body; erythrocytes.

reduced enamel epithelium   Fusion of the ameloblast layer with the outer enamel epithelium.

referred pain   Pain that seems to originate in one area but actually originates in another area.

reflex arc   Sensory message that goes to the spinal cord and meets with a motor nerve to cause an action. The reflex action occurs without the message first reaching the brain to voluntarily cause the action.

reparative dentin   Localized formation of dentin in response to local trauma such as occlusal trauma or caries.

resorption   Physiological removal of tissues or body products, as of the roots of deciduous teeth, or of some alveolar process after the loss of the permanent teeth.

respiratory epithelium   Pseudostratified columnar ciliated epithelium that is found in the nose and most of the rest of the respiratory tract.

rete peg formation   Development of interdigitation between the epithelium and the underlying connective tissue.

reticular fiber   Smaller collagenlike fiber that forms the framework for a number of organs.

retrodiscal pad   Vascular and nerve tissue behind disc of temporomandibular joint.

retromandibular vein   Vein lying behind the mandible. It drains the side of the head and sends blood to both the external and internal jugular veins.

retromolar pad   Pad of tissue behind the mandibular third molars.

retromolar triangle   Triangular area of bone just behind the mandibular third molars.

retropharyngeal   Group of lymph nodes behind the posterior throat wall; refers to the area behind the pharynx.

retropharyngeal nodes   See *retropharyngeal.*

retropharyngeal space   Space behind the pharynx and in front of the cervical vertebrae.

retrusion   Act or process of retraction or moving back, as when the mandible is placed in posterior relationship to the maxillae.

ridge   Long narrow elevation or crest, as on the surface of a tooth or bone.

risorius   Small muscle that lies on the surface of and parallel to the buccinator muscle.

RNA   Ribonucleic acid; the substance in the cell nucleus and cytoplasm that carries the DNA "message" to build other cells or cell products.

rod sheath   Material surrounding the enamel rod. It is slightly more fibrous than the enamel rod.

root   That portion of a tooth embedded in the alveolar process and covered with cementum.

root canal   See *pulp canal.*

root planing   Process of smoothing the cementum of the root of a tooth.

root trunk   That portion of a multirooted tooth found between the cervical line and the points of bifurcation or trifurcation of roots.

rudimentary lobe   Small underdeveloped lobe of a tooth; less than a minor lobe.

rugae   Small ridges of tissue extending laterally across the anterior of the hard palate.

sacral   Relating to the hip region, for example, sacral nerves and vertebrae.

sagittal suture   Suture that extends along the middle of the top of the skull between the parietal bones.

salpingopharyngeal muscle   Muscle that runs from the end of the auditory tube in the nasal pharynx downward into the lateral wall of the pharynx and helps to elevate it in the swallowing process.

sarcomere   Smallest functional unit of a striated muscle fiber, composed of an A band with half an I band at either end and running from Z line to Z line.

sclerotic dentin   Condition in which the tubules have been filled in with dentin because of damage to the odontoblast.

sebaceous glands   Small oil-producing glands that are usually connected to and lubricate hairs.

secondary attachment epithelium   Epithelium of free gingiva that produced mucosal attachment at base of gingival sulcus.

secondary dentin   Dentin formed throughout the pulp chamber and pulp canal from the time of eruption.

secondary dentition   Permanent dentition.

secondary enamel cuticle   Mucopolysaccharide cementing substance secreted by the reduced enamel epithelium that functions in cementing the base of the gingival sulcus to the tooth.

secondary groove   See *supplemental groove.*

secondary nodes   Second group of lymph nodes involved in the spread of infection.

seromucous   Pertaining to a mixture of serous and mucus-secreting cells in the same gland.

seromucous acini   Glandular acini that have both mucous and serous cells.

serotonin   Compound that can affect blood flow in different parts of the body.

serous   Pertaining to thin watery type of glandular secretion, serum.

serous acini   Glandular cells that produce watery secretion.

serous demilunes   Cluster of serous salivary cells that sits, like a cap or half-moon, on a mucous acinus. This acinus therefore secretes both mucus and serum.

Sharpey's fibers   Part of the periodontal ligament; embedded in cementum or alveolar bone.

short palate   Palate of insufficient length to meet the back wall of the throat.

sickle cell anemia   Disease in which the red blood cells are defective and cannot properly carry oxygen.

simple columnar epithelium   Single layer of tall cells found lining the digestive tract and other ducts of the body.

simple cuboidal epithelium   Single layer of square or cubelike cells that line many of the ducts of the body.

simple squamous epithelium   Single layer of flat cells that are found lining blood vessels, chest and abdominal cavities, and many other areas.

single root   Root with one main branch.

skeletal classification   A system of classifying bones based on the position of the maxilla in relation to that of the mandible. This classification does not pertain to the teeth.

skeletal muscle   Striped voluntarily controlled muscle that allows for body movement.

slough   Loss of dead cells from the surface of tissue; pronounced *sluff.*

smooth muscle   Unstriped involuntarily controlled muscle found in the digestive tract and other organs; helps move food along the digestive tract.

soft tissue   Noncalcified tissues, such as nerves, arteries, veins, and connective tissue.

spasm   Constant contraction of muscle.

specialized mucosa   Mucosa found on the top, or dorsum, of the tongue that includes the papillae and taste buds.

sphenoethmoidal recess   Most posterosuperior area of the nasal cavity.

sphenoid bone   Large bone that helps form the base of the skull in front of the occipital bone and part of the side of the skull.

sphenoid sinus   One of the paired paranasal sinuses located in the body of the sphenoid bone.

sphenopalatine artery   See *pterygopalatine artery.*

sphenopalatine nerve   See *pterygopalatine nerve.*

sphere of Monson   Imaginary sphere that theoretically could rest on the mandibular arch.

spillway   See *embrasure.*

spinal nerves   Thirty-one pairs of nerves that exit from the spinal cord at each vertebral level.

spongy bone   Less dense bone in the middle of a bone, frequently referred to as the marrow area. In alveolar bone, the layer between the cribriform plate and the cortical plate.

statoacoustic nerve   Eighth cranial nerve (VIII); related to hearing and balance.

stellate reticulum   Ectodermally and epithelially derived middle layer of the enamel organ. It serves as a cushion for the developing enamel.

sternocleidomastoid muscle   Muscle extending from the mastoid process down and forward in the lateral neck to the sternum and clavicle.

sternohyoid muscle   Infrahyoid muscle from the sternum to the hyoid bone.

sternomastoid muscle   See *sternocleidomastoid muscle.*

sternothyroid muscle   Muscle that goes from the sternum to the thyroid cartilage of the larynx.

stolarized molar   The permanent maxillary first molar is tipped mesially so that the distal marginal ridge of the upper first molar touches the mesial marginal ridge of the lower second molar.

stomodeum   Depression in the facial region of the embryo that is the beginning of the oral cavity.

stratified columnar epithelium   Epithelium that is rather rare but, when seen in large ducts, consists of two rows of columnar cells.

stratified cuboidal epithelium   See *stratified columnar epithelium.*

stratified squamous epithelium   Most common of the multiple-layered epithelia; found as skin and mucosa.

stratum basale   Bottom layer of stratified squamous epithelium; see also *basal layer.*

stratum corneum   Top layer of stratified squamous epithelium.

stratum germinativum   See *basal layer.*

stratum granulosum   Layer above the stratum spinosum in stratified squamous epithelium. Granules in this layer indicate the beginning of cell death.

stratum intermedium   Fourth developing layer of the enamel organ; responsible for aiding ameloblast nourishment.

stratum spinosum   Layer immediately above the basal layer in stratified squamous epithelium. The cells produced in the basal layer move up into the spinous layer.

striae of Retzius   Incremental growth lines seen in sections of enamel.

striated ducts   Salivary intralobular ducts that look like they have stripes at the base of the cells because of infolding of basal cell membrane and mitochondria trapped in between the infoldings.

styloglossus   Extrinsic tongue muscle running from styloid process into the tongue.

stylohyoid muscle   Suprahyoid muscle going from the styloid process to the hyoid bone.

styloid process   Small pointed projection of bone that points downward and forward from the base of the skull just behind the mandible.

stylomastoid foramen   Small foramen between the mastoid and styloid process. The facial nerve exits from the skull here.

stylopharyngeal muscle   Muscle that runs from the styloid process down into the lateral wall of the pharynx; helps to elevate and dilate the pharynx in the swallowing process.

subclavian vein   Vein that drains blood from the arm. It joins with the internal jugular vein to form the brachiocephalic vein.

sublingual caruncle   Small elevation of soft tissue at the base of the lingual frenum that is the opening for the submandibular duct.

sublingual fold   Fold of tissue extending backward on either side of the floor of the mouth; duct of submandibular gland lies below it.

sublingual fossa   Depression for the sublingual gland on the medial surface of the mandible above the mylohyoid line in the canine region.

sublingual gland   Major salivary gland that lies in the floor of the mouth adjacent to the mandibular canines.

subluxation   Dislocation of the mandible.

submandibular   Referring to the region below the mandible; a group of lymph nodes around the submandibular gland.

submandibular fossa   Depression for the submandibular gland on the medial surface of the mandible below the mylohyoid line in the molar region.

submandibular gland   Large major salivary gland that lies beneath the mandible near the angle of the mandible.

submandibular nodes   See *submandibular*.

submental   Area below the chin; a group of lymph nodes beneath the chin.

submental nodes   See *submental*.

submucosa   Supporting layer of loose connective tissue under a mucous membrane.

succedaneous   Permanent teeth that succeed, or take the place of, the deciduous teeth after the latter have been shed, that is, the incisors, canines, and premolars.

sulcus   Long V-shaped depression or valley in the surface of a tooth between the ridges and the cusps. A sulcus has a developmental groove at the apex of its V shape. Sulcus also refers to the trough around the teeth formed by the gingiva.

superior auricular muscle   Muscle extending from above the ear down into the upper part of the ear.

superior constrictor muscle   Muscle that forms the back and side of the upper throat area; see also *superior pharyngeal constrictor muscle*.

superior nasal concha   Small projection of ethmoid bone from the upper lateral nasal wall.

superior nuchal line   Horizontal line on the external surface of the occipital bone for the attachment of neck muscles.

superior orbital fissure   Groove in the upper lateral part of the orbit between the greater and lesser wings of the sphenoid.

superior pharyngeal constrictor muscle   The upper of three muscles that forms the throat wall and helps to move food downward into the esophagus. Part of the muscle joins anteriorly with the buccinator muscle of the cheek.

superior vena cava   Vein that drains blood from the head and arms into the heart.

supernumeraries   Extra teeth in the jaw.

supplemental canal   See *accessory root canals*.

supplemental groove   Shallow linear groove in the enamel of a tooth. It differs from a developmental groove in that it does not mark the junction of lobes; it is a secondary, or smaller, groove.

supplemental tooth   Supernumerary tooth that resembles a regular tooth.

supraeruption   Eruption of a tooth beyond the occlusal plane.

suprahyoid muscles   Muscles above the hyoid bone that attach to it.

supraorbital foramen   Supraorbital notch when it has

a small projection of bone extending across it.

supraorbital notch Small notch in the upper rim of the orbit.

supraperiosteal Tissue lying on the surface of bone.

surfaces Four sides and the top of a tooth.

suture Line where two bones join together.

sympathetic system Part of the autonomic (automatic) nervous system that originates from the thoracic and lumbar levels of the spinal cord.

synovial cavity Epithelium-lined space that secretes tiny amounts of fluid, synovia, and is found in joints that are free moving.

synovial fluid Thin watery fluid secreted in joints that lubricates articulating surfaces.

taste buds Small structures in vallate, fungiform, and foliate papillae that detect taste.

temporal bone Bone that forms part of the side of the skull, including the ear area.

temporal branches Branches of the maxillary artery that serve the temporal muscle.

temporal fossa Large flattened area on the side of the skull that is the origin of the temporal muscle.

temporal muscle Muscle on the side of the head attached to the mandible; elevates and pulls mandible backward.

temporomandibular ligament Thickened part of the temporomandibular joint (TMJ) capsule on the lateral side.

tendon Regularly arranged group of collagen fibers that connects skeletal muscle to bone.

tensor veli palatini Muscle that runs from the auditory tube region downward, forward, and around the lateral side of the hamular process and then turns medially into the anterior part of the soft palate. As its name indicates, when it contracts, it tenses the soft palate in swallowing and speech.

tertiary group See *accidental grooves.*

tertiary nodes Third group of lymph nodes involved

tetracycline staining Discolored teeth that result when an expectant mother or a young child takes the tetracycline antibiotic while tooth crowns are still developing.

therapeutic considerations Treating diseased teeth.

thoracolumbar outflow Another name for the sympathetic nervous system.

thorax (thoracic) Chest region, pertaining to nerves of the chest.

thymus Gland in the chest above the heart that is re-

sponsible for early establishment of immune cells to protect the body.

thyrohyoid muscle Muscle going from the thyroid cartilage of the larynx to the hyoid bone.

thyroid gland Gland in the neck that controls much of the body's metabolic rate.

Tomes' process See *odontoblastic process.*

tongue-tie, tongue-tied Condition when the lingual frenum is short and attached to the tip of the tongue, making normal speech difficult.

tonsillor pillars The vertical folds of tissue that lie in front of and behind the palatine tonsils in the lateral throat wall.

tooth germ Soft tissue that develops into a tooth.

tooth migration Movement of the tooth through the bone and gum tissue.

torus palatinus Large bony growth in hard palate.

trabeculae Interlacing meshwork that makes up the cancellous bony framework.

transitional epithelium Multiple rows of epithelial cells that seem to change in thickness when stretched or relaxed; found in the ureters, urinary bladder, and part of the urethra.

transparent dentin See *sclerotic dentin.*

transseptal fibers Periodontal fibers that extend from the cementum of one tooth to the cementum of the adjacent tooth.

transverse groove of oblique ridge See *oblique groove.*

transverse palatine suture Suture that runs across the posterior part of the hard palate between the maxillae and the palatine bones.

transverse ridge Ridge formed by the union of two triangular ridges, transversing the surface of a posterior tooth from the buccal to the lingual side.

trapezius Muscle at the back of the neck that goes down and out to the lateral part of the clavicle and scapula.

trauma Wound; bodily injury or damage.

triangular fossa Depression formed by the triangular groove between the triangular ridge and the marginal ridge.

triangular ridge Any ridge on the occlusal surface of a posterior tooth that extends from the point of a cusp to the central groove of the occlusal surface.

trifurcation Division of three tooth roots at their point of junction with the root trunk.

trigeminal nerve Fifth cranial nerve (V); supplies motor control to the mandible and sensation to the teeth, oral cavity, and face.

trochlear nerve   Fourth cranial nerve (IV); aids in movements of the eye.

tubercle   Overcalcification of enamel resulting in a small cusplike elevation on some portion of a tooth crown.

tubercle tooth   Very small rudimentary supernumerary tooth.

tuberculum impar   Structure from first pharyngeal arch that forms midline of tongue about one half to two thirds of the way back.

Turner's teeth   Hypocalcification of a single tooth.

ultraviolet radiation   One of the wavelengths in the electromagnetic spectrum; found in sunlight and produced by sunlamps.

united epithelium   Joining of the reduced enamel epithelium with the oral epithelium.

Universal system, Universal Code   System of coding teeth using the numbers 1 to 32 for permanent teeth and the letters A to T for the deciduous teeth.

upper deep cervical   Group of lymph nodes in the upper lateral neck beneath the sternomastoid muscle.

uvula   Small hanging fold of tissue in back of the soft palate.

V_1   First, or ophthalmic, division of the trigeminal nerve.

V_2   Second, or maxillary, division of the trigeminal nerve.

V_3   Third, or mandibular, division of the trigeminal nerve.

vagus nerve   Tenth cranial nerve (X); controls the muscles of the larynx and pharynx, muscles and glands of the digestive tract, and muscle of the heart.

vallate papillae   See *circumvallate papillae.*

vascular   Relating to blood supply.

vasoconstrictor   Substance that constricts blood vessels.

vermilion zone   Red part of the lip where the lip mucosa meets the skin.

vestibule   Space between the lips or cheeks and the teeth.

visceral   Referring to the organs of the body and the structures supplied by involuntary muscle, such as the heart and digestive tract.

viscerocranium   Facial part of the skull.

Volkmann's canals   Blood vessel canal in bone that runs into bone from the outside.

voluntary muscle   Muscle able to be willfully controlled by the person or organism.

vomer   Bone that forms the lower part of the nasal septum.

wedge   Wedge-shaped device that pushes the matrix band tight against the cervical part of the tooth.

white blood cells   Least numerous of the blood cells; responsible for the inflammatory process and other protective functions of the body; leukocytes.

working side   Side to which the mandible is moved.

Z line   Junction between two sarcomeres in skeletal and cardiac muscle.

zygomatic arch   Arch of bone on the side of the face or skull formed by the zygomatic bone and temporal bone.

zygomatic bone   Bone that forms the cheek area.

zygomaticus major   Muscle that extends from the cheek to the corner of the upper lip.

zygomaticus minor   Muscle that extends from the cheek toward the middle part of the upper lip.

Index

Permanent

Maxillary Central Incisors

	RIGHT	LEFT
Universal Code	8	9
International Code	11	21
Palmer notation	1⌋	⌊1
Number of roots		1
Number of pulp horns		3
Number of developmental lobes		4

Location of proximal contact areas
MESIAL: Incisal third
DISTAL: Junction of incisal and middle thirds

Height of contour
FACIAL: Cervical third, 0.5 mm
LINGUAL: Cervical third, 0.5 mm

Identifying characteristics: These incisors are the largest and most prominent incisors. The distoincisal is more rounded than the mesioincisal angle. The lingual surface has a prominent cingulum, broad lingual fossa, and distinct marginal ridges. The pulp cavity is one large single chamber and root canal.

Permanent

Maxillary Lateral Incisors

	RIGHT	LEFT
Universal Code	7	10
International Code	12	22
Palmer notation	2⌋	⌊2
Number of roots		1
Number of pulp horns		1 to 3
Number of developmental lobes		4

Location of proximal contact areas
MESIAL: Junction of incisal and middle thirds
DISTAL: Middle third

Height of contour
FACIAL: Cervical third, 0.5 mm
LINGUAL: Cervical third, 0.5 mm

Identifying characteristics: The lingual anatomical features are similar to those of the central incisors but are more highly developed and have more prominent marginal ridges and deeper lingual fossae. Lateral incisors are more likely to have a lingual pit. The cingulum may be smaller, almost absent. The labial surface resembles that of a central incisor except that the labial surface is more convex. The crown-root ratio is less than in a central incisor because the crown is usually smaller, whereas the root is almost as long. In all other ways the lateral incisors appear as smaller, more rounded versions of the central incisors.

Permanent

Maxillary Canines

	RIGHT	LEFT
Universal Code	6	11
International Code	13	23
Palmer notation	3⌋	⌊3
Number of roots		1
Number of pulp horns		1
Number of cusps		1
Number of developmental lobes		4

Location of proximal contact areas
MESIAL: Junction of incisal and middle thirds
DISTAL: Middle third

Height of contour
FACIAL: Cervical third, 0.5 mm
LINGUAL: Cervical third, 0.5 mm

Identifying characteristics: The maxillary canines are the longest teeth in the mouth. They have a single cusp with mesial and distal ridges forming an incisal edge. A prominent facial ridge is off-center toward the mesial. Cingulum is prominent. The prominent mesiofacial lobe forms this facial ridge of the cusp. The centrofacial lobe forms the lingual ridge of the cusp. This lingual ridge divides the mesial and distal fossae. The distofacial ridge is longer and more rounded than the mesiofacial.

Permanent

Maxillary First Premolars

	RIGHT	LEFT
Universal Code	5	12
International Code	14	24
Palmer notation	4⌋	⌊4
Number of roots		2
Number of pulp horns		2
Number of cusps		2
Number of developmental lobes		4

Location of proximal contact areas
MESIAL AND DISTAL: Just cervical to the junction of occlusal and middle thirds

Height of contour
FACIAL: Cervical third, 0.5 mm
LINGUAL: Middle third, 0.5 mm

Identifying characteristics: These premolars have bifurcated roots. A longitudinal groove is present on the root. The mesial surface shows a developmental fossa. The mesial marginal groove crosses the mesial marginal ridge and extends onto the mesial surface. The facial cusp is wider and longer than the lingual cusp. The mesial ridge of the facial cusp may have a slight concavity.

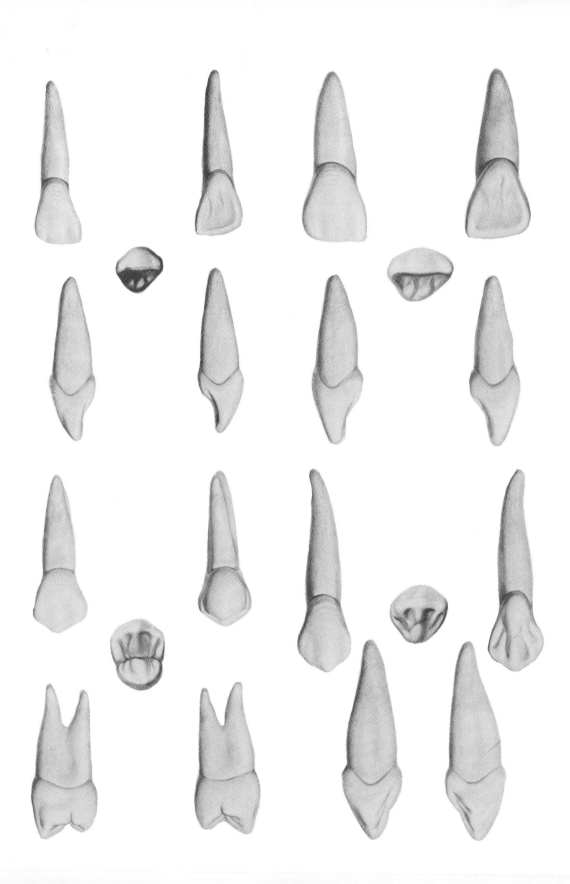

Permanent

Maxillary Second Premolars

	RIGHT	LEFT
Universal Code	4	13
International Code	15	25
Palmer notation	5⌐	⌐5
Number of roots	1	
Number of pulp horns	2	
Number of cusps	2	
Number of developmental lobes	4	

Location of proximal contact areas
MESIAL AND DISTAL: Just cervical to the junction of occlusal and middle thirds

Height of contour
FACIAL: Cervical third, 0.5 mm
LINGUAL: Middle third, 0.5 mm

Identifying characteristics: These premolars usually have a single root. About 40% have two root canals. The buccal and lingual cusps are nearly equal in length. The buccal cusp is shorter than that of a first premolar. The entire crown, especially the occlusal outline, is less angular and more rounded. The occlusal surface has more supplemental grooves. The occlusal developmental grooves are shorter, shallower, and more irregular.

Permanent

Maxillary First Molars

	RIGHT	LEFT
Universal Code	3	14
International Code	16	26
Palmer notation	6⌐	⌐6
Number of roots	3	
Number of pulp horns	4	
Number of cusps	4	
	5 (including cusp of Carabelli)	
Number of developmental lobes	5	

Location of proximal contact areas
MESIAL: Middle third
DISTAL: Middle third

Height of contour
FACIAL: Cervical third, 0.5 mm
LINGUAL: Middle third, 0.5 mm

Identifying characteristics: A cusp of Carabelli may be present. The occlusal outline is square or rhomboidal rather than triangular. The distolingual cusp is well developed. There is a prominent oblique ridge and distal facial and lingual grooves. The crown is nearly as wide mesiodistally as buccolingually. The three roots are widely separated.

Permanent

Maxillary Second Molars

	RIGHT	LEFT
Universal Code	2	15
International Code	17	27
Palmer notation	7⌐	⌐7
Number of roots	3	
Number of pulp horns	4	
Number of cusps	4	
Number of developmental lobes	4	

Location of proximal contact areas
MESIAL: Middle third
DISTAL: Middle third

Height of contour
FACIAL: Cervical third, 0.5 mm
LINGUAL: Middle third, 0.5 mm

Identifying characteristics: These teeth are similar to maxillary first molars except that the fifth cusp is usually absent and the distolingual cusp is less well developed. The oblique ridge is less prominent. The crown is shorter occlusocervically and narrower mesiodistally. It is just as wide buccolingually. The occlusal outline of the crown is rhomboidal to heart shaped. The three roots are less separated.

Permanent

Maxillary Third Molars

	RIGHT	LEFT
Universal Code	1	16
International Code	18	28
Palmer notation	8⌐	⌐8
Number of roots	1 to 4	
Number of pulp horns	1 to 4	
Number of cusps	3 to 5	
Number of developmental lobes	4	

Location of proximal contact areas
MESIAL: Middle third
DISTAL: None

Height of contour
FACIAL: Cervical third, 0.5 mm
LINGUAL: Middle third, 0.5 mm

Identifying characteristics: These teeth vary more in form than any others. They usually do not have a distolingual cusp. The occlusal outline is heart shaped, with three cusps. The roots, usually three, have a tendency to be very close together or to fuse with an extreme distal inclination.

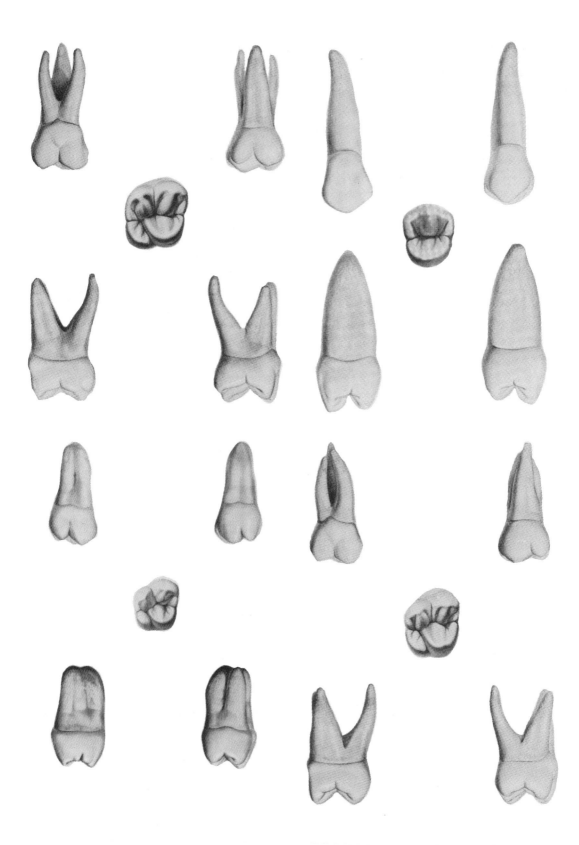

Permanent

Mandibular Central Incisors

	RIGHT	LEFT
Universal Code	25	24
International Code	41	31
Palmer notation	1⌐	⌐1
Number of roots		1
Number of pulp horns		3
Number of developmental lobes		4

Location of proximal contact areas
MESIAL: Incisal third
DISTAL: Incisal third

Height of contour
FACIAL: Cervical third, less than 0.5 mm
LINGUAL: Cervical third, less than 0.5 mm

Identifying characteristics: The distoincisal and mesioincisal angles are nearly identical. The lingual surface is shallow, with no prominent features. The crown is wider faciolingually than mesiodistally. The root is oval shaped in cross section. The incisal edge shows wear on the facioincisal edge. From a proximal view the incisal edge appears to be tilted toward the lingual side.

Permanent

Mandibular Lateral Incisors

	RIGHT	LEFT
Universal Code	26	23
International Code	42	32
Palmer notation	2⌐	⌐2
Number of roots		1
Number of pulp horns		3
Number of developmental lobes		4

Location of proximal contact areas
MESIAL: Incisal third
DISTAL: Incisal third

Height of contour
FACIAL: Cervical third, less than 0.5 mm
LINGUAL: Cervical third, less than 0.5 mm

Identifying characteristics: The crown is similar to that of the mandibular central incisors. The distal lobe is more highly developed than the mesial. The distal incisal ridge angles toward the lingual as if rotating on the root axis. The crown and the root are slightly larger than those of the central incisors.

Permanent

Mandibular Canines

	RIGHT	LEFT
Universal Code	27	22
International Code	43	33
Palmer notation	3⌐	⌐3
Number of roots		1 or 2
Number of pulp horns		1
Number of cusps		1
Number of developmental lobes		4

Location of proximal contact areas
MESIAL: Incisal third
DISTAL: Just cervical to the junction of incisal and middle thirds

Height of contour
FACIAL: Cervical third, less than 0.5 mm
LINGUAL: Cervical third, less than 0.5 mm

Identifying characteristics: The crown is similar to the crown of the maxillary canines but narrower and smoother. It has less prominent lingual features. From a proximal view, the cusp tip is inclined to the lingual. From an incisal view, the distal end of the incisal edge is rotated to the lingual. They have the longest roots in the mandibular arch, with longitudinal grooves on the root.

Permanent

Mandibular First Premolars

	RIGHT	LEFT
Universal Code	28	21
International Code	44	34
Palmer notation	4⌐	⌐4
Number of roots		1
Number of pulp horns		1 or 2
Number of cusps		2
Number of developmental lobes		4

Location of proximal contact areas
MESIAL AND DISTAL: Just cervical to junction of occlusal and middle thirds

Height of contour
FACIAL: Cervical third, 0.5 mm
LINGUAL: Middle third, 1 mm

Identifying characteristics: These premolars have two cusps, one large buccal and one small lingual. The buccal cusps are centered directly over the root. The lingual cusps are centered lingual to the root and are afunctional and nonoccluding. The occlusal surface slopes sharply lingual in a cervical direction. The mesiobuccal cusp ridge is shorter than the distobuccal cusp ridge. It has a mesiolingual developmental groove and one root.

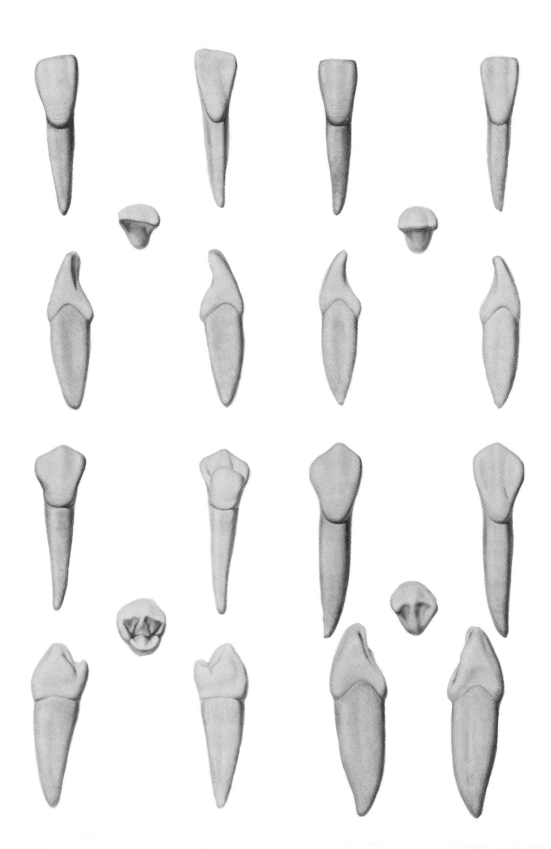

Permanent

Mandibular Second Premolars

	RIGHT	LEFT
Universal Code	29	20
International Code	45	35
Palmer notation	5⌋	⌊5
Number of roots	1	
Number of pulp horns	2 or 3	
Number of cusps	2 or 3	
Number of development lobes	4	

Location of proximal contact areas
MESIAL AND DISTAL: Just cervical to junction of occlusal and middle thirds

Height of contour
FACIAL: Cervical third, 0.5 mm
LINGUAL: Middle third, 1 mm

Identifying characteristics: These premolars have two or three cusps. The buccal cusp is very large. If two lingual cusps are present, the mesiolingual is the larger. Although the lingual cusps are larger than on a first premolar, they are afunctional and do not occlude with the maxillary teeth. A second premolar has more secondary anatomical features and more variation than any other tooth except a third molar. The two-cusp form has a U- or H-groove pattern. A mesiolingual groove is rare and is poorly developed if present. The three-cusp form has a lingual developmental groove between the two lingual cusps. The single root is longer and larger than that of a first premolar.

Permanent

Mandibular First Molars

	RIGHT	LEFT
Universal Code	30	19
International Code	46	36
Palmer notation	6⌋	⌊6
Number of roots	2	
Number of pulp horns	5	
Number of cusps	5	
Number of developmental lobes	5	

Location of proximal contact areas
MESIAL: Middle third
DISTAL: Middle third

Height of contour
FACIAL: Cervical third, 0.5 mm
LINGUAL: Middle third, 1 mm

Identifying characteristics: The five cusps make these the largest mandibular teeth. They are wider mesiodistally than buccolingually. The crown converges lingually and slightly distally. The three buccal cusps are separated by two buccal grooves. The two lingual cusps are separated by one lingual groove. These three grooves converge to form a Y pattern. There are two roots, a mesial and a distal, and three root canals (the mesial root has two root canals).

Permanent

Mandibular Second Molars

	RIGHT	LEFT
Universal Code	31	18
International Code	47	37
Palmer notation	7⌋	⌊7
Number of roots	2	
Number of pulp horns	4	
Number of cusps	4	
Number of developmental lobes	4	

Location of proximal contact areas
MESIAL: Middle third
DISTAL: Middle third

Height of contour
FACIAL: Cervical third, 0.5 mm
LINGUAL: Middle third, 1 mm

Identifying characteristics: These molars have four cusps of nearly equal size. The crown is smaller in all dimensions and has less lingual convergence. There is only one buccal groove and one lingual groove, which join together on the occlusal surface as they bisect the central developmental groove. The groove pattern is therefore a cross (+). The two roots are closer together and incline slightly distally. There is one root canal in the distal root. The mesial root can have one or two root canals.

Permanent

Mandibular Third Molars

	RIGHT	LEFT
Universal Code	32	17
International Code	48	38
Palmer notation	8⌋	⌊8
Number of roots	2 (fused into 1)	
Number of pulp horns	4 or 5	
Number of cusps	4 or 5	
Number of developmental lobes	4 or 5	

Location of proximal contact areas
MESIAL: Middle third
DISTAL: Middle third

Height of contour
FACIAL: Cervical third, 0.5 mm
LINGUAL: Middle third, 1 mm

Identifying characteristics: These are the most variable mandibular teeth in form. They usually resemble the mandibular second molars, with four cusps and a shallower, smaller central fossa, with more secondary and tertiary grooves. A five-cusp form is not unusual. The two roots (mesial and distal) and often fused and inclined toward the distal side.

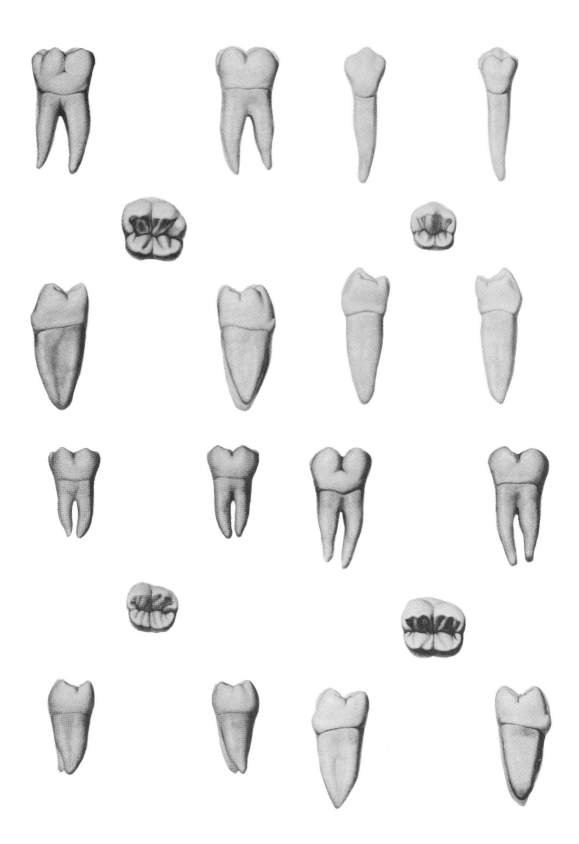

Deciduous

Maxillary Central Incisors

	RIGHT	LEFT
Universal Code	E	F
International Code	51	61
Palmer notation	A⌋	⌊A
Number of roots		1
Number of pulp horns		3
Number of developmental lobes		4

Location of proximal contact areas
MESIAL: Incisal third toward incisal angle
DISTAL: Incisal third toward middle third

Height of contour
FACIAL: Cervical third (more accentuated than permanent teeth)
LINGUAL: Cervical third (more accentuated than permanent teeth)

Identifying characteristics: Crown is wider mesiodistally than longer cervicoincisally. It is more rounded and more bulbous than the permanent central. It is also smaller and constricts more at the cementoenamel junction. Lingual features are more distinct. The facial and lingual height of contours are more convex than the permanent incisors. The pulp horn is larger in relation to the permanent teeth.

Deciduous

Maxillary Lateral Incisor

	RIGHT	LEFT
Universal Code	D	G
International Code	52	62
Palmer notation	B⌋	⌊B
Number of roots		1
Number of pulp horns		3
Number of developmental lobes		4

Location of proximal contact areas
MESIAL: Incisal third toward incisal angle
DISTAL: Incisal third toward middle third

Height of contour
FACIAL: Cervical third (more accentuated than permanent teeth)
LINGUAL: Cervical third (more accentuated than permanent teeth)

Identifying characteristics: The crown is longer cervicoincisally than wider mesiodistally. The crown is smaller and narrower mesiodistally. It is more slender than the primary centrals. The lateral is less squatier and resembles the permanent incisors more closely than the primary maxillary centrals. In proportion to the primary maxillary central the root is much longer. The lingual features are less distinctive, and the cervical constriction is greater.

Deciduous

Maxillary Canine

	RIGHT	LEFT
Universal Code	C	H
International Code	53	63
Palmer notation	C⌋	⌊C
Number of roots		1
Number of pulp horns		3
Number of cusp		1
Number of developmental lobes		4

Location of proximal contact areas
MESIAL: Incisal part of middle third
DISTAL: Incisal part of middle third

Height of contour
FACIAL: Cervical third (more accentuated than the incisors)
LINGUAL: Cervical third (more accentuated than the incisors)

Identifying characteristics: The cusp tip is in the center of the crown from the proximal view. The mesial slope is indented incisally and the distal slope is more rounded (obtuse). The crown is much wider labiolingually than the incisors. The root of the primary canine is proportionally longer than the root of the secondary maxillary canine. The root of the primary canine is long, slender, and tapering and is more than twice the crown length.

Deciduous

Maxillary First Molar

	RIGHT	LEFT
Universal Code	B	I
International Code	54	64
Palmer notation	D⌋	⌊D
Number of roots		3
Number of pulp horns		3
Number of cusps		3
Number of developmental lobes		4

Location of proximal contact areas
MESIAL: Junction of middle and occlusal third
DISTAL: Middle third

Height of contour
FACIAL: Extremely prominent mesiobuccal cervical bulge
LINGUAL: Cervical convexity

Identifying characteristics: Resembles a premolar and a molar. This is a three-cusped molar. The mesiolingual cusp is the largest and sharpest. The most characteristic thing about this tooth is the well-pronounced convexity on the mesiobuccal outline in the cervical third. Three roots—two buccal and one lingual roots.

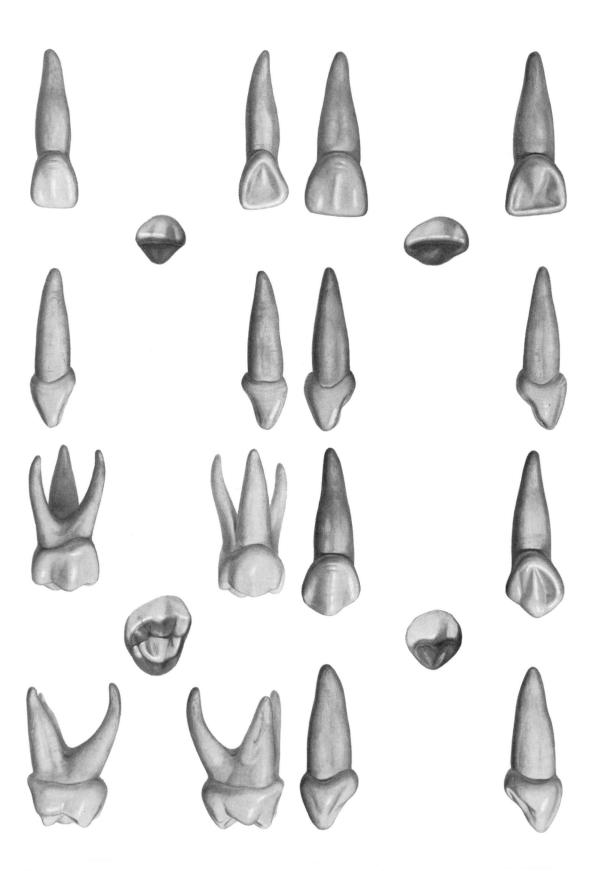

Deciduous

Maxillary Second Molar

	RIGHT	LEFT
Universal Code	A	J
International Code	54	64
Palmer notation	E⌋	⌊E
Number of roots	3	
Number of pulp horns	5 or 4	
Number of cusps	5 or 4	
Number of developmental lobes	5	

Location of proximal contact areas
MESIAL: Junction of occlusal and middle third
DISTAL: Middle third

Height of contour
FACIAL: Junction of occlusal and middle third
LINGUAL: Junction of occlusal and middle third

Identifying characteristics: Resembles permanent maxillary first molar, even has prominent oblique ridge. Three roots—two buccal and one lingual. Roots are long, slender, and flared widely apart. The faciolingual measurement of the crown is greater than the mesiodistal.

Deciduous

Mandibular Central Incisor

	RIGHT	LEFT
Universal Code	P	O
International Code	81	71
Palmer notation	A⌋	⌊A
Number of roots	1	
Number of pulp horns	3	
Number of developmental lobes	4	

Location of proximal contact areas
MESIAL: Incisal angle
DISTAL: Incisal angle

Height of contour
FACIAL: Cervical of crown
LINGUAL: Cervical of crown

The prominences of the facial and lingual at the cervical are as pronounced as any other deciduous teeth and more so than the permanent mandibular incisors.

Identifying characteristics: The incisal ridge is straight from an incisal view. From a facial view the crown is flat. The distal and mesial are almost identical. The crown is wide in proportion to its length in comparison with its permanent successor. The root is long and tapered. It is almost twice as long as the crown.

Deciduous

Mandibular Lateral Incisor

	RIGHT	LEFT
Universal Code	Q	N
International Code	82	72
Palmer notation	B⌋	⌊B
Number of roots	1	
Number of pulp horns	3	
Number of developmental lobes	4	

Location of proximal contact areas
MESIAL: Near incisal angle
DISTAL: Slightly lower than mesial

Height of contour
FACIAL: Cervical third
LINGUAL: Cervical third

As all anterior deciduous teeth, they exhibit pronounced cervical prominences.

Identifying characteristics: The incisal ridge runs slightly toward the distal. The lateral is longer and larger than the mandibular primary central incisor and the root is also longer. The lateral has a more rounded (obtuse) distoincisal angle.

Deciduous

Mandibular Canine

	RIGHT	LEFT
Universal Code	R	M
International Code	83	73
Palmer notation	C⌋	⌊C
Number of roots	1	
Number of pulp horns	3	
Number of cusps	1	
Number of developmental lobes	4	

Location of proximal contact areas
MESIAL: Junction of middle third and incisal third
DISTAL: Junction of middle third and incisal third

Height of contour
FACIAL: Distinct cervical bulge
LINGUAL: Distinct cervical bulge

Identifying characteristics: Similar to primary maxillary canine, except it is slightly shorter and much narrower labiolingually. The mandibular canine also has a shorter root.

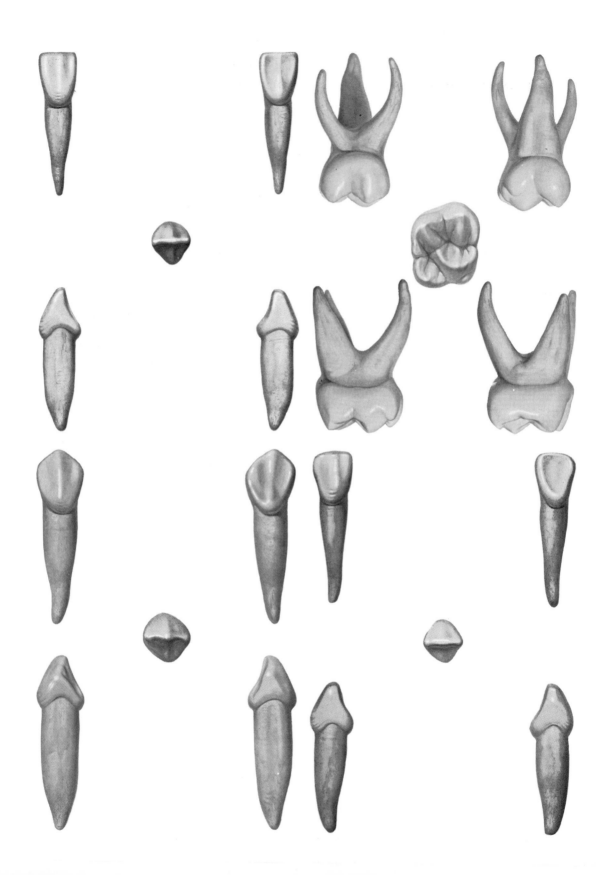

Deciduous

Mandibular First Molar

	RIGHT	LEFT
Universal Code	S	L
International Code	84	74
Palmer notation	D⌉	⌈D
Number of roots	2	
Number of pulp horns	4	
Number of cusps	4	
Number of developmental lobes	4	

Location of proximal contact areas
MESIAL: Middle third
DISTAL: Middle third

Height of contour
FACIAL: An extremely bulbous curvature on the mesiobuccal cervical third
LINGUAL: Middle third

Identifying characteristics: This tooth does not resemble any of the other teeth, deciduous or permanent. This tooth varies so much it appears strange and primitive. The mesial root is much larger than the distal, and the mesial half of the crown is much larger than the distal. The most characteristic thing about this tooth is the extreme convexity on the mesiobuccal at the cervical third. There are two roots, a mesial and a distal.

Deciduous

Mandibular Second Molar

	RIGHT	LEFT
Universal Code	T	K
International Code	85	75
Palmer notation	E⌉	⌈E
Number of roots	2	
Number of pulp horns	5	
Number of cusps	5	
Number of developmental lobes	5	

Location of proximal contact areas
MESIAL: Junction of occlusal and middle third
DISTAL: Middle third

Height of contour
FACIAL: Buccal cervical ridge
LINGUAL: Middle third

Identifying characteristics: Resembles the permanent mandibular first molar. There are three buccal cusps and two lingual cusps; two roots, a mesial and a distal. The roots are longer than the deciduous first molars and flared far apart.

Additional Notes

Additional Notes

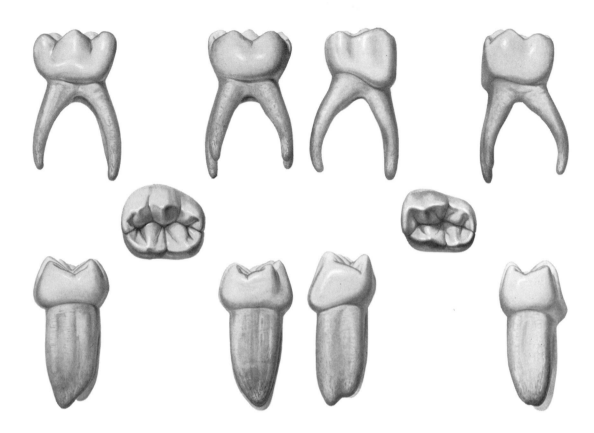